ORTHOPAEDIC ASPECTS OF CEREBRAL PALSY

Clinics in Developmental Medicine Nos. 52/53

Orthopaedic Aspects of Cerebral Palsy

Edited by

ROBERT L. SAMILSON

1975

Spastics International Medical Publications

LONDON: William Heinemann Medical Books Ltd.

PHILADELPHIA: J. B. Lippincott Co.

ISBN 0 433 00000 0

1975 Spastics International Medical Publications

Printed in England at THE LAVENHAM PRESS LTD., Lavenham, Suffolk

This book is dedicated to the memory of

DR. J. WILLIAM HILLMAN (1921-1970)

President of the American Academy for Cerebral Palsy and Professor of the Department of Orthopedic Surgery at Vanderbilt University Medical School, USA.

Contents

PREFACE

The patient with cerebral palsy has many problems. In this era of problem-oriented records and super-specialization, there is a tendency on the one hand to delve into each and every problem, searching for solutions. At the same time, super-specialization has, at times, lost sight of the patient as a total person. In no area of medicine or the social sciences is there a greater opportunity for appreciation of the totality of person than in the management of the patient with cerebral palsy. Medical students and young physicians become far more understanding individuals when they are given the opportunity to participate in the care of cerebral palsied patients.

In 1963, several orthopedic residents at Sonoma State Hospital and the University of California School of Medicine in San Francisco approached me with regard to a reference work that would help them understand the orthopedic aspects of cerebral palsy. I must confess that no volume was available, to my knowledge, which gave a comprehensive understanding of the problems of the cerebral palsied child, as well as the fundamentals of orthopedic examination of such children, and the elements for decision-making in their management.

I discussed the situation with my colleague, the late Dr. J. William Hillman, during an annual meeting of the American Academy for Cerebral Palsy. He was extremely enthusiastic and supportive, and without this, this volume would never have been written. It was felt that a contribution by a single author would not reflect a global attitude towards management. With the expert assistance of Dr. Martin Bax, Editor of Developmental Medicine and Child Neurology, a list of contributors, each accomplished in the area about which he or she was to write, was compiled. All those invited agreed to participate. This was not to be a 'cookbook' of orthopedic surgery and cerebral palsy. Rather, we wish to convey principals of care which would prove useful, keeping in mind the pediatric, neurological, psychological, educational, vocational, and associated problems of the patient with which the orthopedist must be aware in order to truly care for the patient.

No constraints were placed on the contributors, as long as they gave a cogent reason for any opinions which they expressed. All were most co-operative. Without this co-operation, such a multi-authored volume would have been impossible.

The American Academy for Cerebral Palsy has been a most useful and encouraging forum for learning an interdisciplinary approach to the care of cerebral palsied patients. I have had the privilege of serving that organization, as it has served me.

Transatlantic co-operation was fostered by an international conference in Bristol, England, sponsored by the National Spastics Society and superbly managed by Dr. Ronald Mac Keith. Many of the contributors to this volume were privileged to attend this conference on the orthopedic aspects of cerebral palsy.

The United Cerebral Palsy Association has been most supportive in permitting me to train young physicians in the care of cerebral palsied patients. To the Association, my orthopedic residents, and most of all, to my patients, I owe a great deal of gratitude.

Preparation of this volume has taken ten years, and hopefully it reflects time-tested fundamentals, as well as a good deal of progress.

Besides the help of those mentioned above, Miss Lynda Evans, Miss Dian Coley, Miss Dorly Barnsley and Mr. Paul Brooker of the Editorial Office of Spastics International Medical Publications were of immense assistance. Miss Ellen Ross, my secretary, spent many hours typing and re-typing manuscript and correspondence. Mrs. Adele Smith and Miss Mary Halligan of my office were of great help, as well. Mr. John Wehner, Jr. of Lippincott Company in Philadelphia, has been of assistance in United States distribution of the text. Finally, without the forebearance, encouragement, and tolerance of my wife and family, this volume would not have been written.

Robert L. Samilson, M.D.

CHAPTER 1

Historical Notes — the Past Generation

WILLIAM T. GREEN

Orthopedic surgery and orthopedic surgeons have played a very significant rôle in the evolution of our knowledge of and in the treatment of cerebral palsy. If any one person may be said to have been largely responsible for initiating this, it was William John Little of England (1810-1894) (Keith 1919, Bick 1948). Little's interest was stimulated by his own deformity and by tenotomy.

Little, as a young child, had a short febrile illness, apparently anterior polio-myelitis, which resulted in a equinovarus deformity of his foot with a contracted heel cord. This deformity became a major factor in his life. It directed him into medicine. He chose to study at the London Hospital, where he was greatly interested in anatomy and factors relating to deformity. He became a member of the Royal College of Surgeons in 1832, and a lecturer in comparative anatomy at the London Hospital; however after being there for a couple of years, he was passed over for an appointment in surgery, so he decided on further study in Germany with Müller of Berlin, a decision which was influenced by his own deformity.

In 1816 Delpech of Montpellier had performed a tenotomy of the tendo achilles for club foot. He published his experiences in 1823 (Dclpcch 1823). Delpech it was who at this early period stated that, when muscle balance was upset, deformity of the body developed, and that deformities arise due to a lack of balance in the action of muscle groups. Little had consulted him regarding the possibility of a tenotomy to correct his own deformity, but Delpech advised against it because of the high likelihood of post-operative infection in those pre-Listerian days. Little was disappointed in this and while he was in Germany he consulted George Frederick Louis Stromeyer (1804-1876) (Stromeyer 1838, Bick 1948), who at that time was practicing in Hanover and had taken up subcutaneous tenotomy of the tendo achilles in 1831. Stromeyer recommended that he have the procedure, and he did. Little was so enthusiastic about the result that he stayed on with Stromeyer for a period to perfect his technique. He took the procedure back to Berlin, where it was soon adopted, and, in turn, to England. He was soon doing tenotomies for tendons other than the tendo achilles. He had an increasing interest in deformities. With his great popularity arising from his introduction of tenotomy and the results obtained, he was able to raise funds in 1838 to establish the 'Orthopaedic Institution', which later became the Royal National Orthopaedic Hospital. In 1839 he wrote a treatise on the nature of club foot and analogous distortions (Little 1839), and during 1843-44 he gave a series of lectures on 'The Nature and Treatment of the Deformities of the Human Frame', (Little 1843), in which amongst other things he first discussed infantile spastic paralysis which soon became known as 'Little's Disease'. In 1853 he published a treatise on the nature and development of deformities (Little 1853).

As he saw an increasing number of patients with cerebral palsy requiring tenotomy, he became more and more interested in the etiology of cerebral palsy. His crowning contribution was a classic monograph entitled '*On the Influence of Abnormal Parturition, Difficult Labours, Premature Birth and Asphyxia Neonatorum on the Mental and Physical Condition of the Child, Especially in Relation to Deformities*', (Little 1862, Rang 1966). This was first given in part as a lecture to the Obstetrical Society. One only has to consider the title to appreciate how far beyond his time he was in his understanding of etiological factors in the production of cerebral palsy.

With the coming of antisepsis and aseptic techniques, the use of tenotomy grew rapidly. It soon became evident that lengthening of a tendon in cerebral palsy was far preferable to tenotomy, since the spastic muscle retracted markedly, and its needed function might not be restored when healing occurred. Little himself in his later years came to recognize that tenotomy could cause difficulty as well as good, that it could not be used indiscriminately, and, further, that continuity of care afterwards was necessary.

Other operative procedures were added. Selective neurectomies to decrease the spasticity of muscles came into use. Stöffel (1913) first laid stress on the value of neurectomies; in his original contribution he emphasized the geographic localization of various nerve trunks within the peripheral nerves, and recommended division of the appropriate intra-neural columns. This localization of innervation for certain muscles could be recognized, but there was always a risk that paralysis would be produced at operation. The technique that developed and was probably more widely used was to divide appropriate branches of the nerve as they went into the muscle, thus removing a part of its innervation. Other procedures, such as fasciotomies, were added, and arthrodeses increasingly came to be used to correct deformities, provide stability and simplify motor control.

In the beginning there was great enthusiasm for the surgical results, but secondary assessments were often disappointing. Many patients seemed to be greatly improved immediately after surgery, but often they tended to fall back into their former deformity or to develop new ones. Other patients were unimproved, and complications arose which on occasion made them worse. By 1930 many in the field were quite critical of surgical procedures. There seem to have been several reasons for this. In the complex area of cerebral palsy, a lack of experience resulted in an inadequate appreciation of the indications for surgery, its possible benefits and its limitations. Particularly important was the need to appreciate the principles of postoperative care, including the use of proper intermittent splinting and neuromuscular training. Too often it was not recognized that surgical measures were only a step in the total treatment, and that there were only particular indications for their use for patients who met certain criteria. It was obvious that there was much to learn.

These problems stimulated a broader approach to cerebral palsy and its various manifestations. The importance of evaluation of the mental capacity of the child, of the classification of the disease into various types, and of recognition of the prognostic implications, was recognized (Phelps 1932). The use of exercises, muscle training and braces was explored and expanded. Originally this approach was fostered by orthopedic surgeons who had had experience in the treatment of anterior poliomyelitis. This was a time when many orthopedic hospitals were established, and there was a broadening interest in the crippled child by society in general.

During this period in the United States, the late Winfield Morgan Phelps was a leading figure (1894-1971), although he was not alone. Phelps, an orthopedic surgeon, finished his orthopedic training in 1925 at the Children's Hospital, Boston, a hospital with a strong physical therapy tradition in the treatment of poliomyelitis, and where Bronson Crothers was developing the new field of pediatric neurology, taking a particular interest in cerebral palsy. In this specialized treatment clinic, the parents were taught to do exercises by the therapist, and a total program for the evolving child was emphasized.

Phelps became totally interested in cerebral palsy. He became Professor of Orthopedic Surgery at Yale Medical School, but soon resigned to devote himself solely to cerebral palsy; he established The Children's Rehabilitation Institute of Baltimore, and became a consultant to clinics for cerebral palsy in many areas of the United States. He stimulated the formation of such clinics and the general interest of the public in their support.

Parents of patients with cerebral palsy were stimulated to have a greater collective interest in cerebral palsy, and societies were formed to foster treatment, special clinics and research, both on a local and a national level. In the United States, an American Academy for Cerebral Palsy was formed in 1947, which brought together physicians and workers from various specialties and disciplines. Phelps was its first president.

Appreciation of the value of surgery in the treatment was slow to return. Phelps, for example, as late as 1957 was pessimistic as to the value of soft tissue surgery in the growing child, maintaining that the deformity would only recur; later, however, he withdrew from this position and agreed that the poor results on which his assertion was based were probably due to a failure to give the patients the necessary post-operative care. Attention was temporarily diverted away from surgery on many centers by a great enthusiasm for various systems and methods of physical therapy and neuromuscular training. Gradually, the importance of surgery as a fundamental part of the treatment came to be generally appreciated, and its indications and limitations became fully recognized.

Many have contributed to the placing of orthopedic surgical measures in their present perspective.* Important as surgery may be, there is general agreement that it must be considered as an adjunct in the general plan of treatment, and that it has particular indications in particular patients. Training of the motor mechanism is the basic aim of therapy as far as musculo-skeletal function is concerned, and efforts should be concerned from the beginning with developing controlled function and preventing fixed deformity. Surgical measures—by reducing deformity, by changing relative agonist-antagonist action and establishing better balance of muscle power,

---

*Most changes in medicine occur by evolution, and one should be cautious before ascribing credit to particular individuals, even to those who may have made the first written record. Many persons of the past and present have contributed to the whole. I have not named contributors in the present generation lest I omit those who have contributed as much or more.

and by decreasing the spasticity of muscles and simplifying the problems of control—are often an indispensable part of rehabilitation. Operative procedures involving the peripheral neuromuscular system are particularly effective where deformities or deforming tendencies play a major rôle in the disability. They are usually only indicated where spasticity is a factor. Soft tissue procedures, despite statements to the contrary, are most useful in the growing child, provided that the proper indications are present and post-operative care and training are effective and prolonged.

Many factors combine to determine the result to be obtained. The surgical procedure chosen must have a reasonable chance of improving function and reducing deformity. The patient's motor function must meet certain minimal requirements with regard to balance, motion, and control, and his mental status ought to be such that he will be able to use any possible correction that is obtained and be able to co-operate in a post-operative regimen. In particular, the post-operative care must be well-chosen, thorough and long, and include muscle training, splinting and gait training, if appropriate. Simple night-splinting may be necessary in the growing child until growth is completed, unless the desired reciprocal balance in the agonist-antagonist muscles can be established; corrective exercises too may need to be a way of life, at least during the growing period. Before surgery is embarked upon, the family and the patient should understand the implications of the surgery, and must be prepared to give full co-operation in the post-operative regimen.

REFERENCES

Bick, E. M. (1948) *Source Book of Orthopedics, 2nd edn.* Baltimore: Williams & Wilkins. pp. 212, 215, 420, 425, 427.
Delpech, M. J. (1823) 'Tenotomie du tendon d'Achilles.' *in Chirurgie Clinique de Montpellier, ou Observations et Réflexions Tirées des Travaux de Chirurgie Clinique de cette Ecole.* Paris: Gabon. p. 181.
Keith, Sir A. (1919) *Menders of the Maimed.* London: O.U.P. p. 63.
Little, W. J. (1839) *A Treatise on the Nature of Club Foot and Analagous Distortions.* London: W. Jeffs.
—— (1843) 'Lectures on the nature and treatment of the deformities of the human frame.' *Lancet,* **1,** 350.
—— (1853) *On the Nature and Treatment of the Deformities of the Human Frame.* London: Longman, Brown, Green & Longman.
—— (1862) 'On the influence of abnormal parturition, difficult labours, premature birth and asphyxia neonatorum on the mental and physical condition of the child, especially in relation to deformities.' *Transactions of the Obstetrical Society of London,* **3,** 293.
Phelps, W. M. (1957) 'Long-term results of orthopedic surgery in cerebral palsy.' *Journal of Bone and Joint Surgery,* **39A,** 53.
Rang, M. (1966) *Anthology of Orthopedics.* Edinburgh: Livingstone. p. 48.
Stöffel, A. (1913) 'The treatment of spastic contracture.' *American Journal of Orthopedic Surgery,* **10,** 611.
Stromeyer, G. F. (1838) *Beiträge zur operativen Orthopädik oder Erfahrungen über die subcutane Durchschneidung verkürtzter Muskeln und deren Sehnen.* Hanover: Helwing'schen Hof-Buchhandlung.

CHAPTER 2

Differential Diagnosis and Natural History of the Cerebral Palsied Child

MARGARET H. JONES

Definition of Cerebral Palsy

By definition, the term cerebral palsy reflects 'a disorder to movement and posture due to defect or lesion of the immature brain' (Bax 1964).

'The term cerebral palsy does not designate a disease in the usual medical sense. It is, however, a useful administrative term, which covers individuals who are handicapped by motor disorders which are due to non-progressive abnormalities of the brain. The disorder of motor control is only one, and often the least, of the difficulties that face these children. Inevitably, many children with impairment of the brain may have mental irregularities, and some will have convulsions; others will have defects of hearing, eyesight, or other sensory difficulties.' (Crothers and Paine 1959).

Prevalence of Cerebral Palsy

The prevalence of cerebral palsy, as defined above, has been estimated by various investigators in various countries to vary between 0.6 and 5.9 per 1000 births (Schenectady County Study 1949, Henderson 1961, Rutter *et al.* 1970).

Life Expectancy of Patients with Cerebral Palsy

Based on a study of 3108 cerebral palsied patients aged less than 18 years, Schlesinger *et al.* (1959) reported the death rate among cerebral palsied males to be thirteen times higher than among normal boys of the same age, and among cerebral palsied girls to be seventeen times higher than among normal girls. The mortality rate for the severely physically handicapped was 27 to 30 times higher than that for an age and sex matched group from the general population. The mortality rate for those with mild physical involvement was four to five times that expected. Table I is constructed from these data.

TABLE I

Number surviving at different ages (projected)

Age (Years)	Males		Females	
	General pop.	C.P.	General pop.	C.P.
5	1000	1000	1000	1000
20	988	874	994	898
30	972	666	987	779
40	952	406	975	575
45	933	159	964	388

With current supportive therapy, the life expectancy of the cerebral palsied may well be greater than that found by Schlesinger *et al.*

Long-term Prospects for Patients with Cerebral Palsy

Although long-term prospective studies are not available, the predicted outcomes in groups of children have been compared with the actual statuses of different groups of adults. For example, estimates by physicians in Los Angeles of the outcome in a series of 1138 children were compared with the actual statuses of 250 cerebral palsied adults who had been evaluated at a Vocational Training Center (Jones and Maschmeyer 1958). The extent of the physical involvement was similar in the two groups (Table II), as was the severity of the involvement (Table III).

<table>
<tr><td colspan="3">TABLE II
Extent of physical involvement</td><td colspan="3">TABLE III
Degree of severity of physical involvement</td></tr>
<tr><td>Extent of physical involvement</td><td>Children
(n = 1138)
Per cent</td><td>Adults
(n = 250)
Per cent</td><td>Degree of severity</td><td>Children
(n = 1138)
Per cent</td><td>Adults
(n = 250)
Per cent</td></tr>
<tr><td>Quadriplegia</td><td>62</td><td>69</td><td>Severe</td><td>22</td><td>16</td></tr>
<tr><td>Hemiplegia</td><td>22</td><td>16</td><td>Moderate</td><td>45</td><td>47</td></tr>
<tr><td>Paraplegia</td><td>10</td><td>5</td><td>Mild</td><td>33</td><td>26</td></tr>
</table>

About half of each group were of normal intelligence, and five to six per cent were of above average intelligence; 22 per cent of the children and 28 per cent of the adults had intelligence quotients on the borderline of normal. Seizures had occurred in 37 per cent of the children and in 32 per cent of the adults, but had occurred in only 10 per cent of the adults after the age of 16 years. The predicted outcomes for the children and the present statuses of the adults are compared in Table IV.

TABLE IV

Comparison of physicians' estimated outcomes in 1138 cerebral palsied children with the actual statuses of 250 cerebral palsied adults

Predicted outcome or actual status	*Percentage of the 1138 children (predicted)*	*Percentage of the 250 adults*
Almost completely dependent (some self-care possible)	23 per cent	15 per cent
Self-care only (independent at home)	24 per cent	36 per cent
Partly self-supporting	20 per cent	38 per cent
Entirely self-supporting	33 per cent	11 per cent*

*After a period of training and counseling at the Center, the percentage of the 250 adults in full-time employment increased from 11 to 29 per cent. The primary reasons for the previous failure of a number of patients to find employment were identified as (1) a lack of appropriate training, (2) immature attitudes towards work assignments, poor work habits and immature social attitudes and (3) physical disability.

From their study of the final outcomes in cerebral palsied patients who had undergone treatment for their physical disorders, Wortis and Cooper (1957) concluded that factors other than the physical ones played a great rôle in determining the final outcome.

Personality and behavioural factors have been found to play a major rôle in determining eligibility for gainful employment. For example, a survey of cerebral palsied adolescents and adults in Israel revealed that almost half had marked emotional imbalance, social maladjustment or an inability to accept their handicap (Margulec 1966). 38 per cent showed poor work habits, and 70 per cent were reported to have problems in concentration.

Curtis (1951-1953), a vocational counselor, concluded from his attempts to place a group of cerebral palsied adults in employment that the single most important factor was the handling the individuals received from their parents in the very early years of life.

In Scotland, long-term follow-up studies of 67 children who had attended a special school identified 60 per cent who were either gainfully employed or were expected to be so after training (Pollock and Stark 1969). In Denmark, a study of 1127 cerebral palsied patients aged 15 to 31 years revealed that 34 per cent were employed and socially independent, while a further 10 per cent were under training for employment (Hansen 1960). In a survey of cerebral palsied patients admitted to college, follow-up studies revealed that those students who had pursued vocationally-oriented college majors were more often successfully employed and had fewer problems (Hutchinson and Muthard 1969).

In the absence of secondary contractures and deformities, the severity of the physical deficit in patients with a central nervous system lesion tends to remain unchanged, once the early stages of motor development have passed. However, increased disability with age was reported in three patients by Hanson *et al.* (1970). All three showed an acute early episode, after which they were left with a fairly stable mild deficit. It was not until they were somewhere between their 8th and 15th years that they were afflicted by the fairly rapid accession of a more severe extrapyramidal motor disability. No cause for the changing picture was discerned.

Spontaneous improvement has occurred in some cases despite definite spastic quadriplegia or dyskinesia following trauma or anoxia at birth. No clues have yet been identified by which one may recognise those children in whom spontaneous improvement will occur with age (Paine 1964).

Multiple Handicaps in the Child with Cerebral Palsy

In addition to disorders of movement and posture, other neurological abnormalities due to central nervous system lesions are frequent in patients with cerebral palsy, and may be major factors in determining the over-all outcome. For example, Tablan (1970), in a study of 333 cerebral palsied patients, found that 11.7 per cent had two disabilities, 40.0 per cent had three disabilities, 32.0 per cent had four disabilities, 11.7 per cent had five disabilities, 3.0 per cent had six disabilities, and 1.6 per cent had seven disabilities.

Reports vary as to the frequency of different types of associated handicap. In Tablan's (1970) series, 82 per cent had speech problems, 34 per cent had visual defects, 32 per cent showed hyperkinetic behavior, 19 per cent were mentally retarded, 15 per cent were suffering from deafness, and 13.6 per cent showed perceptual deficiencies. In another study (Henderson 1961), 25 per cent had speech problems, 25 per cent epilepsy, 58 per cent visual defects, 50 per cent mental retardation and 23 per cent deafness. The deafness had not been suspected in two thirds of the last-mentioned group prior to audiometric testing. Robinson (1973) found that deafness does not commonly follow perinatal hypoxia unless at least two other associated deficits (*e.g.* grand mal seizures, microcephaly) are present. In general, the incidence of associated physical handicaps tends to increase in proportion to the severity of the motor and mental deficits.

CHARACTERISTICS AND COURSE OF DEVELOPMENT OF DIFFERENT TYPES OF
CEREBRAL PALSY

(1) Spasticity

In patients with spasticity one usually finds (Paine and Oppé 1966):
(1) a loss of control and differentiation of fine voluntary movements;
(2) suppression of normal associated movements;
(3) presence of certain abnormal associated movements;
(4) hypertonus of the clasp-knife type, with give-way following build-up of resistance to passive movement (stretch reflex);*
(5) exaggerated tendon reflexes and possible clonus at the ankle or other joints;
(6) depression of superficial reflexes;
(7) specific abnormality of reflexes referrable to the pyramidal pathway, such as the sign of Babinski.

If the spasticity is restricted to the arm and leg on the same side (hemiplegia), the condition may be either congenital or acquired.

Flexor tone tends to be greater than extensor tone, especially in the upper extremities. Perceptual disturbances are frequent. Imbalance of strength of muscles leads to contractures of spastic muscles and weakness resulting from disuse of their opponents. Flexor-extensor synergies predominate.

Spastic Hemiplegia, Congenital

In infancy, the first signs of congenital spastic hemiplegia are usually asymmetrical use of the of the extremities, a tendency for one hand to be fisted in the prone position more than the other, and a lack of reciprocal kicking. On examination, resistance to passive supination of the forearm and to elbow and finger extension may be greater on one side. Contractures may be evident by the age of one to one and a half years (Byers 1941). A stronger Babinski response on the affected side is to be

---

* Though some muscles show muscular hypertonus of the clasp-knife type, other muscles in the same child may be normal or show hypotonus. It is important to identify the muscle groups involved.

expected. In the second half of the first year, primitive postural and righting responses, such as the buttress or lateral parachute reaction, as well as the forward parachute and placing response in the lower extremities, are poorly performed or slower on the affected side.

Cranial nerves are frequently involved, with resulting concomitant strabismus (Crothers and Paine 1959) and supranuclear involvement of the muscles innervated by the lower cranial nerves, especially paresis of the face (Byers 1941). Tongue muscles may also be involved, but in the hemiplegic child speech and swallowing mechanisms are rarely affected. With persistence of the hemiplegia, somatic undergrowth (greater in the upper than in the lower extremity) may be observed. This is frequently accompanied by proprioceptive or cortical sensory loss, especially in the fingers and hand of the affected side; sometimes the patient shows inattention to objects entering the visual field from the affected side. The degree of motor deficit may be related to the sensory loss (Jones 1960, Paine and Oppé 1966).

Seizures occur at some time in approximately one third of all cerebral palsied individuals, (more frequently in the hemiplegic and quadraplegic) but the onset may be delayed until early childhood. The finding of spike foci on electroencephalography makes the likelihood of seizures greater. Intellectual progress has been found to be unfavorably influenced by the presence of seizures. For example, in a follow-up study of cerebral palsied patients, Glenting (1963) reported satisfactory intellectual development in 82 per cent of those who had had no seizures, but in only 55 per cent of those with seizures. Perlstein and Hood (1956) reported that in their series of hemiplegic children the mean I.Q. of the 76 who had seizures was 70.2, whereas that of the 97 children who had no seizures was 97. As suggested by Carmichael (1961), the principal reason for this discrepancy may be the effect of the heavy doses of drugs administered to patients with seizures.

As regards physical development, three factors appear to be of major importance in determining the course of the condition during growth. The first is the amount of attention paid to the affected hand; the second is somatic undergrowth of the affected side; and the third is the development of contractures, in particular contractures in the pronators of the foreams and the flexors of the elbows, wrists and fingers, or tightening of the tendo achilles, with limitation of both passive and active dorsiflexion of the foot. Contractures are especially likely to become evident during periods of rapid growth, which result in increased muscle imbalance.

Aggressive behavior and frequent temper tantrums are characteristic of hemiplegic children, and may be quite marked and of major importance. No significant difference in the time of development of speech or walking has been reported between right and left hemiplegics (Kastein and Hendin 1951, Hood and Perlstein 1956, Crothers and Paine 1959).

Acquired Spastic Hemiplegia

Hemiplegia may occur during a febrile illness, with or without accompanying seizures, and with or without a past history of abnormal birth. Alternatively, it may develop insidiously. Initial flaccid paresis is followed by the development of spasticity. In acquired hemiplegia, choreiform or other types of abnormal movements may be seen, especially at the time when the initial weakness is beginning to disappear. The aphasia following hemiplegia which affects the dominant side varies in duration.

The diagnostic problems presented by acquired hemiplegia have been discussed in Bax and Mitchell (1962) and, from a neuroradiological viewpoint, in Isler (1971). Definite prognostic statements cannot be made without very long-term follow-up (Crothers and Paine 1959). In Crothers and Paine's (1959) series, the intellectual prognosis was more favorable if the child was over two years of age when the hemiplegia developed.

Spastic Paraplegia and Diplegia

By definition, the paraplegic is the child in whom involvement is present in the legs only. Diplegia refers to the child who has greater spasticity in the lower than in the upper extremeties. Spastic diplegia is the type of cerebral palsy most frequently seen in children who are born small-for-dates or before term. McDonald (1967) reported that 81 per cent of 70 cerebral palsied children whose birthweights had been 4 lbs (1800g) or less had spastic diplegia. McDonald also reported that spastic diplegia occurred more often in single children of low birthweight (6.7 per cent) than in multiple births (1.9 per cent). A possible etiology is cyanotic attacks in the early postnatal period, resulting in arterial hypotension in the areas where the anterior and middle and middle and posterior cerebral arteries supply adjacent zones (periventricular leukomalacia) (Banker and Larroche 1962, McDonald 1967).

In the first six months of life, it is unusual for either physicians or parents to identify any specific abnormality in a premature child's development. In the second half of the first year, increased clasp-knife spasticity in the hip adductors, hip, knee and ankle flexors, and the pronators of the forearms, becomes evident. Reciprocal kicking may not be seen. Sitting is delayed.

Secondary contractures and deformities may develop as early as the second or third year of life. Hip dislocation may occur in association with spasticity in the hip adductors and flexors, whether or not weight-bearing takes place. X-rays of the hips may show flattening or tear-drop formation of the epiphysis of the caput femoris in children of the toddler age group, despite a normal acetabulum (Mathews *et al.* 1963). Because of the difficulty of assessing hand function in the very young child, a premature infant may at first be thought to have only spastic paraplegia, whereas subsequently involvement of the upper extremities is definite (Jones *et al.* 1962).

If no deficit can be detected in the hands, a careful search for spinal lesions is essential before symptomatic treatment is begun. Some children who develop spastic paraplegia or diplegia have a positive family history of a similar problem. Without such a history, it is frequently difficult, if not impossible, to differentiate between non-progressive and progressive spastic paraplegia (Crothers and Paine 1959, Peterson and Coventry 1969).

The term 'double hemiplegia' is sometimes used for children in whom the hands and arms are more seriously involved than the legs, and who have a disorder which has the appearance of hemiplegia except that it affects both sides of the body. Some people would reserve the words 'spastic quadriplegia' or 'tetraplegia' for these children, who are discussed under a separate heading below.

Spastic Quadriplegia or Tetraplegia

Whereas in hemiplegics the arm is usually more involved than the leg, the reverse is frequently true in quadriplegics. Quadriplegics also commonly show deficits resulting from involvement of the supranuclear connections to the lower cranial nerves, *e.g.* a marked lack of facial expression in the lower half of the face, continuously open lips and drooling, and a lack of voluntary control of the tongue, which tends to lie in the mid-line, often protruding, with little movement of the tip and no lateral movement. In addition, they tend to have feeding problems, due to an absence of suck-swallow reflexes, and a failure to integrate feeding with breathing.

During early infancy, hypotonia is the prominent finding in children who will later develop spastic quadriplegia. Signs such as brisk or increased tendon reflexes and the persistence of a strong extensor plantar response are indications that this hypotonia will give way to a strong clasp-knife type of spasticity by the age of two to five years. The evolution of the increased muscle tone in these patients has been separated by Ingram (1964) into (a) the hypotonic stage, (b) a dystonic stage, and (c) a third stage in which rigidity and spasticity are present together in varying degrees. The differential diagnosis of the floppy infant is presented under the heading 'hypotonia' below.

Typically, the spontaneous posture of infants and children with spastic quadriplegia or tetraplegia is characterised by flexion of the trunk, adduction of the shoulders, flexion of the elbows, pronation of the forearms, and a tendency to adduction of the thumbs and flexion of the fingers. There is flexion, adduction and, sometimes, internal rotation at the hips, flexion at the knees, and plantar flexion of the feet, with inversion rather than eversion, and considerable scissoring when the patient is held in vertical suspension. As in patients with spastic paraplegia and diplegia, subluxation of the hips may develop.

With prolonged sitting, standing or lying in abnormal positions, children with spastic quadriplegia are likely to develop kyphosis or scoliosis. From a follow-up study comparing the outcome in treated and untreated patients with spastic quadriplegia, Paine (1962) concluded that among those receiving treatment (physiotherapy), gait was better and contractures were less severe or frequent, although the proportion of patients requiring orthopaedic surgery at a later date was similar in both groups.

Mental retardation and seizures are more common than in patients with spastic paraplegia or diplegia. In Crothers and Paine's (1959) series, patients with bilateral symmetrical quadriplegia appeared to be less intelligent than those with asymmetrical abnormalities.

(2) Dyskinetic Types of Cerebral Palsy—Extrapyramidal

Congenital Athetosis

In children considered as having athetosis, there are alterations in posture, with intermittent assumption of abnormal postural attitudes. Extensor tone tends to predominate. Tension may be little or great, and may vary with changes in emotional state. There is often spasticity as well in some muscles. Movements seen in patients with athetosis may be described under the following headings: athetoid movements; choreo-athetoid movements; dystonic movements; and ballismus.

Athetoid movements (mobile spasms) can be described as involuntary, irregular, coarse and relatively continuous writhing or squirming motions. They may combine flexion, extension, abduction, adduction, pronation and supination, and tend to affect the peripheral musculature of the limbs and the face. Athetoid movements are generally greater distally than they are in the proximal parts of the extremities. They may recur in series, intensified by voluntary motion or tension, but disappear in sleep. Tension frequently develops with increasing age (De Jong 1958).

Choreo-athetoid movements are similar in type to athetoid movements but are more abrupt, brief and jerky, *i.e.* like those seen in Sydenham's chorea.

Dystonic movements (torsion spasms) are similar to athetosis, but involve larger portions of the body (*e.g.* an entire extremity or the trunk) in slow rhythmic movements. There is frequently twisting of the spine, but little, if any, involvement of the digits. Muscles are hypotonic at rest, hypertonic in action.

Ballismus is a rare condition, characterised by large scale violent tossing or flinging movements, usually beginning in the proximal muscles of a limb.

Tremor is characterised by regular alternating movements, which may be fine (nine to ten per second) or coarse (three to five per second), and either static or intentional. Present in infancy, it persists throughout life.

Evolution of Types of Movement in Athetoid Cerebral Palsy

In the newborn period, infants with central nervous system damage from hyperbilirubinemia, for example due to Rhesus incompatibility or other blood incompatibility, most often show opisthotonus (Jones *et al.* 1954). Follow-up studies of older infants indicate a subsequent silent period as regards motor abnormality (Polani 1959, Ingram 1964). Polani (1959), however, found that of 73 patients who later developed athetosis, 25 had been seen by a physician in the first two months of life because of sucking or swallowing difficulty, and another eight at five to seven months when solid foods were introduced. Eleven had had stridor in the first two or three months. After the second month, neurological disturbances were found as follows: (1) developmental delay without other signs in 8; (2) attacks of opisthotonus in 37 floppy infants; (3) hypertonia which relaxed during sleep in 25; (4) striking hypertonia which relaxed during sleep in 25. In 39 of the 56 patients in whom the time of onset was known, the unwanted movements had first been observed before the age of two and a half years; in the remaining 17 the athetoid movements had first been observed at between three and three and a half years of age. In general, no abnormal movements had been detected prior to the end of the first year of life. Children who had shown lingering hypertonus from birth later began to show slow writhing movements of the trunk, whereas those in whom opisthotonus had disappeared early subsequently developed choreoathetosis of the face, tongue and limbs. Paine (1964) found that if athetoid movements were seen early, the child was more likely to develop a mild rather than a severe disability of hand function.

With growth, contractures and deformities are less likely to occur in children with athetosis than in those with spasticity. However, persistent lying, sitting or standing in asymmetrical or abnormal positions may result in contractures and deformities. For example, torticollis, scoliosis and abnormalities of the hips, knees and ankles may be found in severely involved patients. Secondary deformities are particularly to be expected in the presence of persisting strong asymmetrical tonic neck reflexes and if the patient shows dystonic movements or torsion spasms.

Crothers and Paine (1959) found that persistence of an obligate asymmetrical tonic neck reflex tends to interfere seriously with independent walking, although some individuals do learn to walk. Crothers and Paine also reported that, although both spastics and athetoids may show persistent asymmetrical tonic neck response, if a child with hypotonia lacks this reflex, he is likely to have extrapyramidal cerebral palsy. Other signs of extrapyramidal cerebral palsy are a delayed, stiff or disorganized parachute reaction and a delayed or incomplete Landau response.

Speech difficulty may parallel the over-all degree of athetosis. Breath control, as well as motor function of the lips, mandible and tongue, may be affected. There may be dysfunction in one or more of the oral pharyngeal functions.

Except for secondary deformities as indicated above, athetosis, once it has evolved, tends to be static. An increase in emotional tension during adolescence and adult life, in an effort to control the unwanted movements, may result in increased, often painful, muscle spasm.

Rigidity

The term rigidity is used when there is either resistance to passive movement throughout the entire range of motion, either constantly (lead-pipe type) or intermittently (cogwheel type). Rigidity is therefore to be contrasted with the 'clasp-knife' type of response referred to in the section on spasticity. Rigidity is frequently found both in patients with spasticity and in those with athetosis, but may occur alone. It may vary from time to time. Patients with spastic quadriplegia and rigidity show marked opisthotonus. Pathologically, such patients have both basal ganglia and cortical lesions (Christensen and Melchior 1967).

If rigidity predominates in the first two years of life, it may become more intense with age (Ford 1960). In these individuals, tonic fits, with retraction of the head, flexion of the arm and extension of the legs, have been reported. The deep tendon reflexes may be normal or they may be impossible to evaluate because of the rigidity. Bulbar signs and symptoms are usually present. Mental retardation is often found and may be severe.

(3) Ataxia and Ataxic Diplegia

'Ataxia is usually defined as a loss of the power of muscular co-ordination or as inco-ordination of muscular action. To this extent, it could be said to exist in all cerebral palsy, in as much as inco-ordination of movement is common to spastic as well as extrapyramidally involved patients. The word as more properly used implies inco-ordination either of cerebellar origin or based on interference with the proprioceptive system (including the peripheral nerves and the posterior column of the spinal cord). If this definition is adhered to, ataxic cerebral palsy must be a rare phenomenon.' (Crothers and Paine 1959.)

In Ingram's (1964) series of 15 children classified as ataxic, many were reported to have other neurological abnormalities in the limbs, such as an increase in muscle tone or hypotonia or athetosis or tremor. A clinical, pathological study done in Denmark (Christensen and Melchior 1967) did not include any cases diagnosed as having pure ataxia. Ataxia in combination with other types of cerebral palsy was reported in five patients. Neuropathological examination, however, revealed cerebellar abnormalities in 24 out of 69 patients. Christensen and Melchior concluded that clinical ataxia was probably masked in these patients by the presence of spasticity, rigidity and athetosis.

Ingram (1964) and Gustavson *et al.* (1969) have both described a group of children who, following apnea and generalized seizures in the newborn period, are 'floppy' for the first six months, and show delay in developmental milestones, especially in speech; they also have a tendency to hydrocephalus. At about four months of age, the legs show signs of spasticity, and knee jerks, previously difficult to obtain, appear. Intention tremor of the head (especially on side to side motion) and of the hands (especially on reach) also appears. The patient shows gross unsteadiness in walking and a tendency to circumduct the legs. Infrequent swallowing and excessive drooling are also present. Spontaneous improvement occurs over a period of time. Some of these children are retarded mentally. The family history suggests a dominant mode of inheritance in some.

(4) The Floppy Infant

Many cerebral palsied children are hypotonic or floppy as babies; on the other hand, most hypotonic babies do not develop cerebral palsy. The diagnosis of the hypotonic baby is one of the most difficult problems in paediatrics, and only a brief outline of the subject is given here.

'The diagnosis of hypotonia may, to some extent, be a subjective impression, based on the resistance of a limb to passive movement, or even on the postures which the child adopts.' (Dubowitz 1969)

In the initial and subsequent assessment of muscle function in the floppy infant, two positions have been found very useful (Dubowitz 1969). 'In ventral suspension, with the infant supported by a hand under the chest, head control, trunk curvature and control of the arms and legs can be readily assessed. A normal full-term newborn infant will hold his head at about 45 degrees or less to the horizontal; the back will be straight or only slightly flexed, the arms flexed at the elbows and partially extended at the shoulder, and the the knees partially flexed. Even an immature infant will show a variable degree of postural tone, depending on the length of gestation. The floppy infant, in contrast, will have marked head lag and floppiness of the trunk, arms and legs.'

When observed in the supine position, if he can move his limbs against gravity, either spontaneously or in response to a stimulus, or if he is able to maintain an elevated limb, he probably does not have significant weakness.

'The first two questions to be asked when confronted with a floppy baby are:
(1) is this a paralysed child with incidental hypotonia?
(2) is this a hypotonic child without significant muscle weakness? (see Table V).
An answer to these questions will subdivide the cases into two broad groups: the paralytic and the non-paralytic. The distinction can usually be made by careful

TABLE V

Suggested classification of the floppy infant (From Dubowitz 1969)

I. *Paralytic Conditions (weakness with incidental hypotonia)*
  (1) *Proximal spinal muscular atrophies—neurogenic atrophies*
      (a) Infantile spinal muscular atrophy (Werdnig-Hoffmann's disease)
      (b) Benign variants

  (2) *Congenital myopathies*
      (a) 'Structural' ——central core disease
                         nemaline myopathy
                         myotubular myopathy
                         mitochondrial abnormalities
                         miscellaneous
      (b) Metabolic — glycogenoses

  (3) *Other neuromuscular disorders*
      (a) Muscular dystrophy — early onset Duchenne dystrophy
      (b) Congenital muscular dystrophy
      (c) Dystrophia myotonica
      (d) Myasthenia gravis
      (c) Periodic paralysis
      (f) Polymyositis
      (g) Peripheral neuropathies

II. *Non-Paralytic Conditions (hypotonia without significant weakness)*
  (1) *Disorders of the central nervous system*
      (a) Non-specific mental deficiency
      (b) Hypotonic cerebral palsy, athetosis, ataxia
      (c) Metabolic disorders: abnormalities of amino acid metabolism,
                         abnormalities of mucopolysaccharide metabolism,
                         lipidoses
      (d) Mongolism
      (e) Birth trauma, intracranial haemorrhage, anoxia

  (2) *Hypotonia-obesity syndrome (Prader-Willi)*

  (3) *Connective tissue disorders*
          Congenital laxity of the ligaments; Marfan's syndrome;
          Ehlers-Danlos syndrome; osteogenesis imperfecta; arachnodactyly

  (4) *Metabolic, nutritional, endocrine*
          Coeliac disease, hypothyroidism, hypercalcaemia, renal tubular acidosis, rickets

  (5) *Acute illness*
          Infection, dehydration

  (6) *Miscellaneous*
          Congenital heart disease

  (7) *Benign congenital hypotonia; 'essential hypotonia'.*

observation of the floppy infant in the supine position. If he is able to move his limbs against gravity, either spontaneously or following a stimulus to the soles of the feet or the hands, or if he is able to maintain the posture of an elevated limb, he does not have significant weakness.' (Dubowitz 1969.)

In one follow-up study of cerebral palsied children who had shown hypotonia from an early age, all were found subsequently to have acquired normal or lively deep tendon reflexes and athetosis (Crothers and Paine 1959). Paine (1963) followed 112 patients who had first been referred for neurological evaluation between the ages of six months and two and a half years, and had been found to have hypotonia on

15

physical examination. He suggested that patients with 'congential hypotonia' could be divided into three groups.

(1) Patients with a family history of double jointedness, hypotonia, or a delay in learning to walk, without neurological abnormalities, and whose progress is benign apart from some delay in achieving motor milestones.

(2) Patients similar to those in group (1), but without positive family histories. Follow-up of eight such children showed four to be mentally retarded, one to be abnormally clumsy, and three to be normal. Paine concluded that in these patients the early hypotonia was of central origin.

(3) Patients with overt or borderline deficits, in whom the hypotonia of the muscles is a manifestation of abnormal function of the central nervous system. The presence of tonic neck reflexes, even as an isolated neurological sign should make one suspect that a patient belongs to this group rather than to groups (1) or (2).

(5) Mixed Types of Cerebral Palsy

Any of the above types of abnormal movements may be, and often are, combined in the same individual. Early in life it is often very difficult either to determine whether more than one type is present, or to differentiate with certainty between the types. The course will depend on the extent and severity of the involvement.

DIFFERENTIAL DIAGNOSIS

The differential diagnosis of the motor disorder in cerebral palsy involves:

(1) the identification in infancy of the cerebral palsied child as compared to the child with a progressive (possibly remediable) condition;

(2) the classification of the cerebral palsy according to the type of sensory motor involvement;

(3) the differentiation of cerebral palsy from other known syndromes, progressive and/or remediable conditions, in which hyper- or hypotonio are present, with or without spasticity, athetosis, rigidity or ataxia.

The Identification of the Infant with Cerebral Palsy

The following clues are helpful in the identification of the child with cerebral palsy.

(a) As compared to the normal, the developmental sequence of the postural and righting reflexes may be delayed, and roughly parallel intellectual development. However, Walton *et al.* (1962) have identified clumsy children who, at first considered mentally retarded, were found on further study to have developmental apraxia and agnosia. Such children showed a marked discrepancy between their verbal skills and their performances on the Weschler Scale for children.

Deficits in feeding, suck-swallowing reflexes and breathing may be the earliest abnormalities observed in the newborn or young infant who later shows motor abnormalities considered to come under the heading of cerebral palsy. Malfunction in the oral pharyngeal area in infancy may correlate with delay in development and abnormality in speech, as well as with difficulty in feeding in infancy (Bosna 1967, Wolff 1968, Ardran and Kemp 1970, Mueller 1972).

(b) The sequential evaluation of postural and righting reflexes may provide important clues (Milani-Comparetti and Gidoni 1967). As illustrated in Figures 1a to e, muscle tone, deep tendon reflexes (DTR's), tonic neck reflexes (TNR's), neck-righting reflexes (NRR's) and automatisms are directly related to the development of sitting, standing and walking balance (Paine 1964).

(c) There may be evidence of peripheral neuropathy in patients with genetic disorders which will develop later. Nerve conduction times will need to be measured for diagnosis (Philippart 1973, personal communication).

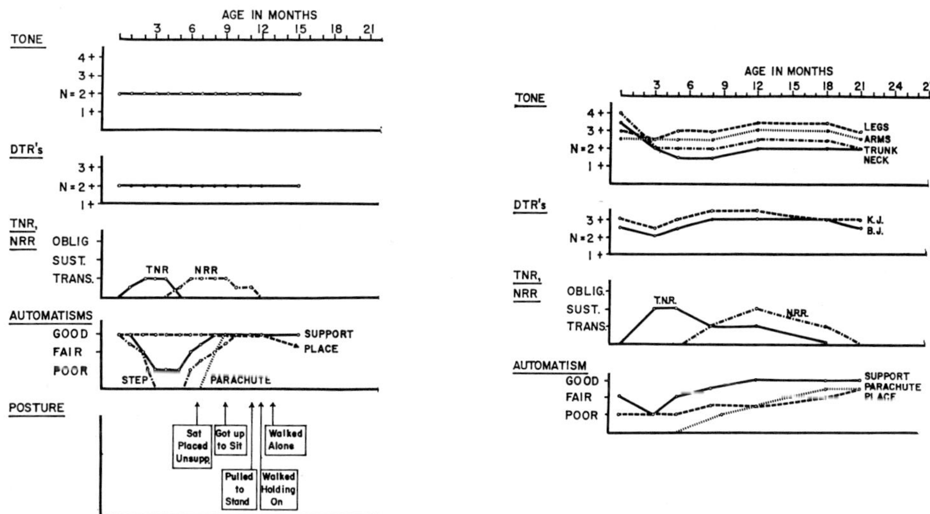

Fig. 1a (*left*). Evolution of signs in a normal infant, including muscle tone and tendon reflexes (on scale of 0 to 4+, 2+ being normal), tonic neck and neck righting reflexes (obligate sustained, or transient*), stepping, supporting, placing and parachute responses and postural maturation. Note that stepping and supporting reactions are suppressed at about three months and later re-emerge, as appears to take place in most but not in all normal babies. (From Paine 1964)

Fig. 1b (*right*). Evolution of spastic tetraparesis presumably based on anoxia at birth. Neonatal hypertonus and hyperreflexia disappear and later return, the tone increasing in the extremities before the trunk and neck. Both appearance and disappearance of tonic neck and neck righting reflexes are delayed. Supporting reaction is more effective than parachute. (From Paine 1964)

*In Figures 1a to e 'obligate sustained' indicates a tonic neck reflex imposable for an indefinite period and obtained on every trial; 'sustained' indicates an imposable pattern maintained for more than 30 seconds but subsequently broken down by the infant; and 'transient' indicates an imposable pattern broken through in less than 30 seconds.

17

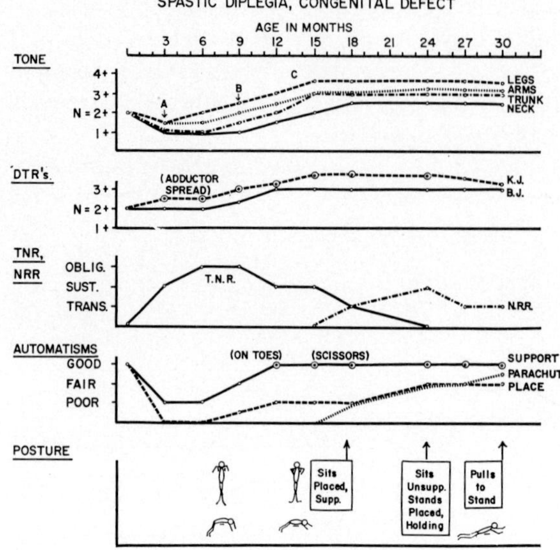

Fig. 1c. Evolution of spastic tetraparesis associated with cerebral dysgenesis but not manifestly abnormal in the newborn period. Note phase of hypotonia at three months. Posture in vertical and horizontal suspension in space is also indicated by line drawings. (From Paine 1964)

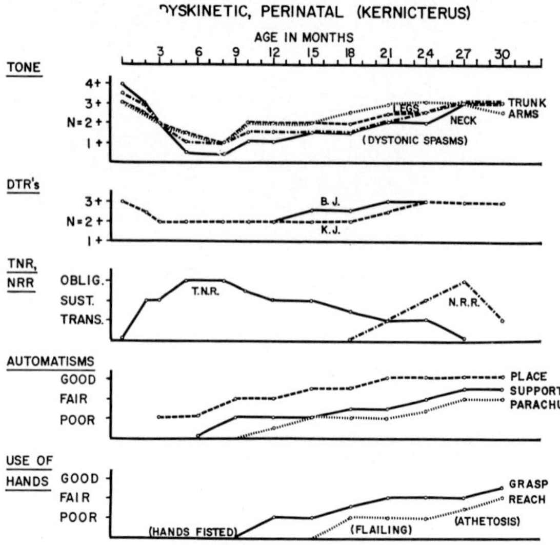

Fig. 1d. Evolution of one patient who developed dystonia and athetosis. Kernicterus, as in this example, produces a rigid newborn who later becomes hypotonic for a considerable period. (From Paine 1964)

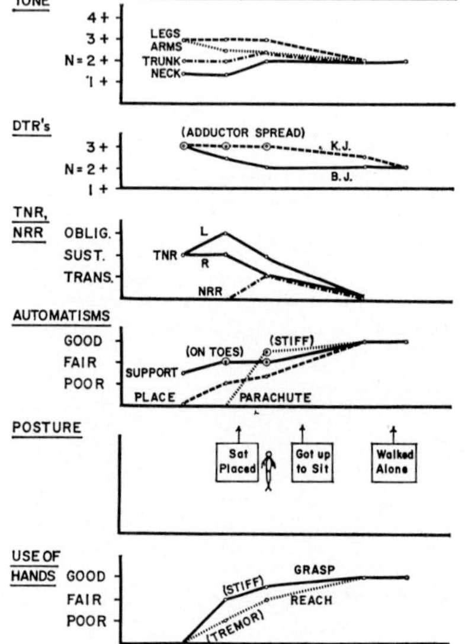

Fig. 1e. Evolution of signs following anoxic birth. Baby appeared to have probable spastic tetraparesis in first year of life, but no abnormal motor signs could be detected subsequent to age 19 months. (From Paine 1964)

Differentiation of Type of Cerebral Palsy

The characteristics of the two most common types of cerebral palsy, spasticity and athetosis, are compared in Table VI. It is essential to remember that assessment is difficult, often erroneous, unless the infant or young child is fully relaxed.

TABLE VI

Comparison of characteristics of spasticity and athetosis (from Gillette 1969).

	Spasticity	*Dyskinesia (asthetosis included)*
Muscle response to stimulus	Exaggerated stretch reflex	Continuum of reflexive movement
	Short stretch augments tone, long stretch inhibits	Short stretch inhibits tone, long stretch augments
Tone	Greatest in flexors of arms, extensors of legs	Extensor tone predominates throughout
Synergy	Flexor-extensor synergies predominate	Labyrinthine and neck reflexes predominate
Orientation	Perceptual disturbances	No perceptual disturbances
Strength	Imbalance of power due to constant unbalanced tone, contractures and weakness of disuse	Imbalance of power due to response to labarynthine and righting reflexes

Muscular relaxation is just as important as muscular contraction in determining the action of muscles. Holt (1966) finds that reliable predictions about the functional activity of muscles cannot be made from observation or from the action of muscles in response to voluntary motion. Clinical spasticity is a complex phenomenon, and apparently similar 'spastic' muscles do not always act the same way as expected.

Figure 2 shows two children with cerebral palsy, of similar age and type of deformity. Electromyograms from these two children (Fig. 3) show that, in spite of the apparent similarities, their neuromuscular involvement differed considerably. One has marked activity in the hamstrings and gastrocnemius muscles, while in the other these muscles are relatively quiet and the quadriceps and anterior tibial muscles are the most active (Holt 1966).

Figure 4 is a walking electromyographic record which was taken to find out why this girl was failing to make progress. She was extremely floppy, and the therapists reported that she made no effort to use her muscles to stand. The record shows that despite the clinical impression to the contrary this girl's muscles were in fact in constant strong activity (Holt 1966).

On the basis of this electromyographic evidence, Holt proposed the following statements.

(a) 'The state of activity of the muscles cannot be predicted reliably from inspection and clinical examination.'

(b) 'The functional activity of a muscle may be different from its action in response to conscious effort.'

19

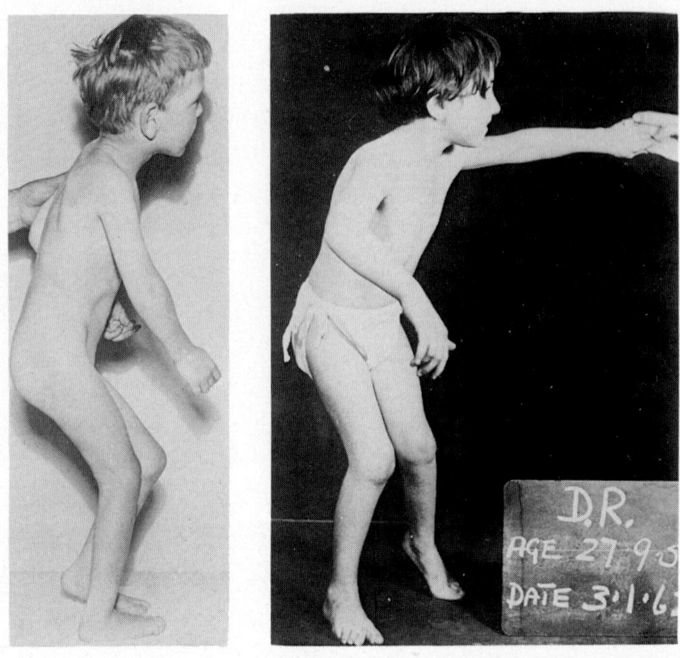

Fig. 2. Two children with apparently similar type of involvement. (From Holt 1966.)

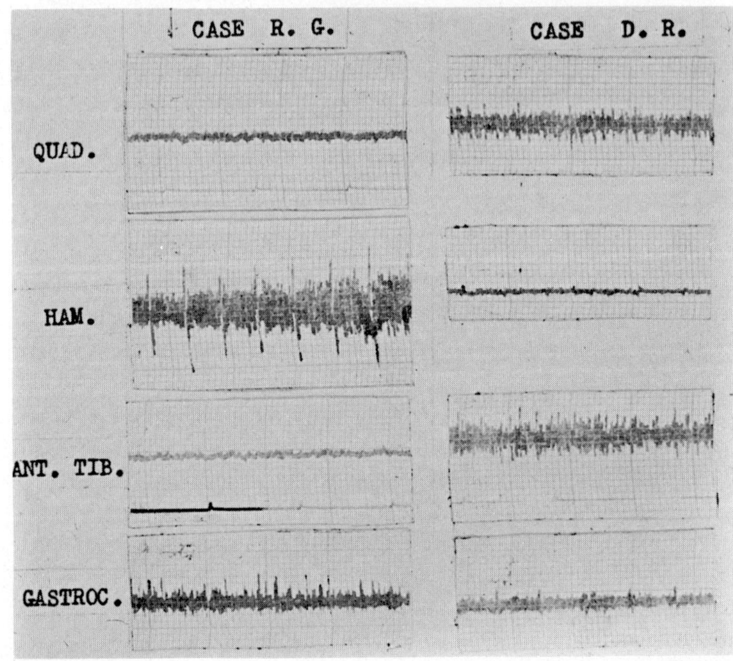

Fig. 3. Electromyograms of children in Figure 2, showing differences in neuromuscular involvement.

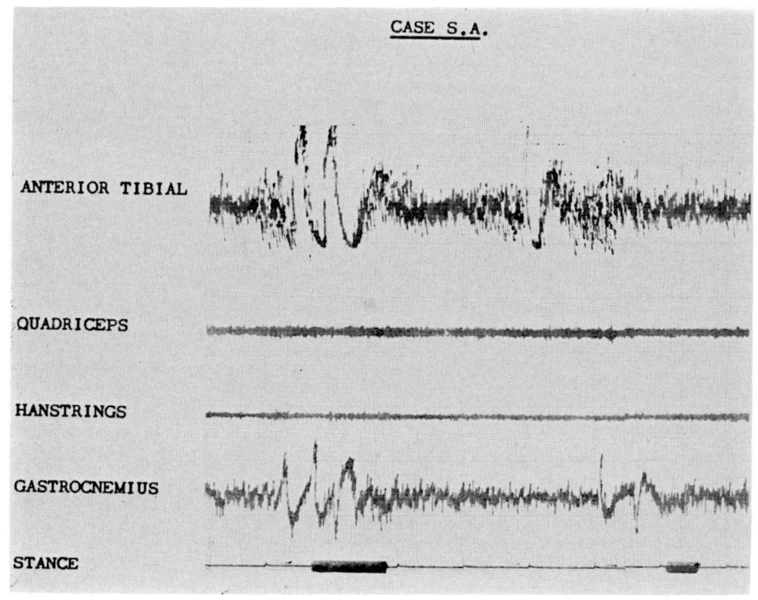

Fig. 4.
(From Holt 1966)

Differentiation of Cerebral Palsy from Other Known Syndromes and from Progressive and/or Remediable Conditions

A list of known syndromes presenting with hypotonia, hypertonia or ataxia is set out in Table VII (From Smith 1970).

As indicated by Dubowitz (1969) (see Table V), many conditions which have to be differentiated from cerebral palsy are characterized by muscle weakness with incidental hypotonia (for example the proximal muscle spinal atrophies, congenital myopathies and other neuromuscular disease). In this (the 'paralytic') group (Group I), diagnostic procedures are directed towards establishing the presence and nature of any underlying neuromuscular disorder, muscle biopsy being the most useful investigation. Table VIII lists some examples of studies to be considered for the diagnosis of some of the conditions listed in Group I. The most significant for diagnosis are underlined.

In the 'non-paralytic' group (Group II), muscle biopsy is not, in general, useful, although in borderline cases, especially if other factors such as intellectual impairment accompany some degree of muscle weakness, it may be helpful.

Differentiation of Cerebral Palsy from 'Non-paralytic' Disorders with Mental Retardation

The following screening procedures are suggested (Philippart 1973, adapted from Dubowitz 1969).
(a) Scrum electrolytes: to exclude such conditions as hypercalcemia, hypernatremia, hypo- or hyperkalemia, and renal acidosis.
(b) Urine or blood amino acid chromatography: to exclude some inborn errors of metabolism.

TABLE VII (from Smith 1970)

Syndromes with central nervous system deficits resulting in hypotonia, hypertonia or ataxia

	Frequent in	*Occasional in*
Hypotonia	Achondroplasia	Aminopterin-induced syndrome
	Cerebro-hepato-renal syndrome	Blepharophimosis
	Down's syndrome	Cri-du-chat syndrome
	Generalized gangliosidosis	Hypercalcemia—peculiar facies—supravalvular aortic stenosis
	Lowe's syndrome	myotonic dystrophy
	Marfan's syndrome	13 trisomy syndrome
	Marinesco-Sjögren syndrome (with or without weakness)	
	Oculo-cerebro-renal syndrome	
	Prader-Willi syndrome	
	Rieger's syndrome	
	XXXXY syndrome	
	No. 18 long arm deletion syndrome	
Hypertonia	Cornelia de Lange syndrome	Incontinentia pigmenti
	Menkes' syndrome	Sturge-Weber syndrome
	Sjögren-Larsson syndrome	X-linked hydrocephalus
	18 trisomy syndrome	13 trisomy syndrome
	No. 21 long arm deletion syndrome	
Ataxia	Ataxia-teleangiectasia (onset one to five years)	
	Biemond's syndrome	
	Cockayne's syndrome	
	Marinesco-Sjögren syndrome	

(c) Urine analysis for aryl sulphatase A: to exclude metachromatic leucodystrophy.

(d) Serum or leucocyte analysis for alpha glucosidase: to exclude Pompe's disease Type II.

(e) Serum protein bound iodine and boneage: for diagnosis of hypothyroidism.

(f) Skull radiography: for intracranial calcifications, craniostenosis, and increased intracranial pressure.

(g) Chromosome studies: especially if the patient has obvious malformations.

(h) Lumbar puncture: for abnormalities such as increased CSF protein.

Conclusions

The term cerebral palsy refers to a heterogeneous group of individuals, three quarters of whom have had the condition from birth, and one quarter from early life. Many cerebral palsied patients have visual, hearing or tactile deficits. About one third have seizures at some time, and about 10 per cent have epilepsy continuing into adult life. Prediction of the natural history for an individual child is complicated (a) by the difficulty of making an early definitive diagnosis, (b) by the knowledge that in a

22

TABLE VIII

Examples of investigations for 'paralytic' group (weakness with incidental hypotonia) (Adapted from Dubowitz 1969 and Walton 1969, with assistance from A. Philippart and R. Groover)

Studies	Infantile muscle atrophy	Morphologically distinct congenital myopathies	Muscular dystrophy pseudohypertrophy	Dystrophia myotonia	Myasthenia gravis	Periodic paralysis	Polymyositis	Peripheral* neuropathy
Clinical clues	Generalized or proximal muscle weakness	Generalized weakness, proximal, distal	Proximal weakness Early shoulder and pelvic girdle weakness	Facia. diplegia, may appear normal in infant delay in opening eyes after crying	May appear normal after rest, weakness with exercise	Normal between attacks. Chronic weakness may develop later	Associated with acute illness—often muscle tenderness	Normal or loss of DTR and distal muscle weakness
Muscle biopsy	Denervation atrophy	Abnormal characteristic morphological changes in muscle	Myopathic changes	Myopathy. Special stains may reveal some characteristic changes.	n. or focal denervation	Abnormal + −	Myopathic with inflammatory changes	Denervation
Serum enzymes	n. or slightly ↑	usually normal	CPK ↑ LDH ↑ SGOT ↑	usually normal	n.	usually normal CPK may be elevated in attack	CPK usually increased often quite high	CPK usually normal may be slightly elevated
Immune glob.	n.	n.	n.	(linked with secretor gene) IgG ↓	n.	n.	n.	n.
Electromyography	Denervation	May be normal or "myopathic"	"Myopathic"	Abnormal sound patterns ± characteristic pattern of myotonia	Rapid fatigability of muscle to repeated stimulation	May be normal but isoelectric if during attack	'Myopathic'	Denervation
Nerve conduction velocity	normal or minimally slow	n.	n.	n.	n.	n.	n.	Usually slowed
Nerve biopsy	not helpful	not helpful	not helpful	not helpful	not helpful	not helpful	not helpful	Degen. changes (sural nerve usually studied)
Genetics**	AR	AR or AD	X-linked AR	AD	NF except in congenital type	AR	NF	depends on type

*The possibility of peripheral neuropathy due to genetic disorders which will develop later needs to be kept in mind.
**AR—autosomal recessive, AD—autosomal dominant, NF—non-familial.
Most important tests underlined.

small percentage (possibly 10 to 20 per cent) the motor problem present in infancy will improve, and (c) by the knowledge that long-term outcome depends probably more on how the children are handled in their early lives and on social and environmental factors than on the basic sensory-motor deficits. Optimally, between one quarter and one third become entirely self-supporting in adult life.

BIBLIOGRAPHY

Ardran, G. M., Kemp, F. H. (1970) 'Some important factors in the assessment of oropharyngeal function.' *Developmental Medicine and Child Neurology,* **12,** 158.

Banker, B. Q., Larroche, J. C. (1962) 'Periventricular leukomalacia of infancy—a form of neonatal anoxic encephalopathy.' *Archives of Neurology,* **7,** 386.

Bax, M. C. O. (1964) 'Terminology and classification of cerebral palsy.' *Developmental Medicine and Child Neurology,* **6,** 295.

—— Mitchell, R. G. (Eds.) (1962) *Acute Hemiplegia in Childhood. Clinics in Developmental Medicine No. 6.* London: Spastics International Medical Publications with Heinemann Medical.

Beintema, D. J. (1968) *A Neurological Study of Newborn Infants. Clinics in Developmental Medicine, No. 28.* London: Spastics Society with Heinemann.

Bosna, J. F. (1967) 'Human infant oral function.' *in Symposium on Oral Sensation and Perception.* Springfield, Ill.: C. C. Thomas.

Brazelton, T. B. (1961) Psychopathologic reactions in the neonate. I. The value of observation of the neonate.' *Journal of Pediatrics,* **58,** 508.

Byers, R. K. (1941) 'Evolution of hemiplegia in infancy.' *American Journal of Diseases of Children,* **61,** 915.

Carmichael, E. A. (1961) 'Hemiplegia and hemispherectomy.' *in Hemiplegic Cerebral Palsy in Children and Adults. Little Club Clinics in Developmental Medicine, No. 4.* London: Spastics Society with Heinemann, p. 132.

Christensen, E., Melchior, J. (1967) *Cerebral Palsy —A Clinical and Neuropathological Study. Clinics in Developmental Medicine, No. 25.* London: Spastics Society with Heinemann.

Crothers, B., Paine, R. S. (1959) *The Natural History of Cerebral Palsy.* London: O.U.P.

Curtis, L. W. (1951-1953) *Vocational Placement in Cerebral Palsy.* New York: United Cerebral Palsy Association.

De Jong, R. N. (1958) *The Neurological Examination.* New York: Hoeber-Harper.

Denhofe, E. (1967) *Cerebral Palsy—The Preschool Years.* Springfield, Ill.: C. C. Thomas.

Dubowitz, V. (1969) *The Floppy Infant. Clinics in Developmental Medicine, No. 31.* London: Spastics Society with Heinemann.

Foerster, O. (1910) 'Der atonische-astatische Typus der infantilen Cerebrallähmung.' *Deutsche Archiv für klinische Medizin,* **98,** 216.

Foley, J. (1968) 'Deterioration in the EEG in children with cerebral palsy.' *Developmental Medicine and Child Neurology,* **10,** 287.

Ford, R. R. (1960) *Diseases of the Nervous System in Infancy, Childhood and Adolescence. 4th Edn.* Springfield: Ill.: C. C. Thomas.

Gillette, H. E. (1969) *Systems of Therapy in Cerebral Palsy.* 'Springfield, Ill.: C. C. Thomas.

Glenting, P. (1963) 'Course and prognosis of congenital spastic hemiplegia.' *Developmental Medicine and Child Neurology,* **5,** 252.

Gustavson, K. H., Hagberg, B., Sanner, G. (1969) 'Identical syndromes in cerebral palsy.' *Acta Paediatrica Scandinavica,* **58,** 330.

Hansen, E. (1960) 'Cerebral palsy in Denmark.' *Acta Psychiatrica et Neurologica Scandinavica,* Suppl. 146.

Hanson, R. A., Berenberg, W., Byers, R. K. (1970) 'Changing motor patterns in cerebral palsy.' *Developmental Medicine and Child Neurology,* **12,** 309.

Henderson, J. L. (Ed.) (1961) *Cerebral Palsy in Childhood and Adolescence.* Edinburgh: Livingstone.

Holt, K. S. (1966) 'Facts and fallacies about neuromuscular function in cerebral palsy as revealed by electromyography.' *Developmental Medicine and Child Neurology,* **8,** 255.

Hood, P. N., Perlstein, M. A. (1956) 'Infantile spastic hemiplegia. V. Oral language and motor development.' *Pediatrics,* **17,** 58.

Hutchinson, J., Muthard, J. E. (1969) 'College and the C.P.' *Developmental Medicine and Child Neurology,* **11,** 253. (*Abstract.*)

Ingram, T. T. S. (1964) *Paediatric Aspects of Cerebral Palsy.* Edinburgh: Livingstone.

Isler, W. (1971) *Acute Hemiplegias and Hemisyndromes in Childhood. Clinics in Developmental Medicine Nos. 41/42.* London: Spastics International Medical Publications with Heinemann Medical.

Jones, M. H., Maschmeyer, J. E. (1958) 'Childhood Aims and Adult Accomplishments in Cerebral Palsy.' *International Record of Medicine,* **171,** 219.

Jones, M. H., Sands, R., Hyman, C. B., Sturgeon, P., Koch, F. P. (1954) 'Study of the incidence of central nervous system damage following erythroblastosis foetalis.' *Pediatrics,* **14,** 346.

—— Wenner, W. H., Toczek, A. M., Barrett, M. L. (1962) 'Prenursery school program for children with cerebral palsy.' *American Medical Women's Journal.* **17,** 713.

Kastein, S., Hendin, J. (1951) 'Language development in a group of children with spastic hemiplegia.' *Journal of Pediatrics,* **39,** 476.

Kendall, R. H., Bissell, E. M., Pedder, R. A. (1964) 'Deterioration of the cerebral palsied in adolescence.' *Developmental Medicine and Child Neurology,* **6,** 80.

McDonald, A. (1967) *Children of Very Low Birth Weight.* Spastics Society with Heinemann.

Margulec, J. (1966) *Cerebral Palsy in Adolescence and Adulthood.* Jerusalem: Academic Press.

Mathews, S. S., Jones, M. H., Sperling, S. C. (1953) 'Hip derangements seen in cerebral palsied children.' *American Journal of Physical Medicine,* **32,** 213.

Milani-Comparetti, A., Gidoni, E. A. (1967) 'Pattern analysis of motor development and its disorders.' *Developmental Medicine and Child Neurology,* **9,** 625.

Mueller, H. A. (1972) 'Feeding and prespeech development.' in Pearson, P. H. (Ed.) *Physical Therapy in the Physical Disabilities.* Springfield, Ill.: C. C. Thomas.

Paine, R. S. (1962) 'On the treatment of cerebral palsy. The outcome of 177 patients, 74 totally untreated.' *Pediatrics,* **29,** 605.

—— (1963) 'The future of the "floppy infant": a follow-up study of 133 patients.' *Developmental Medicine and Child Neurology,* **5,** 115.

—— (1964) 'The evaluation of infantile postural reflexes in the presence of chronic brain syndromes.' *Developmental Medicine and Child Neurology,* **6,** 345.

—— (1966) 'Cerebral palsy: symptoms and signs of diagnostic and prognostic significance.' *Current Practice in Orthopedic Surgery,* **3,** 39.

—— Oppé, T. E. (1966) *The Neurological Examination of Children. Clinics in Developmental Medicine, Nos. 20/21.* London: Spastics Society with Heinemann.

Perlstein, M. A., Hood, P. M. (1956) 'Infantile spastic hemiplegia, intelligence, oral language and motor development.' *Courrier,* **6,** 567.

Peterson, H. A., Coventry, M. B. (1969) 'Long-term results of surgical treatment of adults with cerebral palsy.' *Developmental Medicine and Child Neurology,* **11,** 35.

Philippart, M. (1973) *Personal communication*

Polani, P. E. (1959) 'The natural history of choreoathetoid cerebral palsy.' *Guy's Hospital Reports,* **32,** 108.

Pollock, G. A., Stark, G. (1969) 'Long-term results in the management of 67 children with cerebral palsy.' *Developmental Medicine and Child Neurology* **11,** 17.

Prechtl, H. F. R. (1965) 'Prognostic value of neurological signs in the newborn infant.' *Proceedings of the Royal Society of Medicine,* **58,** 3.

Roberts, C. J. (1970) 'Visual handicaps in congenitally deaf children.' *Developmental Medicine and Child Neurology,* **12,** 32.

Robinson, R. O. (1973) 'The frequency of other handicaps in children with cerebral palsy.' *Developmental Medicine and Child Neurology,* **15,** 305.

Rutter, M., Graham, P., Yule, W. (1970) *A Neuropsychiatric Study in Childhood. Clinics in Developmental Medicine,* Nos. 35/36. London: Spastics International Medical Publications with Heinemann Medical.

Schenectady County Study. Report of the New York State Joint Legislative Committee to study the problem of cerebral palsy (1949). *A Survey of Cerebral Palsy in Schenectady County.* New York Legislation Document 55, Section 2.

Schlesinger, E. R., Allaway, N. C., Pelton, S. (1959) 'Survivorship in cerebral palsy.' *American Journal of Public Health,* **49,** 343.

Smith, D. W. (1970) *Recognizable Human Malformations.* Philadelphia: W. B. Saunders.

Tablan, D. J. (1970) 'Clinical analysis of the brain-damaged child. An analysis of 333 cases in the Philippines.' *Paper presented at the International Society for Rehabilitation of the Disabled, Dublin.*

Walton, J. N. (1969) *Disorders of Voluntary Muscle. 2nd edn.* London: Churchill.

—— Ellis, E., Court, S. D. M. (1962) 'Clumsy children: developmental apraxia and agnosia.' *Brain,* **85,** 603.

Wolff, P. H. (1968) 'The serial organization of sucking in the young infant.' *Pediatrics,* **42,** 943.

Wortis, H., Cooper, W. (1957) 'Life experience of persons with cerebral palsy.' *American Journal of Physical Medicine,* **36,** 328.

CHAPTER 3

The Paediatric Rôle in the Care of the Child with Cerebral Palsy

MARTIN C. O. BAX and RONALD MAC KEITH

The main theme of this book is the care of the child who has been found to have cerebral palsy, but, apart from his concern with all aspects of the care of such children and their families, the paediatrician is also concerned with the prevention of cerebral palsy and with ensuring its early identification. There is no need to talk here about the prevention of cerebral palsy, for Mitchell (1971) has reviewed what can be done; this is very considerable. We wish, however, to emphasise the importance of early identification of cerebral palsy, because this affects the extent to which the child will require orthopaedic surgery. The child who is identified by the paediatrician at six months as having cerebral palsy and gets continuing care thenceforward, may not require the extensive surgery often needed by children brought late to the attention of the specialists.

With rare exceptions, children with cerebral palsy can be identified within the first year of life, but for this to be achieved all children should be given regular periodic developmental assessments under the supervision of a paediatrician. This assessment can be done in ten minutes. Various schemes for such examinations have been put forward, those of Frankenburg and Dodds (1967) and Egan *et al.* (1969) being but two examples. We shall not detail here the methods used, but simply report that in the clinic with which we are associated 90 per cent of the local cerebral palsied children arrive for treatment before the age of one year. Of the ten per cent of older children, most are recent arrivals in the district, while some are children who when still under one year old had only minor and uncertain signs of cerebral palsy and were therefore not in urgent need of physiotherapy.

Diagnostic problems are occasionally caused by unusual forms of normal development (Robson and Mac Keith 1971). In this paper, one of us has described the influence of the hitching or bottom shuffling trait on the natural history of cerebral palsy, showing that the emergence of signs of cerebral palsy could be delayed until the second or third years of life. In the first year, some cerebral palsied children show only generalised delay in development, but the periodic developmental examinations and the natural concern about the child lead eventually to the diagnosis. The child under one year of age who is suspected of having cerebral palsy presents some special difficulties in management which we shall not discuss here. We shall limit ourselves in this chapter to discussing the rôle of the paediatrician in the care of the overt and clear-cut case of cerebral palsy.

Assessment

Babies with cerebral palsy reach the specialist paediatrician either for observation, because they are considered to be at risk following a difficult delivery or seizures in the perinatal period, or, at a later age, because developmental delay has been recognised or suspected. The paediatrician examines the child, confirms the motor delay, does a general paediatric assessment, and then identifies the underlying motor disorder. He also carries out such diagnostic tests as he feels appropriate to identify, where possible, the cause of the disorder. Sometimes this is traceable. It is of genetic origin, the parents will be guided to seek genetic advice. The child with pure hemiplegia and paraplegia will be carefully studied to eliminate the possibility of a cerebral or spinal neoplasm. The methods used in the neurological study of children are well known; they have been set out by Paine and Oppé (1966).

Assessment of the child with developmental delay must be comprehensive. This is for two reasons. Firstly, any delay in motor development can be due to a variety of reasons; there might be cerebral palsy, but the delay might be due mainly to associated mental handicap. The other reason for comprehensive assessment is that if a child is found to have one chronic neurological deficit the chances are that there is another; the finding of one should be a stimulus to complete a comprehensive evaluation. Having made the general paediatric assessment, found the cause of the neurodevelopmental deficits, and ascertained the extent and severity of underlying disorders, the paediatrician's first task is to explain to the parents his comprehensive diagnosis. He must ensure that they have taken it in. He must help them to understand the nature of the tragedy which has overtaken them, so that they neither over-nor under-estimate it. Then he must give them ways in which they can help the child in his daily life. The task of informing parents that they have a handicapped child is a difficult one, and needs to be done by experienced doctors with the understanding which has been suggested elsewhere (Mac Keith 1973).

The non-orthopaedic management of the handicapped child can be discussed under eight main headings, which are as follows.

Motor function; visual function; auditory function; speech and language; school and learning; drive and powers of concentration; emotional state and social situation; general physical health.

These headings are to systematize and guide one's thinking, and must not distract the paediatrician from the whole child and his family. After the initial full assessment, the need is to make a provisional plan of comprehensive long-term action for helping the child. This plan should be open to review at any time, and should allow for periodic comprehensive re-assessment of the child. It is important to begin management quickly; usually the best way to begin is to offer the parents some immediate practical advice about what they themselves can do. We believe that management of the cerebral palsied child should always be sensitive to the needs of the parents, who should be offered explanation, support and help, not only initially, but repeatedly thereafter. The burdens of the parents of handicapped children are varied; they include physical labour, financial burdens, additional anxieties and, in many cases, social isolation.

Non-orthopaedic Management

The Motor Disorder

Other sections of this volume deal extensively with the orthopaedic management of the motor disorder in cerebral palsy, and various forms of physical treatment are also outlined. The orthopaedic surgeon and the paediatrician will work closely together, and with colleagues in physical medicine and in physiotherapy, occupational therapy and speech therapy, to advise the parents about management of the child's various disorders, for cerebral palsy is usually a 'symposium' of disorders and all need care. In severe cases, physical therapy and other treatments are of occasional value. Although the child may be on drugs for other reasons, we are not particularly impressed with the value of drugs for specific treatment of the physical disorder.

The paediatrician's main rôle is often in helping the parents to place the child's several problems in perspective, and to sort out the conflicting advice given to them by enthusiasts of different methods of physical therapy. There are numerous schools of thought at the moment, and widely differing forms of therapy are recommended. Although we each feel that the practice of our own physical therapists is indeed optimum, it is idle to deny that others would disagree with this.

Vis-à-vis the parents, at the moment our rôle is to make them aware that brain damage once sustained cannot be cured, but that much can be done to help; we must help parents understand that, although the physical disorder can be ameliorated, some motor deficit is likely to be permanent, although its nature will not be unchanging. A parent may feel that an orthopaedic surgeon is over-anxious to operate on a child, and may not be convinced that good results are likely to be obtained. The paediatrician must therefore, be familiar with his orthopaedic colleagues' approach and techniques; he must be prepared to interpret the plans of the surgeon for the parents, and discuss with them the merits of the procedure suggested and the chances of benefit.

The planning and timing of surgical procedures should fit in with the over-all management of the child; for example, it is not a good idea to submit a child to major surgery during his first term at a new school, or shortly after a move. A child and his parents need to be consulted, and the optimum moment selected for the operation, bearing in mind that the full benefit of surgery is often not apparent until several months have passed, and that, even with the best physiotherapy, there is often a period after an operation when the patient's activities have to be restricted and, for one reason or another, his abilities are temporarily diminished (Holt 1965, Holt and Reynell 1967).

The paediatrician stands back a little from the enthusiastic efforts of his colleagues in managing the physical disorder, and is likely, therefore, to be in a better position to decide how treatment can be best directed to the over-all benefit to the child. Thus, after discussion with the child's parents, he will help decide when, how much and how long physical therapy should be used. Our own feeling is that by the time child has reached school age, he should no longer have to attend for daily hour-long physical therapy sessions. Rather than interrupt the child's schooling, physical management should take the form of physical education within an ordinary school curriculum, albeit of a specially planned and well thought-out nature.

The motor disability in cerebral palsy is the most overt and obvious sign of the child's dysfunction. It is not, perhaps, the most disabling, in so far as other problems of communication and of learning may be more significant in terms of the child's over-all function. It may be wiser to pay more attention to these problems than to spend too much time attempting to achieve the impossible in physical therapy. Perhaps the order of importance of abilities is being able to communicate, being able to sit, being independent in dressing and toiletting, and then walking.

Visual Function

It has repeatedly been shown that visual disorders are more common in children with cerebral palsy than in the normal population. Alas, it has also been shown repeatedly that the diagnosis and treatment of visual handicap has commonly been overlooked. Techniques for the assessment of visual acuity in handicapped children at a very early age have been evolved by Dr Mary Sheridan (Sheridan 1969, 1973). These allow assessment of vision, even in the most severely physically handicapped child.

Strabismus is very common in the cerebral palsied child, and when detected in any child over the age of six months, even if it is only intermittent, should be brought immediately under the supervision of an ophthalmologist. We regularly check the visual acuity of our own patients when they attend, and refer to ophthalmological colleagues the earliest sign of any deficit. The ophthalmologist is expert on the structure of the eye; but it is the responsibility of the paediatrician to supervise testing of whether and how well an infant or young child can see.

The cerebral palsied child may have, apart from the visual defects that commonly appear in ordinary children, peculiar difficulties with vision; eye movements may be disorganised, and the child may have difficulty holding the eyes still. Electro-oculograms (EOGs) may demonstrate these difficulties, and, although we do not carry out EOGs routinely, the possibility of using these techniques should always be borne in mind when assessing a child who presents with learning disorders.

Auditory Function

Hearing loss also is more common in cerebral palsy than in the ordinary population. There is a well-known association between high tone loss and the athetosis consequent on hyperbilirubinaemia. All children with cerebral palsy must therefore have full testing of their hearing capacity in the everyday situation, especially of spoken sounds, and, if this is impaired, they should be referred to the ear, nose and throat surgeon. In testing, it should be remembered that listening requires not only normal auditory acuity, but also the ability to attend to the spoken word. The child's response to the spoken voice should always be assessed as well as his response to pure tone audiometry. We always use either the Reed* or the Stycar* test to tell whether the child can hear quietly spoken words clearly from a distance. Young cerebral palsied children sometimes have difficulties of auditory attention or of

*The Reed test is available from the Royal National Institute for the Blind, 224 Great Portland Street, London W.1.; the Stycar test is available from the National Foundation for Educational Research in England and Wales, The Mere, Upton Park, Slough, Bucks.

perception of speech. It is important to identify the child with problems of auditory attention; when spoken to by an adult, such a child will respond best if the speaker is sufficiently close for him or her to be able to fixate on the speaker's face.

Speech and Language

Speech and language disorders are common in cerebral palsy, and the routine comprehensive assessment will include receptive and expressive language. We have outlined the language and speech assessment for the handicapped elsewhere (Bax and Mac Keith 1972). From an early age we encourage the mother of the cerebral palsied child to pay particular attention to talking to him at a close distance, so that he 'learns his mother tongue at mother distance'. We can stress that the development of communication by receptive and expressive language is more important to the cerebral palsied child than learning to walk. Parents are often obsessed with the child's motor disorder ('Doctor, when will he walk?'), and fail to pay attention to promoting the child's developing skills of communication. Colleagues from speech therapy help us with the assessment of speech and language and with making plans for the treatment of the child's speech or language disorder. These plans should be explained to the parents, and integrated into any other therapeutic programme that may be going on. Parents can, with encouragement and guidance, do a great deal.

School and Learning Disorders

As the child reaches three, four or five years of age, a crisis of anxiety arises for the parents as they wonder where the child will go to school. They hope that their child will be able to go to an ordinary school. The doctor must encourage them to think about this problem realistically as soon as possible. Many, but not all, handicapped children benefit from nursery school experience, and the family also may get a more realistic view of their child from watching him in the company of other non-handicapped children. Parents' fears about their child going to a special school, whether it is for physically handicapped children or for slow-learning children, can often be overcome by encouraging them to visit it before the child is due to go there, and the school will usually co-operate with this. The educational facilities available vary from country to country, from state to state and from city to city. The merits of the different types of facility that are available for specifically handicapped children are a matter for debate. The child may go for part of each day to a special class in an ordinary school, or he may go all day. Some believe that special units attached to ordinary schools are better than special schools because they prevent the development of an over-protective attitude towards the handicapped child, and allow him to develop, much more realistically, an idea of his own potential. Others believe that such units cannot provide the special facilities and help which the child may benefit so much from, and believe that all cerebral palsied children should be in special schools. The paediatrician will have his own views on these topics, but he should remember that there is little solid research basis for different approaches at the moment (see, however, Anderson 1973). The parents' and the child's wishes should be very much to the fore when the decision about school is made, and the possibility of revision expressed.

The child with cerebral palsy commonly has special specific learning difficulties. A full psychological assessment should be made at around the time he goes to school. As education proceeds, special help may or may not be needed. It is a mistake to over-emphasise the correlation between failure on one individual item in a psychological battery, and consequent failure at learning. The teacher's comments on what the child actually does should always be considered in the psychologist's assessment of what he or she thinks the child will do. The paediatrician will again play an interpretive rôle with the parents, when necessary, helping them to understand the ideas and suggestions which have been put forward by the educationalists, and often meeting the teachers with whom lies the decision on school placement and methods of teaching.

'Drive' and Powers of Concentration

The child with cerebral palsy may have difficulties as regards attention, concentration and 'drive'. This last is difficult to define, but describes the child's innate curiosity and the over-all interest with which he interacts with his environment. This varies greatly in cerebral palsy. The athetoid child, who, despite extraordinary motor difficulties and appalling speech defect, nevertheless thrusts himself forward into every activity, contrasts with the spastic diplegic child who, with a relatively high I.Q., sits lethargically in a wheel chair and seems to play very little part in any daily activity. Although these different types are clinical impressions (the athetoid may possibly seem to show more interest because of his much greater lability of facial expression) and have not been solidly documented, they are familiar to most of us who have worked with cerebral palsied children.

We are not over-impressed with the use of medication to help the under-active child, but prefer to try and motivate him by providing, from an early age, a rich and stimulating environment. Some believe that the under-active, spastic child is a particularly suitable target for programmed learning. The over-mobile athetoid child may conversely benefit from a more restricted environment, so that specific tasks can be presented to him without distraction. One of us has recently discussed the highly active school child and some elements in his management (Bax 1972). A small number of brain-damaged children present with 'true' hyperkinetic syndrome. Here the child is persistently distractable, impulsive and highly active, both at home and at school, despite the presence of adults who can usually limit the activity of the 'simple' over-active child. In these children, the drug of choice at the moment seems to be methylphenidate. Some of these 'true' hyperkinetic children react paradoxically by becoming less active on stimulant drugs, while barbiturates, particularly phenobarbitone may make them more active. The child who has epilepsy and cerebral palsy, is best treated not with phenobarbitone but with phenytoin as the drug of first choice. The calming effect of stimulant drugs is attributed to their increasing the brain's power to suppress some of the incoming stimuli.

Emotional and Social Health of the Child

Rutter et al. (1970) have recently shown conclusively that children with brain damage, as evidenced by cerebral palsy or epilepsy, have four to five times as much behaviour disturbance as ordinary children. Except for the hyperkinetic syndrome, however, the types of psychiatric disorder diagnosed in these children are the same as those diagnosed in the normal population, and are brought about by the influence of the same types of environmental factors. A pessimistic attitude towards a child's disturbed behaviour, on the basis that it is due to the brain damage and not susceptible to treatment is, therefore, no longer valid. Awareness that such children are particularly likely to behave badly will alert the paediatrician to the early signs of disturbance, and he will work closely with his psychiatric colleague. We feel that the psychiatrist can help greatly, both by advising the paediatrician about his handling of the child by sometimes taking on the child himself for individual therapy.

In the framework of the emotional and social disorders of the handicapped child, come the problems of his parents. Their feelings and the way in which these affect their behaviour have been recently reviewed by one of us (Mac Keith 1973). We can anticipate three or four common crisis periods in the family life. The first of these is the early period when the cerebral deficits are first suspected or diagnosed. The second is when the time for schooling approaches, and parents wonder if their child will go to an ordinary school. The third is towards the end of schooling, when the parents begin to think of the period after school and the difficulties for the handicapped person in open employment, and when the patient, now adolescent, wonders if he will be independent, have a job and get married. Finally, the time of the sudden realisation by the parents that they will soon no longer themselves be able to provide the care and attention which they feel their child, now adult, needs. Preparing the parent in advance for these decisions is probably one of the most helpful things the paediatrician can do. Ample time for discussion with the parents must always be set aside, and it is also important that the paediatrician should always be accessible for immediate consultation if a crisis suddenly blows up within the family. The disorder is chronic, but some of the problems it produces do at times require urgent consultation.

General Physical Health

While he is wrestling with the problems of the child with cerebral palsy, the paediatrician does not forget his paediatric rôle and his ordinary job with any child. Coughs and colds and minor chest infections are as common, or more common, among the cerebral palsied population, and the misery of the child whose nose is running when he is unable to wipe it effectively hardly bears thinking upon. The child also may not be able to complain adequately of particular aches and pains, and familiar disease entities present in handicapped children in bizarre ways.

Treatment too may need modification. For example, the child who spends his whole day in a wheel chair does not want to receive an injection in the buttocks and will be much better off having it in the arm.

Nutritional Problems

Obesity and under-nutrition can both present in cerebral palsy. The immobile child in a wheel-chair can rapidly develop obesity, and once this has been established it may be extremely difficult for the child to lose weight. Children should be regularly weighed, and appropriate dietary restriction imposed at an early stage. Athetoid children who have difficulty eating and swallowing may have difficulty in acquiring an adequate calorie intake. High calorie diets presented in an easily assimilated form are a theoretical solution, but are not always successful in practice.

Dental Care

Dental care is as important for the cerebral palsied child as it is for the ordinary child, and special clinical facilities should be made available, with a dental team interested in and sympathetic to the problems of such children.

Cerebral palsied children tend to have more enamel defects in their primary and secondary dentition, as they have often had tetracyclines in the neonatal period. The parents often think that these defects and stains are caries, and need reassuring about this. Probably, cerebral palsied children do not have a high prevalence of dental caries and periodontal disease, but they certainly have fewer *treated teeth*. This reflects the difficulties that dentists have with these children.

The evidence about malocclusion in cerebral palsy is rather uncertain, though athetoids are said to have proclined upper incisors and an anterior bite. Some forms of scoliosis are also associated with more dental decay. Bruxism (teeth grinding) is a particular problem in athetoids, and they may need to wear a protective shield.

Good oral hygiene, which really means regular tooth brushing, may prove difficult for these children to achieve themselves. Parents need to be shown how to help. Being regular visitors to doctors and behavioural psychologists, cerebral palsied children may too often be rewarded with sweets, and develop a liking for them.

Epilepsy

The commonest neurological disorder associated with cerebral palsy is epilepsy. The treatment and management of epilepsy are complex problems in themselves, which we cannot discuss here. All those concerned with the cerebral palsied child should be on the alert for the occurrence of fits, and it is particularly important to be alert to the occurrence of minor seizures, which may pass unnoticed in an individual whose motor function is abnormal, but which may be making him highly distractable and seriously impairing his ability to learn.

Acknowledgement. The authors are grateful to J. N. Swallow, M.D.S., for his assistance in the preparation of the section on dental care.

REFERENCES

Anderson, E. M. (1973) *The Disabled School Child.* London: Methuen.
Bax, M. C. O. (1972) 'The active and the over-active school child' *Developmental Medicine and Child Neurology,* **14,** 83. (Annotation.)
—— Mac Keith, R. C. (1972) 'The paediatric role in the study of children with communication disorders.' *in* Rutter, M., Martin, J. A. M. (Eds.) *The Child with Delayed Speech.* Clinics in Developmental Medicine No. 43. London: Spastics International Medical Publications with Heinemann Medical. p. 168.
Egan, D. F., Illingworth, R. S., Mac Keith, R. C. (1969) *Developmental Screening 0 to 5 years.* Clinics in Developmental Medicine No. 30. London: Spastics International Medical Publications with Heinemann Medical.

Frankenburg, W. K., Dodds, J. B. (1967) 'The Denver Developmental Screening Test.' *Journal of Pediatrics,* **71,** 181.

Holt, K. S. (1965) *Assessment of Cerebral Palsy.* London: Lloyd Luke.

—— Reynell, J. K. (1967) *Assessment of Cerebral Palsy II. Vision, Hearing, Speech, Language, Communication and Psychological Function.* London: Lloyd-Luke.

Mac Keith, R. C. (1973) 'The feelings and behaviour of parents of handicapped children.' *Developmental Medicine and Child Neurology,* **15,** 524. (Annotation.)

Mitchell, R. G. (1971) 'The prevention of cerebral palsy.' *Developmental Medicine and Child Neurology,* **13,** 137.

Paine, R. S., Oppé, T. E. (1966) *Neurological Examination of Children.* Clinics in Developmental Medicine Nos. 20/21. London: Spastics International Medical Publications with Heinemann Medical.

Robson, P., Mac Keith, R. C. (1971) 'Shufflers with spastic diplegic cerebral palsy: a confusing clinical picture.' *Developmental Medicine and Child Neurology,* **13,** 651.

Rutter, M., Graham, P., Yule, W. (1970) *A Neuropsychiatric Study in Childhood.* Clinics in Developmental Medicine Nos. 35/36. London: Spastics International Medical Publications with Heinemann Medical.

Sheridan, M. D. (1969) 'Vision screening procedures for very young or handicapped children.' *in* Gardiner, P., Mac Keith, R. C., Smith, V. (Eds.) *Aspects of Developmental and Paediatric Ophthalmology.* Clinics in Developmental Medicine No. 32. London: Spastics International Medical Publications with Heinemann Medical. p. 39.

—— (1973) 'The Stycar graded balls vision test.' *Developmental Medicine and Child Neurology,* **15,** 423.

The Orthopaedic Assessment in Cerebral Palsy

ROBERT L. SAMILSON and JAQUELIN PERRY

Realistic planning, based on careful, detailed serial evaluations, is the keynote for successful management of the patient with cerebral palsy. The manifestations of peripheral malfunction are myriad, and improved function is a compromise, at best, since irreversible brain damage precludes normality. Making the best of what is left requires the application of an integrated knowledge of anatomy, neurophysiology, biomechanics, developmental medicine and orthopaedic surgery.

Much time, effort and frustration on the part of the patient, the family, and the treating physician are involved in the management of cerebral palsy. How much less frustrating and more efficacious would our efforts become if we applied the knowledge already available to us to predict what the functional and motor capabilities of our cerebral palsied patients would be in the future? How much expenditure of energy, funds and talent is misdirected into teaching a child to walk who does not and will not have the capacity to do so? How much time and money goes into the making of braces for children who can never use them? How many patients, their families, and well-meaning physicians are disappointed by surgical procedures which were not indicated?

Cerebral palsy presents an unfamiliar orthopaedic situation. It challenges the clinician to modify normal peripheral structures, to accommodate for their distorted control in order to improve function. The basic lesion in the brain is permanent, hence central control will never be normal. There will be some change as remaining functional tissue matures. The child is hypersensitive to his environment and may respond differently in a strange, highly stimulative environment, such as a clinic or examining room. The child sensitive to his environment has a limited tolerance to the examining procedure, and a single assessment may lead to faulty conclusions. The key to successful management is realistic planning based on careful detailed, serial evaluations.

The purpose of this chapter is to enumerate some of the useful tests which enable us to make reasonable predictions of the patient's maximum functional capacity, and so direct our energies, and the patient's energies, to the fulfilment of a realistic goal for each cerebral palsied individual (Samilson 1966, 1970).

The motor performance of each patient depends on the developmental state of the central nervous system. Basic to the examination is accurate differentiation between normal maturational changes and the effects of the cerebral palsy lesion.

The normal changes are a consequence of the brain being incompletely formed at birth. Axon myelinization, dendrite expansion and final cell migration continue postnatally for a considerable period of time. As a result, the newborn displays reflex patterns which are serially modified, lost, or replaced with more complex and precise motor responses. When the brain has been damaged, this normal progression is delayed, distorted and prematurely terminated, commensurate with the severity of the damage. In addition, the cerebral palsy lesion permits more primitive forms of motor control to emerge, leading to spasticity, hypertonic responses to limb and body position and simplified reciprocal control.

The orthopaedic surgeon has three basic goals: to make a child appear normal by preventing or correcting deformity, to improve ambulation, and to gain optimum hand function. He is accustomed to focusing on the malfunctioning extremity (or extremities) as an independent unit, or looking at the trunk for its deformed appearance. In mild cases this approach is not inappropriate. With more severe involvement, however, initial concern must relate to the availability of sufficient head and trunk control to permit sitting or standing. Only when these postures can be maintained is planning for walking or productive hand function appropriate.

Hence the patients fall into three groups: standers, sitters, and lyers. These reflect levels of neurological maturation far more than local extremity impairment. As a result the reflex responses indicative of neurological age become significant to the orthopaedist.

Insults to the central nervous system, and/or its failure to develop, place limitations on maximum motor performance. Persistence of certain primitive reflex patterns which are normally present at birth, and the failure of other developmental milestones to appear in an orderly fashion, leads to an inability to walk, stand, sit, maintain head and trunk balance, and use the hands for functional purposes. Recognition of these abnormalities on serial examinations is of extreme importance in making realistic predictions of the patient's future.

The value of orthopaedic surgery in the fulfilment of realistic goals for the individual cerebral palsied patient can also be determined from certain useful tests, readily available to the examining physician.

Normal and Aberrant Neurological Maturation

Recognition of the abnormal requires a familiarity with normal development and its variants. Gesell and Amatruda (1947), Bobath and Finnie (1958), Bobath (1959, 1965), Denhoff and Robinault (1960), Fiorentino (1963), Peiper (1963), Holt (1965), Paine (1965) and Paine and Oppé (1966) have all delineated the normal sequential development of the infant, and the significance of persistent aberrations in development (see this volume Chapter 2). No *single* reflex should be interpreted as a strong prognostic sign, but the assessment of many of them will serve to predict the future.

Normal neurophysiological maturation has been characterized as a progression of dominance from the spinal cord to the brain-stem to the mid-brain, and finally to cortical control (Fiorentino 1963). In an excellent monograph, Fiorentino describes these levels of development, and the imposition they place on motor performance (Fig. 1). Although over-simplified, these functional levels and their characteristics serve a useful purpose in prognosis. Some believe this classification arbitrary, and relate neurological abnormalities to delays or halts in maturation of the cerebrum.

Functionally, however, Fiorentino's classification is useful in defining limitation of activity.

The most primitive level of maturation is at the spinal level, and results in total flexion or extension responses. This is incompatible with motor activity more advanced than prone or supine lying. Normally, this phase lasts during the first two months of life. The crossed extension reflex, which is characterized by adduction of the opposite thigh and plantar flexion of the opposite ankle on tapping the medial aspect of the contralateral thigh, is characteristic of this level of development. This reflex may be a variant of a strong crossed adductor reflex. Its strong persistence past two months of age bodes ill for any motor activity other than total bed care.

Brain-stem dominance normally persists to four to six months of age. Persistence of brain-stem reflexes also predicts a need for permanent bed care. The asymmetrical tonic neck reflex is an example of such a reflex. In the supine position, turning the head to one side will cause the limbs on the side to which the head is turned to extend, whilst the other limbs flex (Fig. 2). Persistence of this reflex past six months of age is incompatible with ambulation. The symmetrical tonic neck reflex, if it persists past six months of age, is also of significance. Extension of the neck obliges the upper limbs to extend and the lower limbs to flex (Fig. 3), whilst flexion of the neck results in flexion of the upper limbs and extension of the lower limbs (Fig 4). Thus crawling or ambulation is difficult or impossible.

Levels of C.N.S. Maturation	Corresponding Levels of Reflexive Development	Resulting Levels of Motor Development
Spinal and/or Brain Stem	Apedal Primitive Reflexes	Prone-lying Supine-lying
Midbrain	Quadrupedal Righting Reactions	Crawling Sitting
Cortical	Bipedal Equilibrium Reactions	Standing Walking

Fig. 1. Levels of neurological maturation (from Fiorentino 1973).

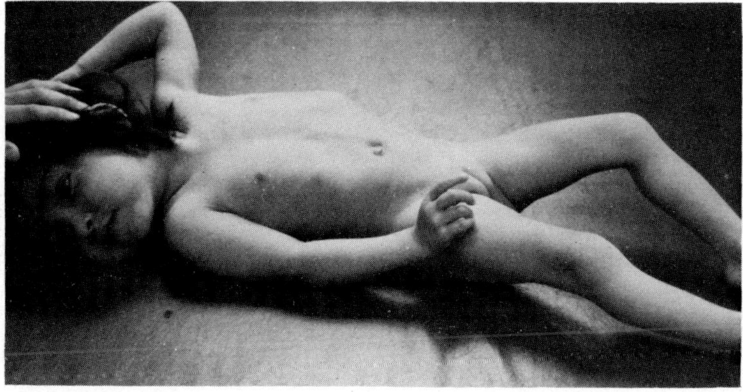

Fig. 2. Asymmetrical tonic neck reflex.

Mid-brain dominance is essential for a quadripedal existence, *i.e.* for such behaviours as crawling and sitting. The righting reactions are characteristic of this level of control. The neck-righting reaction is performed with the child in the supine position, arms and legs extended. Rotation of the head to one side results in rotation of the body in the same direction (Fig. 5). A negative response after one month of age raises a suspicion of delayed neurological development (Fig. 6). The labyrinthine (Fig. 7) and optical righting reflexes are also characteristic of this level of development, as is the amphibian reaction which is essential to crawling. To test for the latter, the child is placed prone with both arms and legs extended. Elevation of the pelvis on one side results in flexion of the arm, hip and knee on the same side. Failure to show this reaction after six months of age is another indication of delayed maturation, and a persistently negative response is probably incompatible with walking (Fig. 8).

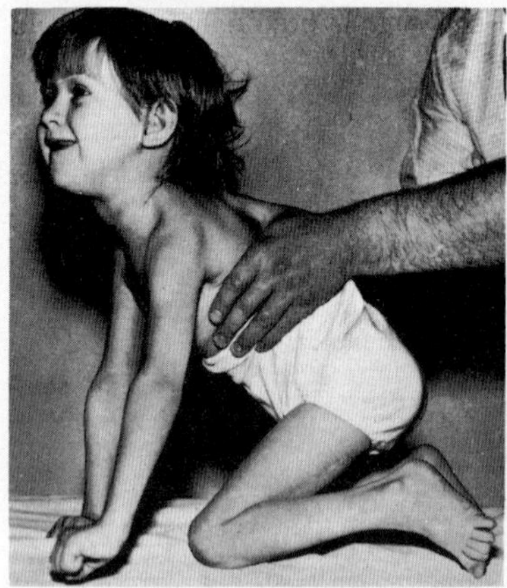

Fig. 3. Symmetrical tonic neck reflex with neck in extension (from Holt 1965).

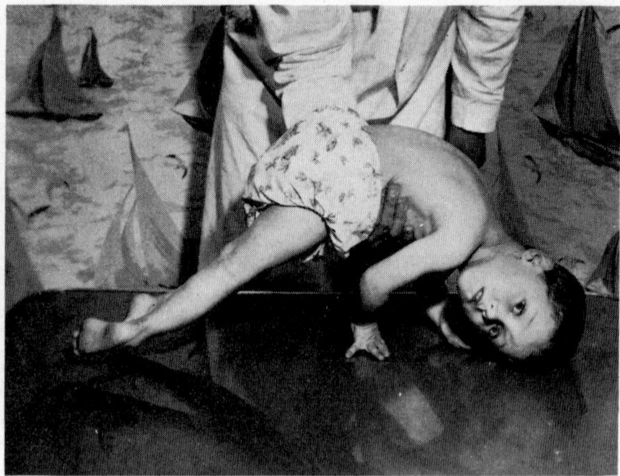

Fig. 4. Symmetrical tonic neck reflex, response to neck flexion (from Holt 1965).

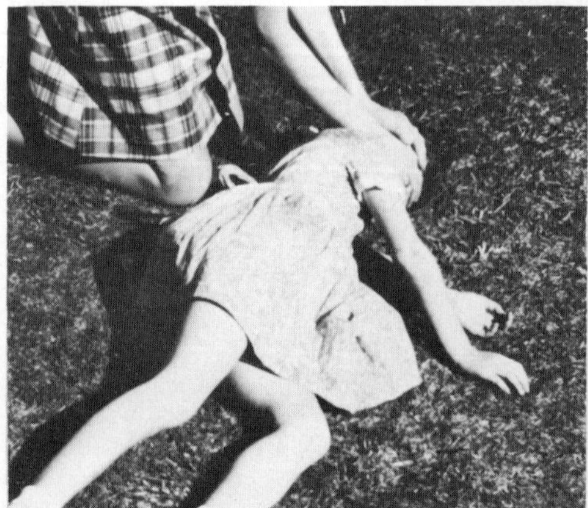

Fig. 5. Neck-righting response. Body follows head.

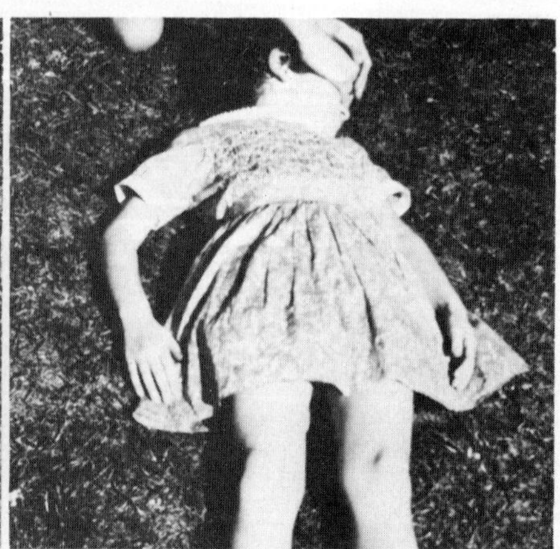

Fig. 6. Negative neck-righting response.

Finally, cortical control is essential to a bipedal existence (standing, walking). The equilibrium reactions are characteristic of this level. Sitting balance should be tested. When the patient is tilted to one side, the arm and leg on the raised side should be abducted and extended and the head and thorax should right themselves (Figs. 9 and 10). Fore-foot kneeling is another equilibrium reaction in the quadruped position (Fig. 11). Failure of these reactions to occur after eight months of age is pathological and makes independent ambulation difficult.

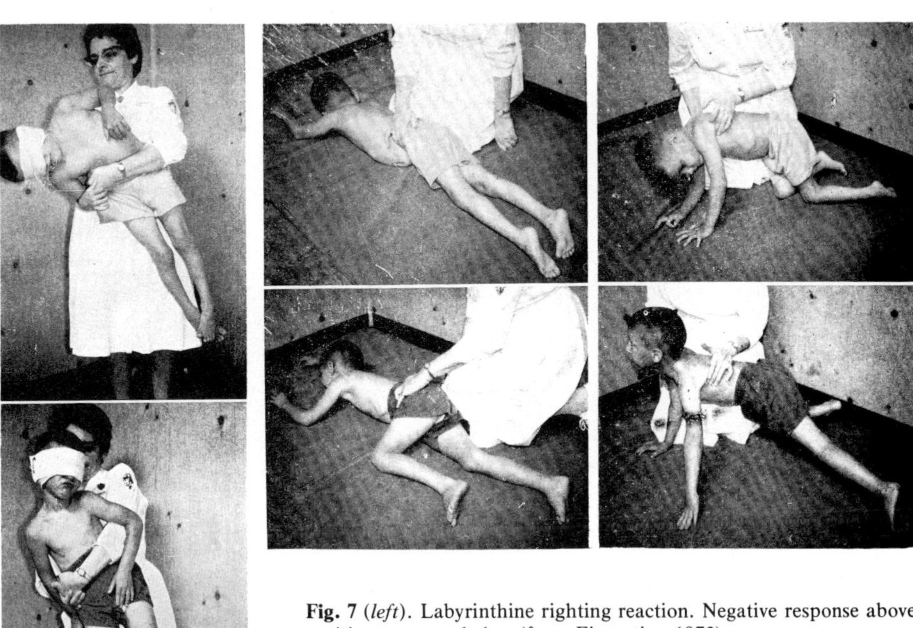

Fig. 7 (*left*). Labyrinthine righting reaction. Negative response above, positive response below (from Fiorentino 1973).

Fig. 8 (*above left*). Amphibian response. Negative response above, positive response below (from Fiorentino 1973).

Fig. 11 (*above right*). Fore-foot kneeling. Negative response above, positive response below (from Fiorentino 1973).

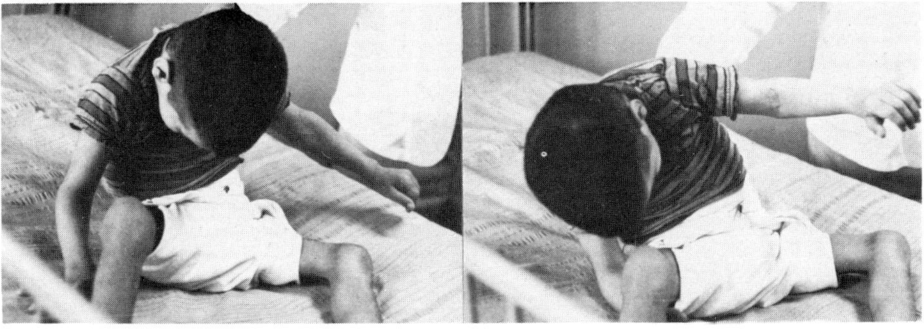

Fig. 9. Equilibrium reaction, sitting position.

Fig. 10. Failure of equilibrium reaction.

So-called 'automatic movement reactions' which persist after they should disappear are also abnormal. The Moro or startle reflex is elicited with the patient supine with arms and legs extended. A sudden noise results in abduction of the arms and movement in other parts of the body (Fig. 12). A positive reaction after six months of age is abnormal. The Landau reflex is obtained by holding the child in the prone position in space supported by the thorax. The head is raised and the spine and legs extend. Such a reaction after two and a half years of age reflects delayed neurological maturation. The parachute reaction is of significance as regards the development of reaching activity with the arms. The child is held head-down and suddenly moved towards the floor. The arms should extend and abduct, and the fingers should extend to protect the head (Fig. 13). Absence of this reaction after six months of age bodes ill for hand function. The incurvatum (Galant) reflex (Fig. 14) may be of some import in the prediction of scoliosis in cerebral palsy if it persists asymmetrically. Stroking the flank results in convex curvature of the spine

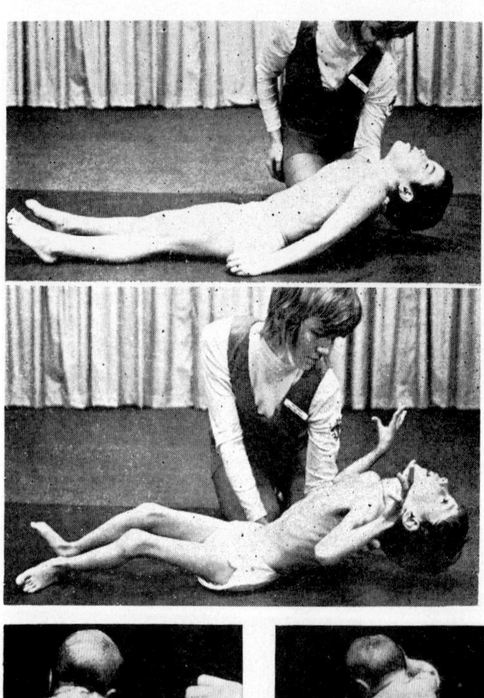

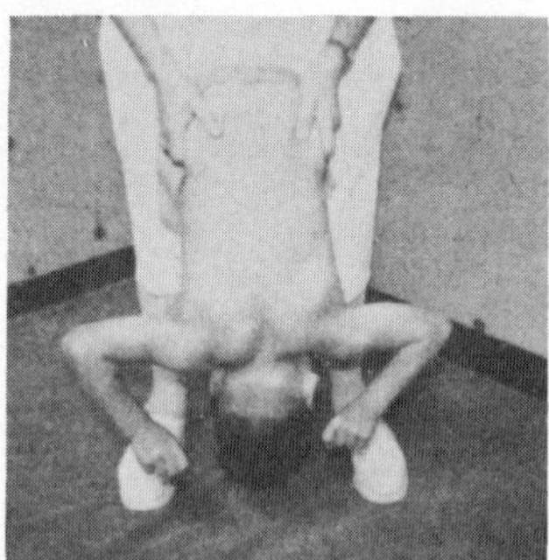

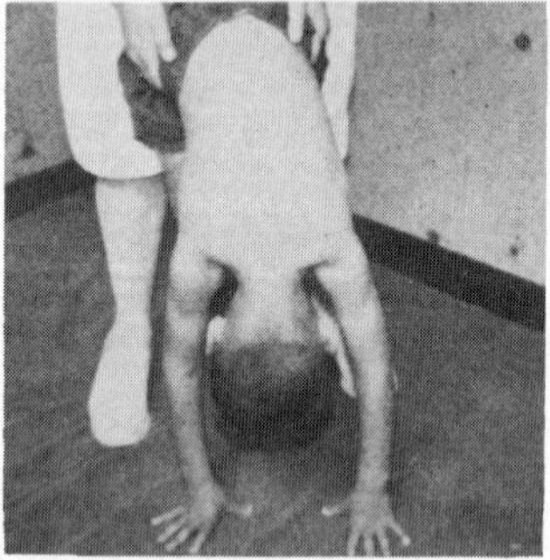

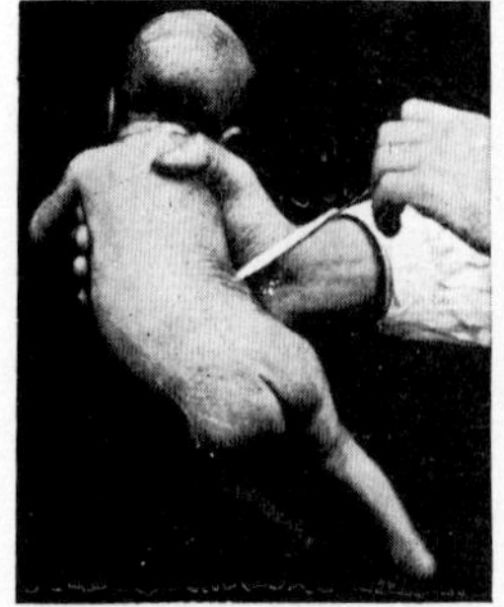

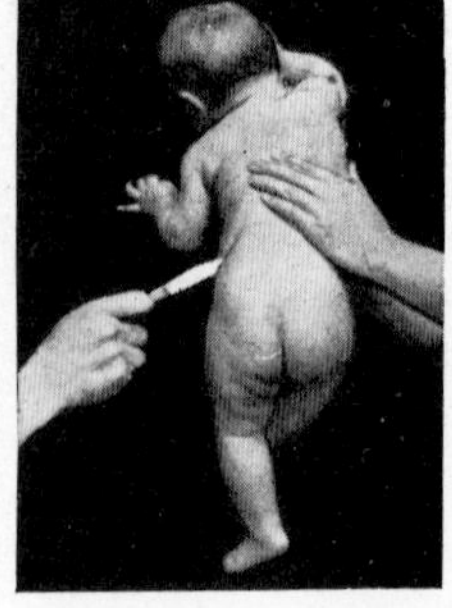

Fig. 12 (*above left*). Moro (startle) reaction (from Fiorentino 1973).

Fig. 13 (*above right*). Parachute reaction. Negative response above, positive response below (from Fiorentino 1973).

Fig. 14 (*left*). Galant or incurvatum reflex (from Peiper 1963).

away from the side stroked, with 'wind blowing' of the hips towards the concavity of the curve.

In summary, the persistence of primitive reflexes which normally disappear, and the failure to appear of other more mature reflexes, are of prognostic significance. Motor performance is strictly limited by the level of maturation of the central nervous system. At spinal level, total bed care is the maximum to be expected. At mid-brain level, crawling and sitting are possible, but ambulation, even assisted, is not. Cortical control is essential to ambulatory activity.

Associated Defects

The orthopaedic surgeon must understand the incidence and implications of associated defects in the cerebral palsied patient. Concentration on musculo-skeletal aberrations to the exclusion of these associated defects will lead to disaster.

Readers are referred to an excellent monograph by Holt and Reynell (1967) for a more thorough discussion of associated defects.

Strabismus is the most common ocular defect in cerebral palsy, and occurs in 40 to 45 per cent of cases (Holt and Reynell 1967). Blindness, partial or complete, occurs in 15 per cent. Nystagmus is present in 10 per cent and optic atrophy in 7 per cent. Obviously, all of these defects will affect hand-eye co-ordination and the ability to ambulate independently.

Deafness occurs in 6 to 16 per cent of cerebral palsied patients (Holt and Reynell 1967), and affects the ability of the patient to co-operate with any form of management until the deficit is recognised and allowances for it are made.

Another defect affecting communication is a defect of speech (Crothers and Paine 1959), which is present in 89 per cent of athetoids, 85 per cent of ataxics, 72 per cent of rigidity patients, and 52 per cent of spastics. Recognition and referral to speech therapists is essential. Mental retardation in association with cerebral palsy is not a contra-indication to surgery, *per se*; but management of the mentally retarded cerebral palsied patient is difficult, and the prognosis less favorable. Crothers and Paine have indicated that 36 per cent of hemiplegics, 70 per cent of quadriplegics and 31 per cent of athetoids have intelligence quotients below 70. With this is mind, we must ask ourselves whether it is the major motor impairment, the mental retardation, or both, which mitigate against more advanced motor performance.

Seizures occur and persist four times as frequently in children with postnatal head injuries (55 per cent) as in the most severely involved cerebral palsied quadriplegics (13 per cent Crothers and Paine 1959). Seizures must be controlled, for fractures frequently occur if they are not. Ambulation and the ability to co-operate are sometimes impaired by the lassitude induced by anticonvulsive medication, as well as by the seizures themselves.

Sensory deficits are a major source of difficulty in the management of the cerebral palsied patient. Astereognosis, perceptual and conceptual defects affect hand function and co-ordination, particularly in the hemiplegic. Forty-two per cent of cerebral palsied children studied by Tachdjian and Minear (1958) had one or more sensory deficits in the hand.

Some Neurophysiological Aspects of Spasticity

Spastic cerebral palsy is characterized by increased stretch reflex mediated through the gamme neuron system (Rushworth 1960). Stretch receptors in the intrafusal fibers of skeletal muscle are responsive to both length and velocity changes. When these intrafusal fibers are stretched, a monosynaptic reflex results in increased alpha motor neuron activity and extrafusal fiber contraction in response to the stretch (Figs. 15 and 16). Golgi tendon organs respond to tendon stretch by an inhibition of alpha motor neuron activity, and thus muscle relaxation. However, this is a slower, polysynaptic reflex, and is overwhelmed by the greater population of gamma stretch receptors.

Spasticity is characterized further by disorganized, synchronous muscle activity. Thus flexors are active in extension as well as flexion, and the usual phasic bursts of electrical activity during brief portions of movement are replaced by continuous electrical activity not corresponding to the function which the tested muscle performs normally.

Motion of the so-called 'normal side' in hemiplegia will result in increased frequency and amplitude of electrical response on the affected side. Purposeful movement thus makes the neurological deficit more apparent, and throws suspicion on whether hemiplegia is truly hemiplegia.

Normally, for any given muscle, the fascicles composing the muscle do not all fire off synchronously, except under certain conditions such as fatigue or heavy effort. However, in cerebral palsy all the fascicles comprising a given muscle do seem to contract at the same time.

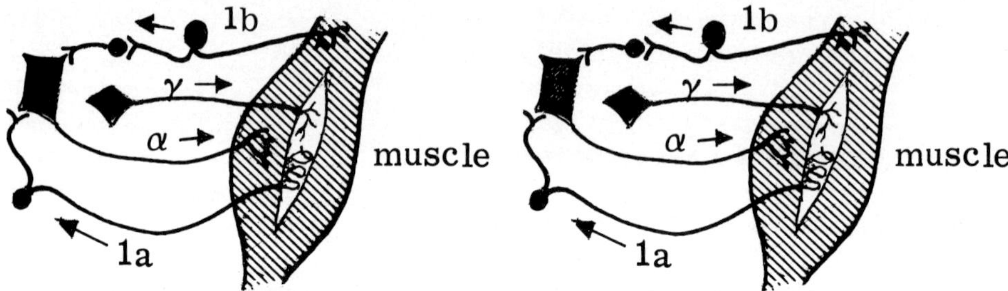

Fig. 15. Stretch reflex. Part I.
Ia fiber fires at 20/second, Ib fibers not firing. (SLIGHT STRETCH OF MUSCLE.)
Momentary Ia silence then Ia fibers start acting again due to gamma activity. (STIMULUS TO MOTOR NERVE PRODUCING A TWITCH OF MUSCLE WITH SUDDEN SHORTENING.)
Ia fibers increase rate of firing (facilitation of motor neuron). (FURTHER STRETCH OF MUSCLE.)
Ia fibers increase rate of firing further and Ib golgi fibers start firing. (INCREASING FURTHER PULL OF MUSCLE.)

Fig. 16. Stretch reflex. Part II.
Ib fiber activity becomes pronounced (harder pull still), inhibiting *a* motor neuron activity. At the same time there is a slowing of Ia activity from the spindle (autogenetic inhibition).
Finally, the muscle gets slack and Ia and Ib firing decreases (lengthening reaction of muscle).
Unless spindles are on a certain degree of stretch, there is failure of spindle Ia activity.
The gamma system resets the level of excitability of motor neurons.

The speed at which a muscle contracts is dependent on its length. Short muscles (*e.g.* interossei) are much slower acting than longer ones (*e.g.* flexor sublimi and profundi). Excursion of a muscle also varies with its length. Force exerted depends on muscle cross-section. These are all-important considerations in choosing an adequate and comparable tendon transfer in the upper limb.

The length-tension diagram for a muscle is of significance in that maximum tension is developed close to midlength (Fig. 17). A muscle that is already short or long cannot exert adequate tension. This explains why finger extensors long-stretched by a palmar flexed wrist in cerebral palsy are usually weak and ineffectual. However, if the wrist is braced or fused in functional position, finger extensor power may improve spontaneously as the long extensors assume midlength.

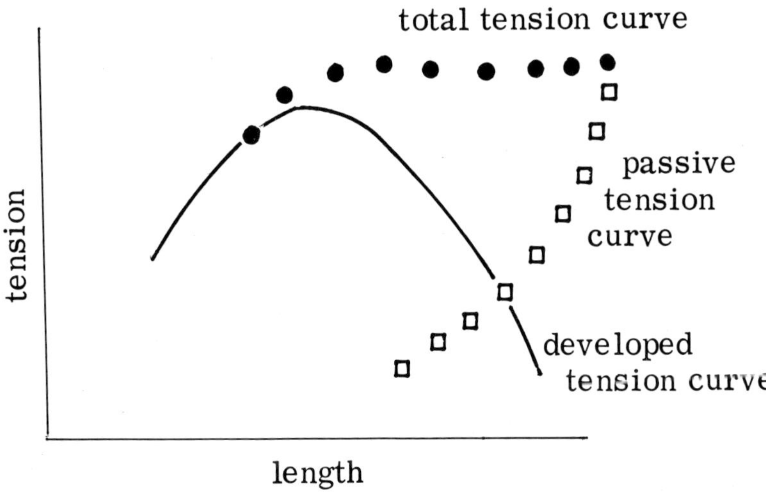

Fig. 17. Magnus-Blix length-tension diagram.

In summary, the neurophysiological characteristics of spasticity are as follows (Mac Keith 1960, Rushworth 1960, Ralston, H., personal communication).
(1) Increased tone in limbs, but decreased tone in neck and trunk. The increased tone is shown by increased resistance to passive movement, often more marked in one direction of movement.
(2) Exaggerated contracting response of muscles subjected to stretch, and hence lowered threshold to stretch reflex.
(3) During passive movement there is often a sudden increase of resistance and, on continued pressure, a sudden decrease.
(4) Clonus and hyperactive tendon reflexes with increased reflexogenic area.
(5) The position of the limb is in part set by postural mechanisms in the brain and in part by the response of muscles to stretch by gravity.
(6) Synchronous electrical activity of agonist/antagonist muscle groups without regard to the function which the muscle performs.
(7) Voluntary contraction commences simultaneously in all parts of a spastic

muscle, and peaks of activity are frequently encountered at the same time in different parts of a muscle. Voluntary contractile activity in normal muscle is asynchronous, so that different parts of muscle contract at different times.

(8) Tendency to repetition, synchronization and irradiation of impulses.

(9) Persistance of primitive neonatal reflexes.

(10) Perceptual and conceptual deficits.

(11) Paresis is proportional to spasticity.

(12) Lack of selective control.

(13) Slowness of voluntary movement.

(14) Failure of integration of 'what's left'.

(15) Diminished or absent stereognosis, two-point discrimination, and position sense.

A recognition and an understanding of these neurophysiological changes in spasticity will permit more intelligent treatment planning. In view of these changes it is understandable why most tendon transfers in spastic upper limbs are tenodeses rather than active transfers, and why long-stretched muscles are weak and ineffectual motors.

Biomechanical Aspects of Cerebral Palsy

The biomechanical results of the neurophysiological changes in cerebral palsy are contracture, malalignment, instability and imbalance. Reciprocal innervation is lacking, and normal agonist/antagonist relationships are lost. The loss of phasic activity and asynchronous electrical potentials in agonist and antagonist muscles helps to explain the so-called 'spasmus mobilis' occasionally seen following flexor ulnaris transfer to wrist or finger extensors, where continued electrical activity in the new position results in reverse deformity. This may also explain the occasional 'athetoid shift', which is not nearly as common as was formerly thought.

One of the characteristics of alterations in muscle action in cerebral palsy is the observation that contracture of a muscle, (such that full passive joint motion is impossible) results in dissipation of antagonistic muscle force on joints proximal or distal to the point of contracture. For example, with wrist flexion contracture, finger extensors do not help to extend the wrist, but dissipate most of their force on the metacarpo-phalangeal joints, resulting in attempted hyperextension of these joints. This is particularly true in the presence of ineffectual intrinsics, which ordinarily would oppose metacarpo-phalangeal extension. One only has to review the interesting work of Stack (1962) on muscle function in the fingers in order to be impressed by the complexity of normal finger motion.

The principles underlying successful tendon transfer must be kept in mind in the evaluation of the cerebral palsied child. Briefly, they are as follows.

(1) Never transfer unless fixed deformity is corrected first. Contractures must be released prior to transfer.

(2) Every tendon which is to be transferred should be evaluated as to its suitability for the job it is expected to do. It is foolhardy to utilize a thin muscle with short excursion to do the work of a thick muscle with long excursion. Boyes (1962) has outlined specific factors necessary for success in this regard, and he rates

brachioradialis and flexor carpi ulnaris as the two muscles with the greatest work capacity in the forearm, and flexor sublimis and flexor profundis in the hand. Amplitude averaged 3.3 cm in wrist motors, 5.0 cm in digital extensors and long thumb flexor, and 7.0 cm in long finger flexors.

(3) A weak muscle always becomes weaker when transferred.

(4) When possible, transplant tendon to bone, rather than to tendon.

(5) Transfers should have as straight a direction of pull as possible to their new position.

(6) Proper tension after the transfer is important. A transfer put in too tightly will result in reverse deformity. A transfer put in too loosely will be ineffectual.

PRINCIPLES OF ASSESSMENT OF THE UPPER LIMB IN CEREBRAL PALSY

Normal and Abnormal Development of Hand Function

It is important to understand the natural development of hand function in the early months and years of life, in order to detect abnormalities in function consequent to brain damage (Gesell and Amatruda 1947; Bobath and Finnie 1958; Bobath 1959, 1965; Fiorentino 1963; Paine 1965). The normal newborn has a characteristic attitude at rest. The arms are adducted to the trunk with elbows flexed. The hands are fisted, the thumbs adducted, the forearms pronated, and the ulnar fingers are more active than the radial fingers. The upper limb resists passive extension, but will extend automatically in the startle or Moro reflex (Fig. 12). The neck-righting reaction is present, so that passive turning of the head to one side will result in rotation of the trunk to the same side (Fig. 5). Head control is poor. Equilibrium reactions are absent. Arm position is rarely affected by change in head position.

The asymmetrical tonic neck reflex gradually becomes apparent, so that turning the head to one side results in extension of the limbs on that side and flexion of the limbs on the opposite side (Fig. 2). This reaction is normal up to six months of age. Persistence past that time is abnormal. At from one to three months of age the infant continues to grasp in pronation, particularly the ulnar fingers. At about four months of age, the head can be held in the mid-line, and the first signs of hand-eye co-ordination become manifest. His two hands can meet in the mid-line, and he looks at them. Hand to mouth activity begins, and he can suck his fist. There is no evidence of hand dominance as yet. When an object is placed in the infant's hand, he grasps with his palm rather than with the ulnar fingers (Fig. 18). He will support himself on his fore-arms in the prone position at about four months of age.

At about the sixth to the eighth month, the infant gradually develops labyrinthine righting reflexes (Fig. 7) and optical righting reactions (Samilson 1966). Until this time, he has moved with total flexion or extension patterns against gravity, so sitting has been impossible. At about the sixth month he begins to alternate flexion and extension patterns, so that he can sit with flexed hips and extended trunk, supporting himself on his extended arms. Later, kneeling and crawling become possible, as the result of abolition of total flexion or extension patterns. The body righting reaction at the sixth or the seventh month permits the infant to turn from supine to prone. The parachute reaction or protective extensor thrust normally develops at about six months of age and remains throughout life (Fig. 13). This is elicited by holding the child face downwards by the waist in horizontal suspension, and suddenly lowering the child toward the floor. Immediate extension of the arms with abduction and extension of fingers denotes a positive reaction. Failure of this response to occur by six months of age bodes ill for hand function in later life (Fig. 14).

Transfer of objects from one hand to another is possible at seven or eight months of age. Now for the first time the infant can reach and grasp with an extended elbow, and his grasp is supinatory and radially oriented (Fig. 20). However, the thumb is not yet opposed to the fingers. Large objects are graspable, but not small ones.

At eight months of age, thumb pinch becomes manifest as pulp-to-side of index finger. The index finger becomes more active and is used for poking and prying. Pulp-to-pulp pinch begins between thumb and index finger at about nine months, and smaller objects are graspable. Release of grasp is still not facile.

At one year of age, thumb opposition is better developed, and is accompanied by grasp with the wrist extended rather than flexed. Release of grasp is more facile, and is accomplished by finger extension. Release of small objects is still difficult.

By eighteen months of age, the child develops proper grasp and release. At two years, he can hold a crayon with the fingers rather than with the whole hand. At three years of age he can put on shoes, and at five years he can use his hands for acquired skills such as drawing and writing. Finite skills require a highly developed sense of proprioception, stereognosis, two-point discrimination and touch.

Reflect for a moment on the difficulties of the cerebral palsied child (Bobath and Finnie 1958; Bobath 1959, 1965). Irreversible brain damage results in the persistence of primitive reflex patterns and the failure of appropriate appearance of developmental milestones. Sensation is impaired (Tachdjian and Minear 1958). Persistence of total flexion pattern in the upper limb results in the typical upper limb attitude, with adducted internally rotated shoulder, flexed elbow, pronated

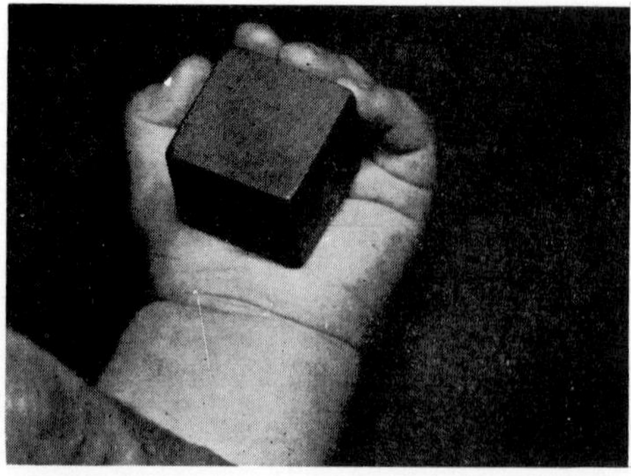

Fig. 18. Mid-palmar grasp (from Illingworth 1962).

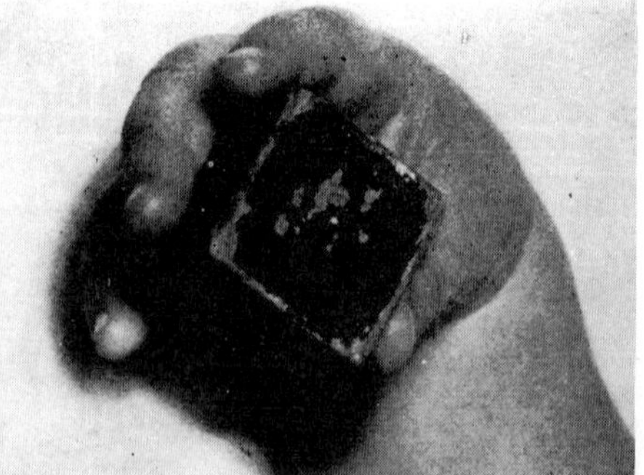

Fig. 19. Radially oriented grasp (from Illingworth 1962).

forearm, flexed wrist, and finger-flexed, thumb-clutched hand. Associated visual impairment prevents hand-eye co-ordination and optical righting responses. Persistence of primitive reflexes, such as the tonic neck reflex, causes the upper limb to respond to head direction (Fig. 2). Perceptual and conceptual impairments are common. Failure of appearance of the parachute or protective extensor reaction and persistence of the Moro reflex make impossible the purposeful pattern necessary for reaching out for an object in space (Carroll 1958). Failure of emancipation of the upper limbs from the lower limbs persists if malfunction in the latter obliges the former to assist in ambulation. No wonder that normality never can be achieved. The early emergence of hand dominance suggests hemiplegic involvement in cerebral palsy, as does a persisent asymmetric tonic neck reflex. Jensen and Alderman (1963) describe the seven most common characteristics of the cerebral palsied hand in attempted grasp. These are: (1) hyperabduction of the fingers; (2) hyperflexion of the wrist; (3) hyperextension of the metacarpo-phalangeal joints, with flexion at the inter-phalangeal joints; (4) hyperextension of the index finger; (5) low arc approach to grasp; (6) the whole hand and thumb oppose in grasp; and (7) slow speed. Reflecting again on retention of primitive patterns which characterize the cerebral palsied child, all the above criteria are explainable. For example, hyperextension at metacarpo-phalangeal joints may be the outcome of ineffectual wrist extension and the use of finger extensors to perform the task. Relative skeletal undergrowth of the involved hemiplegic limb is common, and when it occurs it is almost always accompanied by major sensory deficits.

Phylogenetic aspects of hand function (Bunnell 1964) are interesting, and may be applicable. The intrinsic muscles of the hand are ancient and date back to early fishes. Thus the hand precedes the arm phylogenetically. In amphibians, all digits are motivated by short muscles of the hand, and no finger flexors or extensors originate above the wrist. In reptilia, the flexor profundus is the only forearm muscle which crosses the carpus to motivate the digits. Finally, in mammals, the long muscles of the forearm become continuous with the brevis muscles of the hand.

General Prerequisites for Upper Limb Surgery in the Cerebral Palsied

Motivation is the most important prerequisite for successful upper limb surgery in cerebral palsy as far as the patient is concerned. It is absolutely necessary in postoperative rehabilitation. The individual who has already disassociated his upper limb from bodily functions is not a candidate for reconstruction. Such a patient often does not even express a desire for cosmetic improvement.

Intelligence as measured by standard means in severely handicapped individuals is often misleading. Mental deficiency thus measured is not considered as being a contra-indication to surgery, if the willingness and the ability to co-operate are present. Frequently, such patients do better than those with superior intelligence who are subjected to the frustrations of a knowledgeable life. Gains in function seem to be of more import to the patient in quadriplegics than in hemiplegics. Perhaps this is because having one functional limb results in psychological and physical disassociation of the hemiplegic limb, thereby impeding functional use of whatever gains are achieved.

Age is a consideration. Wrist fusion should be delayed until age twelve years, and metacarpo-phalangeal fusion of the thumb until age seven years. Tendon transfers should be delayed until age seven years. Age is also important in its relationship to motivation and past experiences. Frequently, the older cerebral palsied individual will have disassociated himself from his disabled limb and will have adjusted accordingly. Provided that adequate motivation is present, better results can be expected in younger children. In our experience, athetosis is not *per se* a contra-indication to surgery.

The Surgeon

Patience, fortitude and realism are required of the surgeon who deals with limb reconstruction in cerebral palsy. To expect normal function is foolhardy, and it results in frustration and pessimism. The surgeon must really know the patient, not only his upper limb. This is achieved only after serial examinations. He must know the various surgical procedures available to improve the upper limb, their indications and contra-indications, and must be ingenious enough to make adaptive changes where necessary. Technical proficiency is essential. Patience, firm gentleness and an encouraging attitude toward the patient and his family in the postoperative period are important. If best use is to be made of occupational and physical therapeutic measures before and after surgery the surgeon must be familiar with what is available.

The Environment

Parents and professional personnel involved in the pre-operative and the postoperative care of the patient should have a general knowledge of the problem and not be too impatient. Realistic parents do not expect normal results, and have the capacity to encourage their children to make continual use of what is left. Nursing personnel should be sympathetic and encouraging. Realistic encouragement and persistent opportunity to use the reconstructed upper limb have enabled many patients to improve. Fear is a major emotional stimulus to increased spasticity; gentle patient handling, repeated examinations and friendly surroundings will minimize this impediment to rehabilitation.

Aids to Assessment of the Upper Limb

Motion Pictures

Serial recordings on motion picture film are invaluable in pre-operative and postoperative assessment. The routine adopted for the first recording should be repeated at each subsequent session. We prefer 16-millimeter color film and record the following:

(1) position of both upper limbs at rest;
(2) relationship of upper limbs to lower limbs in gait (when feasible);
(3) use of hands in crutch-walking, mobilization of wheelchair, tying shoes, using spoon and fork, picking up large and small objects, pulling, pushing, grasp and release;
(4) active and passive motion of all of the joints of the upper limb, and tenodesis

effect of wrist position on grasp and release;
(5) wrist motion with fingers flexed;
(6) wrist motion with fingers extended;
(7) recording of finger motion (grasp and release) with and without braces, casts or splints;
(8) recording of wrist and finger motion with and without selective procaine block, and with and without selective electrical stimulation.

Braces, Splints and Casts

Plaster casts are very important not only in treatment but also in pre-operative and post-operative assessment. Casting the palmar flexed wrist in a more functional neutral or slightly dorsiflexed position may improve finger extensor power. Serial observations in this regard are necessary over a three-month period. In contemplating wrist fusion, the optimum position for arthrodesis can be gauged pre-operatively by casting and observing grasp and release in various wrist positions.

After operation, casts should be worn for about 12 to 16 weeks for wrist arthrodesis, and eight to ten weeks for carpo-metacarpal or metacarpo-phalangeal thumb fusion. Tendon transfers are casted for five to six weeks post-operatively, and are supported by light splints or braces for night use for an additional three to six months.

Swanson (1960) has emphasized that the flexor muscles should not be stretched by hyperextending the finger joints, because this can lead to the development of swan-neck deformities. He advises extending the wrist rather than the fingers. Well formed opponens splints are valuable for thumb training. Small aluminium splints may be used for the fingers after correction of swan-neck deformity. Other splints and braces are described in Swanson (1960) and Stamp (1963).

Local Procaine Block

Local one per cent procaine block may be useful in diminishing flexor spasticity so that true extensor strength may be gauged. Dilute procaine is said to block the gamma system without abolishing alpha motor neuron activity.

Electromyography

In a previous paper (Samilson and Morris 1964), we discussed electromyographic changes in the upper limb in cerebral palsy.

Zuh (1961) has recognized four different groups of electromyographic changes in cerebral palsy.
(1) Monoplegia or hemiplegia, with remaining muscles 'physiologic'. The electrical potentials in the extensors are prolonged, and the patient is minimally involved clinically.
(2) Increased spasticity, with spontaneous electrical activity of all muscles. Contractures are usually absent, but if they exist they are minimal. The amplitude of electrical activity in the performing muscles is greater than in the antagonists. Prognosis for surgical correction is reasonable.
(3) Extreme spasticity with tonic contractures. Low amplitude activity because of

tonic contractures. Organization of muscle phasic activity is barely perceptible. Electrical potentials are increased on attempted voluntary activity or on stretch. Prognosis fair for improvement.

(4) Most severe involvement. No increase in electrical activity on attempted voluntary contraction, but increased activity on stretch sensory stimulation, or motion of the opposite limb. Synchronous tremor present. Prognosis poor.

Zuh (1961) stated that 'where continuous activity occurs on both flexion and extension, prognosis for surgical correction is better'.

Taping

Duncan (personal communication) has observed that wrist extensors can be improved functionally, when the finger extensors are disassociated by flexing the meta-carpo-phalangeal joints. We have utilized his suggestions and have found that taping metacarpo-phalangeal joints in flexion and allowing a mobile wrist frequently results in improved voluntary wrist extension. This can be used as a training device. Perhaps the flexed position of the metacarpo-phalangeal joints serves to reduce the tightness of long finger flexors.

Hand Evaluation Sheet

We have utilized a hand evaluation sheet in serial examinations of the cerebral palsied upper limb (Table 1). Any standard form is useful, so long as the same observations are made on serial examinations.

Electrical Stimulation

Electrical stimulation may be used as a training device in teaching the patient to use wrist and finger extensors. It may also be used to determine activity in muscles which clinically appear to be paretic.

Physical Examination of the Cerebral Palsied Upper Limb

The frequent use of many of the procedures already described responsibly recorded and realistically evaluated, comprises much of the physical examination.

Observation of the limbs at rest will usually reveal adduction, internal rotation at the shoulder, flexion of the elbow, pronation of the forearm, palmar flexion of the wrist, and a thumb-clutched hand with spastic finger flexors. All of these aberrations are increased on attempted voluntary motion or under stress. The lack of reciprocal upper/lower limb swing in gait is characteristic of the mild hemiplegic, and is more apparent in children with greater brain damage. Skin temperature changes, hair growth, rubor, cyanosis or blanching should be recorded, and vascular abnormalities detected. Sensation is tested, in the knowledge that 75 per cent or more of these children can be expected to exhibit astereognosis, poor two-point discrimination and poor positional sense. Although this is not a contra-indication to surgical improvement, a better prognosis is to be expected when sensation is intact.

The effect of one joint position on another is analyzed. For example, is wrist dorsiflexion more efficient with the elbow in flexion or extension? The tenodesis effect of joint motion is studied, paying particular attention to the influence of wrist position on grasp and release. The degree and extent of any hypermobility at the meta-carpo-phalangeal joint of the thumb or the proximal inter-phalangeal joints in the fingers is observed and recorded.

Any muscle contractures are detected and recorded. The range of motion of each of the joints of the upper limb, both active and passive, is recorded. The speed of voluntary control is measured, and the clinical degree of spasticity is stated. Thumb position is analyzed, and pinch is described. The effect of wrist position on thumb position is recorded.

Finger motion is carefully analyzed (see Table 1). Muscle power is graded.

Finally, the functional use of the hand is recorded, both in writing and on motion pictures.

Specific Clinical Observations and their Applications

In considering the possibilities for operative improvement of the cerebral palsied upper limb, several monographs are available for review (Cooper 1952; Goldner 1955, 1961; Carroll 1958; Stelling and Meyer 1959; Swanson 1960; Green and Banks 1962; Samilson and Morris 1964; Keats 1965). All agree that most children do not require surgical treatment. All agree that functional training of the upper limb should precede surgery and in some instances may preclude it.

Generally, the first step must be to release contractures. Particularly common are pronation contractures, thumb adductor contractures, flexor sublimis contractures and flexor carpi ulnaris contractures.

Tendon transfers should precede arthrodesis, and frequently obviate the latter. This is true particularly with flexor carpi ulnaris transfer to radial wrist extensors.

The tenodesis effect of joint motion on pluri-articular muscles is of great importance. Release of grasp may be possible only if the wrist is in full palmar flexion, thus exerting a tenodesis effect on the finger extensors. To arthrodese such a wrist without first supplementing finger extensor power by tendon transfer would be disastrous.

Cooper (1952) has discussed how the tenodesis effect of ulnar deviation of the wrist on thumb abductors permits the thumb to remain out of the palm. Also of interest as regards pluri-articular muscles are cases in which release of the sublimis flexors is followed by flexor transfer to the common finger extensors. In such cases, ineffectual flexor power in the presence of relatively increased finger extensor power may result in swan neck or intrinsic-plus deformities at the proximal inter-phalangeal joints.

Picture for a moment the typical severely palmar-flexed wrist in cerebral palsy, and reflect on how it resembles the position of the wrist in Phalen's test for carpal tunnel syndrome (Fig. 20). Median nerve conduction studies in cerebral palsy might prove to be interesting, and may possibly help to explain the characteristic thenar palsy with ineffectual thumb intrinsics.

Finally, arthrodesis should be preceded by pre-operative casting for determination of optimum position and effect on function.

TABLE I

CEREBRAL PALSY HAND EVALUATION

NAME   I.Q.

UNIT NUMBER   WARD

SPASTIC ( )   ATHETOID ( )   BOTH ( )

Drugs (type, dosage, frequency)
Ambulatory ( )   Wheelchair ( )   Bed care ( )
Function in lower limbs e.g. use of crutches
Surgery on lower limbs and effect on upper limbs
O.T.—Type and degree of activity
P.T.—Type, frequency   Parental Attiude
( ) Hand use—self-help   crutches ( )   pushes ( )
                                 clothing ( )   chair   ( )
                                 bathroom ( )   food   ( )
( ) Cosmesis (hand appearance)
     Splinting—type, frequency   Casting—type, frequency
     Psychiatric evaluation
     Follows directions well ( )   fair ( )   not at all ( )
( ) Sensation-protective ( )   pain-touch ( )   sterognosis ( )
( ) Grasp-release   Grasp-strength ( )   Release ( )
     Motion pictures (showing muscle stimulation)
EMG (a) Electrically active finger extension
    (b) Electrically active wrist extension
    (c) Flexor carpi radialis
    (d) Flexor carpi ulnaris
    (e) Extensor pollicis longus, extensor carpi radialis longus and brevis
    (f) Abductor pollicis brevis or extensor pollicis brevis
    (g) Synchronous activity   at rest   on motion
Muscle stimulation as checked on EMG
Voluntary initiation of electrical activity correlated with function
        Strength (trace-excellent)
        (a) Flexor carpi radialis
        (b) Flexor carpi ulnaris
        (c) Extensor digitorum communis
        (d) Extensor carpi radialis longus and brevis
        (e) Extensor pollicis longus
Previous surgery—type and dates and results
        Shoulder motion—active
                        passive
                        contracture
        Elbow motion   —active
                        passive
                        contracture
        Wrist motion
        (a) wrist motion with fingers flexed   —active   flex   extend
                                                passive   flex   extend
        (b) wrist motion with fingers extended—active   flex   extend
                                                passive   flex   extend
        (c) ulnar deviation—amount—fixed or not
        (d) active and passive radial deviation
        Radio-ulnar motion—active   Pro.   Sup.
                           passive   Pro.   Sup.
                           contracture

52

TABLE I (CONTINUED)

    Effect of elbow motion on wrist position —active
                                               passive
    Effect of elbow motion on finger position—active
                                               passive
( ) Positioning hand in space
( ) Thumb motion
     (a) free voluntary control—abduction
                                extension
     (b) adduction or flexion contractures
     (c) opposition
     (d) pulp to pulp pinch
     (e) distance from 2nd M/C head to M/P joint of thumb
     (f) distance thumb misses 5th M/C head on adduction
     (g) lateral pinch (present or not)
     (h) effect of wrist motion on thumb position—ulnar deviation
                                                  flexion
                                                  extension
     (i) thumb in palm occasionally ( )   frequently ( )   always ( )
( ) Finger motion—
     (a) tenodesis effect—grasp and release
     (b) effect of wrist position (flexion, extend, radial deviation, ulnar deviation)
     (c) effect of elbow position, effect of radioulnar position
     (d) effect of thumb position
     (e) voluntary closing
     (f) voluntary opening
     (g) intrinsic function
     (h) swan neck deformity—effect of wrist position on
     (i) I/P joint deformity—contracture
     (j) M/P joint deformity—contracture
     (k) palm hygiene
     (l) sublimis tightness
     (m) index pinch—lateral or pulp to pulp

SAMILSON, CLASSIFICATION   (points)
     (a) Function—grasp, release, thumb pinch, wrist extension (one point each)   (   )
     (b) Cosmesis—absence of contractures of wrist, fingers, elbow, radioulnar (one point
         each)   (   )
     (c) Environmental use—eating, tying shoes, wheelchair, crutch or lift, satisfaction (one
         point each)   (   )

GREEN CLASSIFICATION(from Green and Banks 1962)
( ) *Poor*—paperweight only, poor or absent grasp and release, poor control
( ) *Fair*—helping hand without effectual use in dressing, fair control, grasp and release slow—not
     effective
( ) *Good*—good, helping hand, good grasp and release, good control
( ) *Excellent*—good use in dressing, eating, general activities, effectual grasp and release, excellent
     control

53

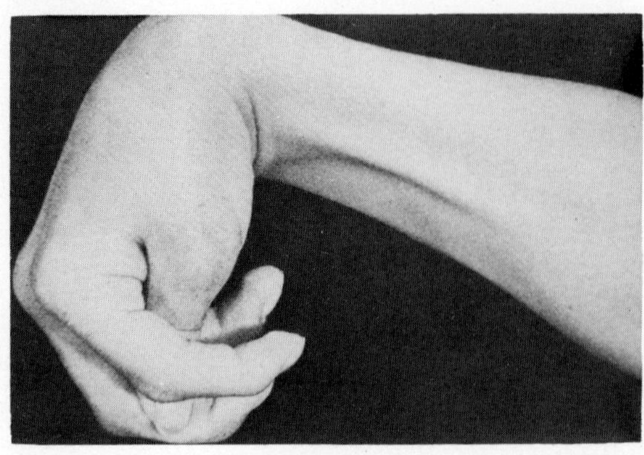

Fig. 20. Pronated fore-arm, flexed wrist and thumb-clutched hand (from Chapchal 1972).

ASSESSMENT OF THE LOWER LIMBS

From the foregoing discussion, it is apparent that isolated consideration of one portion of the body to the exclusion of the others in cerebral palsy is fruitless and misleading. However, for the sake of orderly presentation, we shall consider the hip, knee, ankle and foot separately, at the same time relating one to the other. It is recognized that there are many other tests of prognostic significance other than those which have been and will be described here. We have reported those which we consider to be of most value. The tests described will be subdivided into clinical and laboratory categories, although the latter have helpful clinical significance.

The Hip—Clinical Tests

The most common hip deformities in cerebral palsy are flexion, adduction, and internal rotation contractures (Fig 21a), femoral anteversion, and paralytic hip dislocation (Baker *et al.* 1962, Pollock 1962, Samilson *et al.* 1967).

Hip flexion contracture is of great significance, and is usually due to iliopsoas and/or rectus femoris spasticity. The *Thomas test* (Fig. 21b) is a time-tried clinical test for iliopsoas contracture, and is performed by fixing the pelvis with one thigh flexed firmly on the abdomen, while the patient lies supine with the lumbar lordotic curve obliterated. The amount of hip flexion contracture is calculated by measuring the angle between the contralateral thigh and the examining table. Increased lumbar lordosis and/or knee flexion deformity may accompany hip flexion contracture. Prior to reinforcing hip extension with an Eggers hamstring transfer, it is essential that the hip flexion contracture be corrected. A cardinal principle of tendon transfer is that a fixed deformity, against which the transfer will work, must be corrected first.

The *prone rectus test* (Fig. 22) is carried out with the patient prone. The examiner flexes the patient's knee on the extended thigh, and if the buttocks rise from the examining table on the side tested the rectus femoris is contracted. Adduction contracture is tested in the supine position by determining the degree of passive abduction obtainable. The medial hamstrings frequently contribute to adduction

54

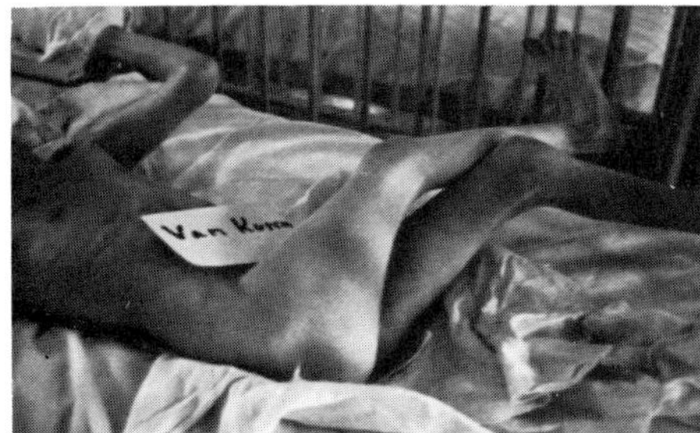

Fig. 21a. Flexion; adduction and internal rotation deformity of hip.

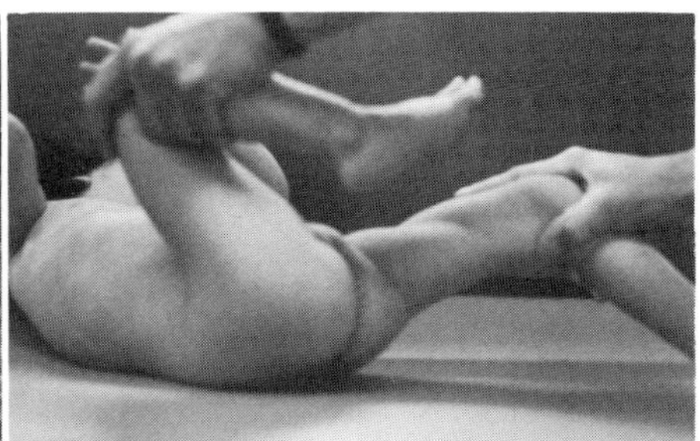

Fig. 21b. Thomas test for hip flexion contracture.

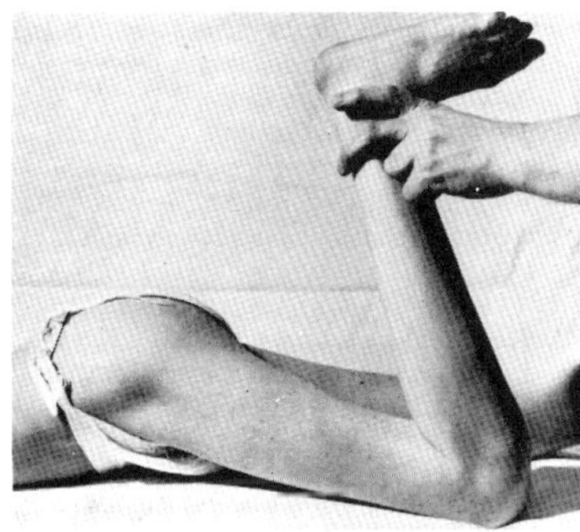

Fig. 22. Prone rectus test (from Holt 1965).

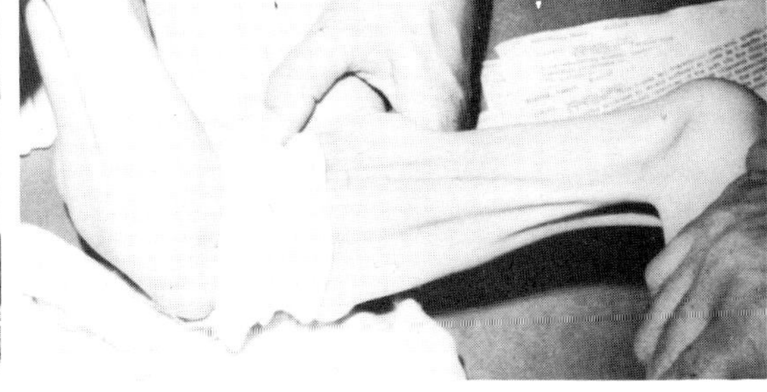

Fig. 23. Phelps-Baker test. Note bowstringing of medial hamstring.

deformity of the hip, and should be tested by the *Phelps-Baker test* (Fig. 23). The basic testing position is the same as for the Thomas test. The contralateral hip is then passively abducted as far as possible with the knee flexed. The knee is then extended, causing the thigh to adduct, if the medial hamstrings are contributing to adduction contracture, palpation of the medial hamstrings will reveal bowstringing.

Tightness of the iliotibial band is evaluated by the *Ober test*. The child lies on his side with the tested side up. The lower thigh is flexed on the abdomen to fix the pelvis. The upper thigh is extended with the knee flexed, and the number of degrees between this thigh and the examining table represents the amount of contracture of the iliotibial band. Frequently, a valgus deformity of the knee accompanies such a contracture. *Pelvic tilt* downwards on the same side may be present also.

Femoral anteversion (Lewis *et al.* 1964) may be gauged clinically by determining the degree of relative internal and external rotation of the hip. If internal rotation far exceeds external rotation, increased femoral anteversion is present. If the reverse is true, femoral retroversion is present. Another test for *femoral anteversion estimation* is performed with the child supine. The examined hip is flexed to 90 degrees with the knee flexed. The examiner places his finger on the most prominent portion of the greater trochanter with the thigh neutrally rotated (Fig. 24). The number of degrees of internal rotation of the thigh required to bring the most prominent portion of the greater trochanter to a mid-lateral position represents a clinical estimation of anteversion.

Push-pull instability in the Thomas test position is of value in recognizing paralytic dislocation. The degree of instability in spastics is not nearly as noticeable as in congenital hip dislocation or myelodysplasia dislocations. The infrequent *anterior dislocation* may present as a prominent bony bulge in the inguinal region (Fig. 25). Shortening of the thigh, and adduction and flexion deformity frequently accompany spastic hip dislocation.

The incidence of dislocated hips (Samilson *et al.* 1972) in cerebral palsy is greatest in severely involved spastic and/or rigid quadriplegics. Coxa valga and femoral anteversion are important factors in the genesis of the deformity, as are retained asymmetrical neonatal reflexes, such as the incurvatum or Galant reflex (Fig. 14) (see this volume Chapter 8). The co-existence of scoliosis and hip dislocation in a large number of cases of cerebral palsy strongly supports this theory (Samilson *et al.* 1972, Samilson and Bechard 1973). Recognition—and correction—of coxa valga and femoral anteversion is essential to the prevention, management and retention of reduction of dislocated hips in cerebral palsy.

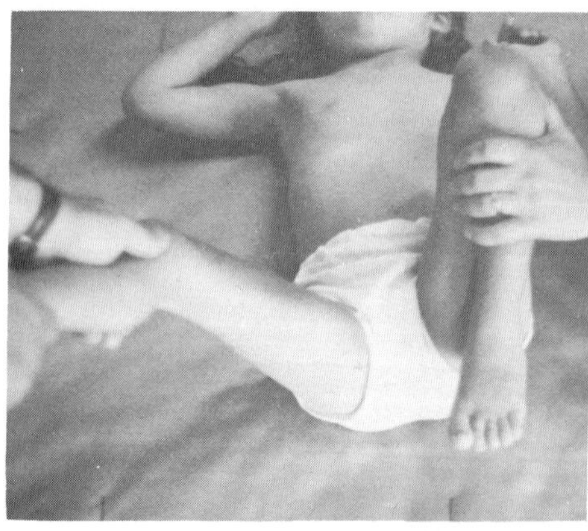

Fig. 24. Clinical testing for femoral anteversion.

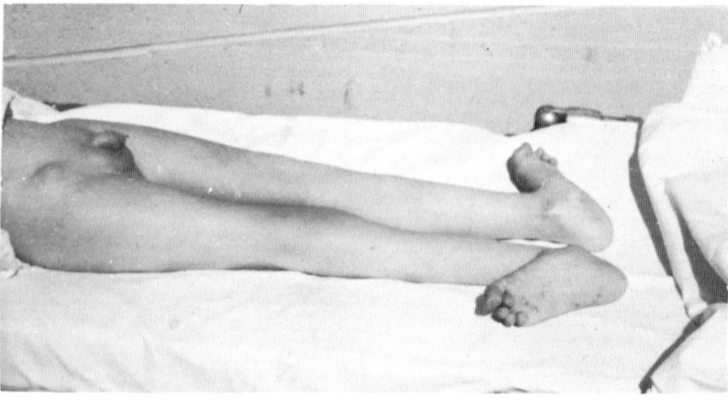

Fig. 25. Anterior hip dislocation. Note femoral head in right groin.

Muscle testing, particularly for *abduction* and *extension* strength, is important. This can be combined with local procaine block of the spastic over-active adductors, where necessary for evaluation.

Standing and walking, when possible, will reveal scissoring, characteristic of adductor spasticity, increased lumbar lordosis, characteristic of hip flexion contracture, and internal rotation, characteristic of anteversion, to name just a few.

Hip Tests—Laboratory

X-ray evaluation can provide useful information concerning hip disabilities in cerebral palsy. A *standing antero-posterior* view of the pelvis will demonstrate pelvic obliquity, which may be due to abduction contracture, shortening of one lower limb, or persistent incurvatum reflex. A supine antero-posterior view, with the patellae facing directly upwards, may reveal relative coxa valga (Fig. 26*a*). This may be true or apparent, but is almost always a sign of co-existent anteversion. X-ray determination of anteversion by the *Ryder-Crane* (Ryder and Crane 1953) or *McGilligan* methods will assist in determining the degree of derotation necessary at corrective osteotomy. *Arthrography* of the hip, using 30 per cent renograffin solution is of value, since an interposed limbus may indicate some difficulty in closed reduction. (Fig. 26*b*). *Scanograms* are of value in leg-length inequality problems in the growing ambulatory hemiplegic child.

Electromyography and electrical stimulation are additional laboratory aids which assist particularly in the evaluation of hip extensors and abductors. Unapparent abductor strength may be uncovered by gentle electrical stimulation, particularly in the face of strong adductors.

Local one per cent procaine block of the obturator nerve will obviate adductor spasticity and permit more accurate abductor testing. Similarly, local block of the femoral nerve will obviate rectus femoris spasticity temporarily, and permit more accurate diagnosis.

Motion pictures of the physical tests performed, of standing and, where possible, of gait will provide an objective recording of the patient's status during various phases of treatment, and is of inestimable value in reviewing long-term results.

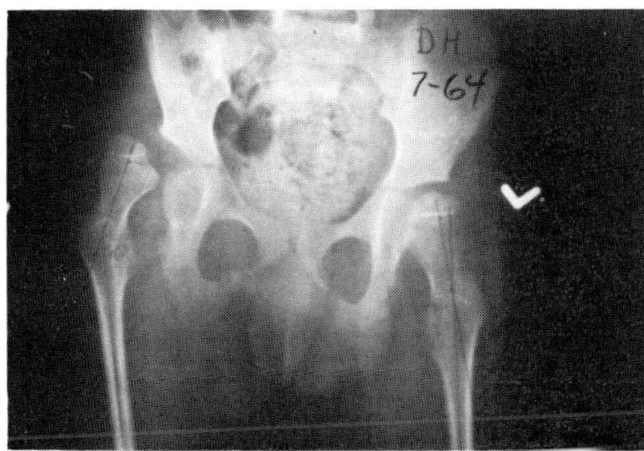

Fig. 26*a*. Bilateral coxa valga, femoral anteversion and dislocation of right hip.

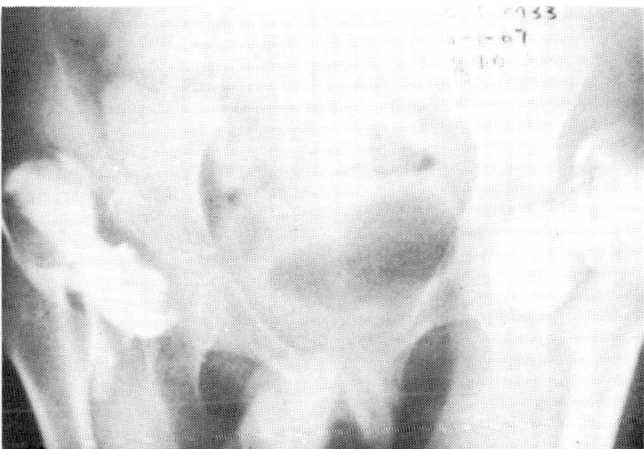

Fig. 26*b*. Hip arthrograms with bilateral dislocations and interposed limbi.

Knee Tests—Clinical

Obviously, many of the tests described above for the hip, also have application to the knee. The Thomas test, Phelps-Baker test (Baker *et al.* 1962), and Ober test are just a few of these.

In addition, the *crossed-adductor spread* of the knee jerk is a bad prognostic sign for ambulation. The *prone extension test* (Banks and Green 1958) (Figs. 27 and 28) is performed with the child lying prone, the hips flexed off the table, and the knees extended. Simultaneous extension of the hip and knee on each side independently is a good prognostic sign for the success of Eggers' hamstring transfer to the femoral condyles (Eggers and Evans 1963). To successfully extend the hip and knee in this way the patient must have good hip extensors and little, if any, hip flexion contracture.

Patella position should be determined. A high-riding patella often accompanies quadriceps-femoris spasticity (Fig. 29*a*), and a characteristic knee-extension kick gait. Lateral patellar position occurs in recurrent patellar dislocation, which is sometimes seen concurrently. Absence of the patella may signify accompanying arthrogryposis multiplex congenita.

The effect of *knee position on ankle position* is of extreme importance. Eggers has pointed out how talipes equinus may be corrected by hamstring transfers (Eggers and Evans 1963), but an objective prognostic test in this regard would be very worthwhile (Fig. 29*b*). Such a clinical test is performed simply by using a *walking cylinder* with the knee in complete extension (Fig. 30). If any spastic equinus that was previously present is corrected, the prognosis for Eggers' procedure to retain this correction is excellent. Similarly, if the ankle can be dorsiflexed past neutral position with the knee flexed (soleus) (Fig 31), but not with the knee extended (gastrocnemius), (Fig. 32), prognosis for gastrocnemius aponeurotic lengthening (Strayer, Vulpius, Baker) is good, and heel cord lengthening is unnecessary. On the other hand, the ankle which cannot be dorsiflexed with the knee flexed or extended under general anesthesia, can only be corrected by lengthening of the Achilles tendon and/or posterior capsulotomy of the ankle.

Muscle testing for quadriceps and hamstring strength should be recorded, and *gait observed* where possible.

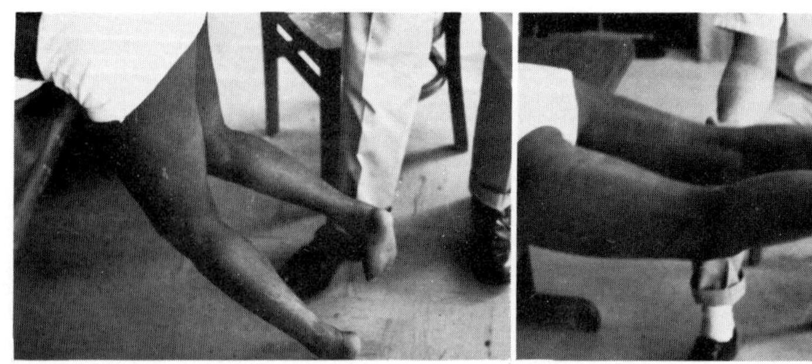

Fig. 27. Prone rectus test. Starting position.

Fig. 28. Prone rectus test. Final position.

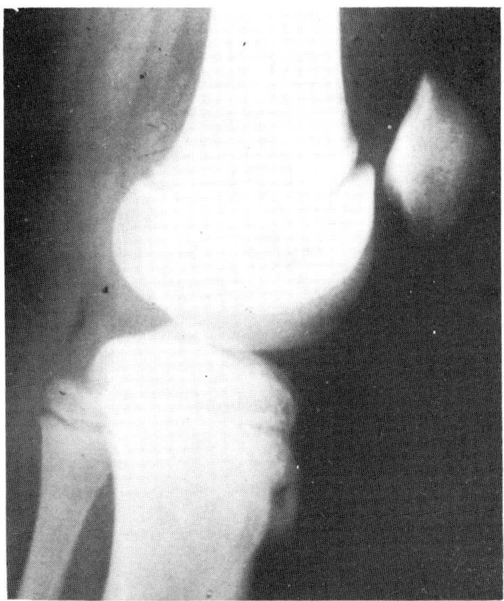

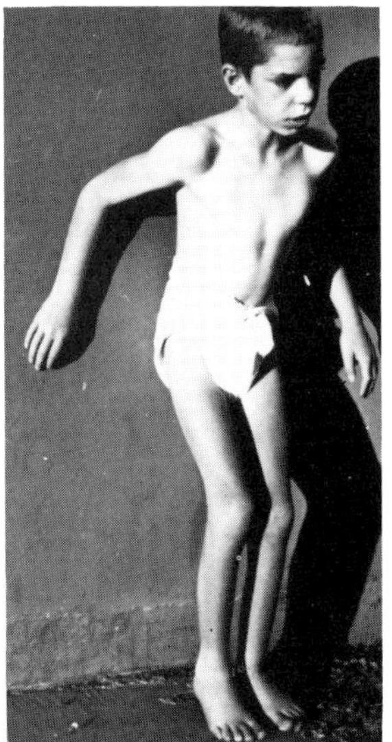

Fig. 29a (*above left*). High patella may mean spastic rectus femoris or rectus femoris contracture.

Fig. 29b (*above right*). Combined hip flexion, knee flexion and equinus.

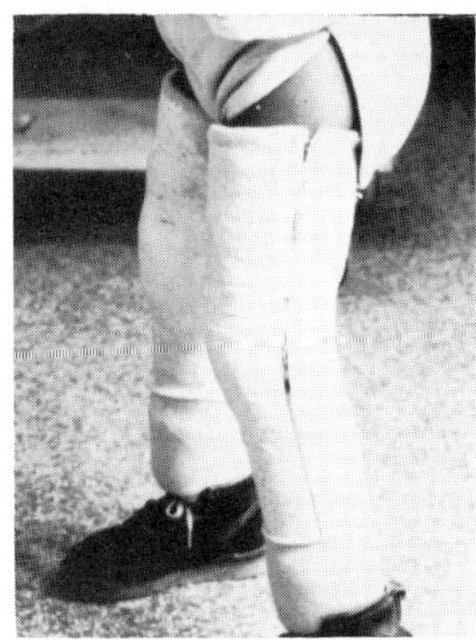

Fig. 30. Cylinder casts in maximum knee extension. Note effect on equinus.

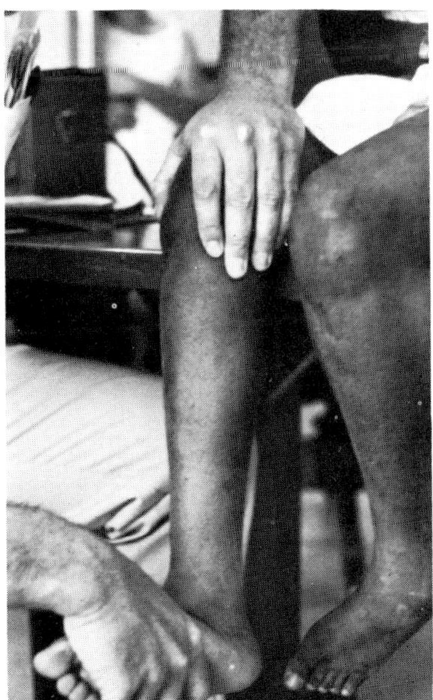

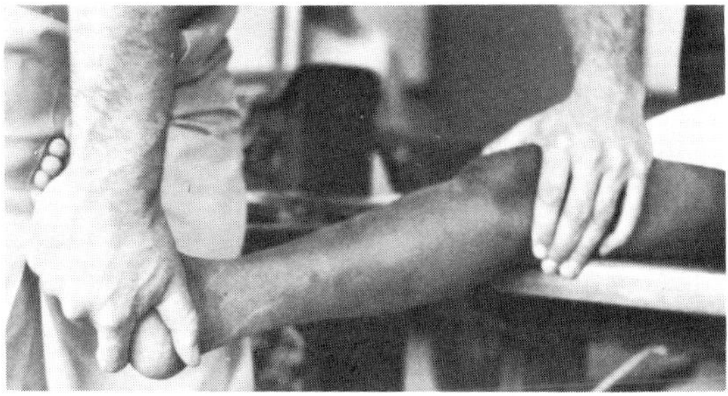

Fig. 31 (*above left*). Ankle dorsiflexion with knee flexed. Subtalar is inverted so that all dorsiflexion occurs at the ankle instead of the mid-tarsus.

Fig. 32 (*above right*). Ankle dorsiflexion with knee extended.

Knee Tests—Laboratory

X-ray evidence of a high-riding patella or patellar dislocation is self explanatory. Bony blocks to full knee extension contra-indicate soft tissue operations until the bony block is corrected. Scanograms, when indicated, are useful.

Electromyography, in our experience, is a good objective prognostic test for the correction of spastic (non-fixed) equinus by hamstring transfer. Electrodes are placed in the gastrocnemius/soleus muscle mass and the child stands in place. Constant high-amplitude recordings are made from the muscle. The hip and knee are then passively extended rapidly by the examiner, whilst a constant electromyographic recording from the calf is made. Sudden cessation of electrical activity from the calf muscles, which lasts as long as the hip and knee are kept extended, is a good prognostic sign for the correction of spastic (non-fixed) equinus by Eggers' procedure. Similarly, lengthening of the Achilles tendon in such a circumstance may result in an iatrogenic calcaneus deformity.

Local procaine block of hamstrings and/or quadriceps may provide additional information on the deforming musculature, and assist in prognosis for improvement.

Again, *motion picture recording* of the examination and gait are of great value in later review.

Ankle Tests—Clinical

The importance of the effect of knee position on ankle position has already been discussed along with appropriate tests (Banks and Green 1958, Martz 1960, Pollock 1962, Eggers and Evans 1963). In passively testing dorsiflexion at the ankle, it is important to invert the foot (Figs. 31 and 32), thus locking the subtalar joint, so that all the dorsiflexion which is achieved occurs at the ankle, rather than at the subtalar and mid-tarsal joints.

The production of iatrogenic calcaneus deformity by injudicious operations on the calf has already been discussed. An additional problem which requires mention is the mentally retarded quadriplegic or diplegic who habitually walks in equinus. Testing reveals that he has no fixed deformity, and he will stand in a plantigrade position on command. The mechanism of the equinus in these cases is not well understood, but it seems that calf muscle operations are contra-indicated. Duncan's (1960) monograph on reflexogenic areas on the plantar aspect of the foot should be reviewed, and tested appropriately.

Tibial torsion can be estimated with the child sitting on the edge of the examining table with the knees flexed at 90 degrees. The difference between the transcondylar axis of the femur and the bimalleolar axis represents the approximate degree of tibial torsion.

Posterior tibial over-activity is most apparent in the swing phase of gait, and is characterized by inversion and plantar flexion (Fig. 33). In the presence of weak dorsiflexion, a non-fixed equinus and demonstrated posterior tibial over-activity, consideration should be given to transfer of the posterior tibial tendon through the interosseous membrane to the middle cuneiform.

Elevation in stance of the plantar aspect of the foot at the base of the fifth metatarsal indicates *peroneal spasticity and over-activity* (Fig. 34). Occasionally, we have seen actual peroneal dislocation over the fibular malleolus in cerebral palsy. When this occurs, the peroneals may become dorsiflexors of the fore-foot, and contribute to rocker-bottom foot deformity (Fig. 35).

Oftentimes, evaluation of active dorsiflexor power is difficult. The *dorsiflexion confusion test* is of value in determining whether or not active dorsiflexion is possible. The child sits on the edge of the table with knees flexed at 90 degrees, and is asked to flex the hip against the resistance of the examiner's hand on the thigh; active ankle dorsiflexion becomes apparent with this maneuver (Fig. 36). Unfortunately, this activity may not be present in gait, even though a positive dorsiflexion confusion test is present.

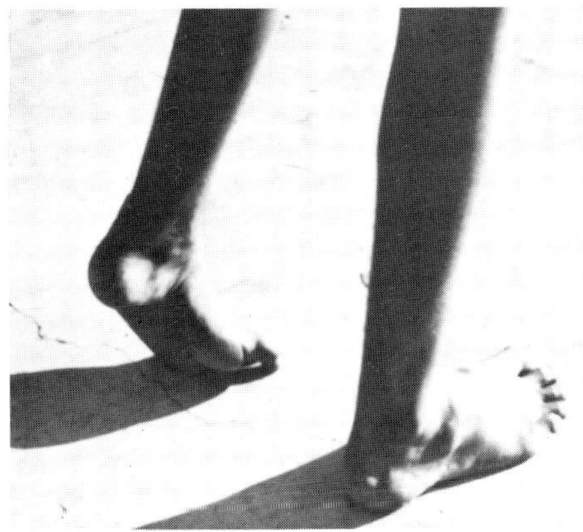

Fig. 33. Posterior tibial over-activity.

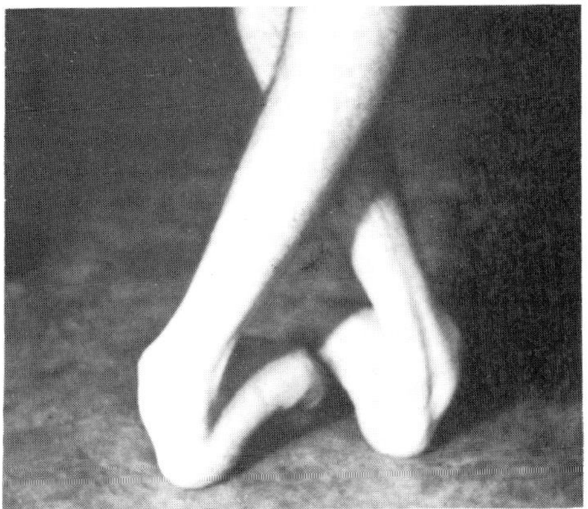

Fig. 34. Peroneal spasticity. Peroneals have dislocated anterior to fibular malleolus and dorsiflexed the fore-foot.

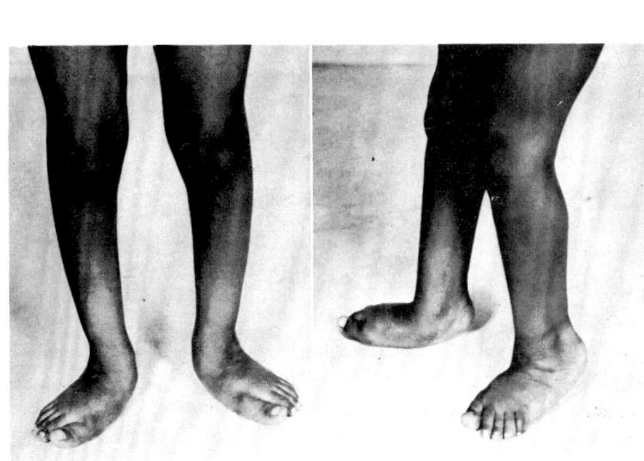

Fig. 35. Rocker-bottom foot (from Bassett 1966).

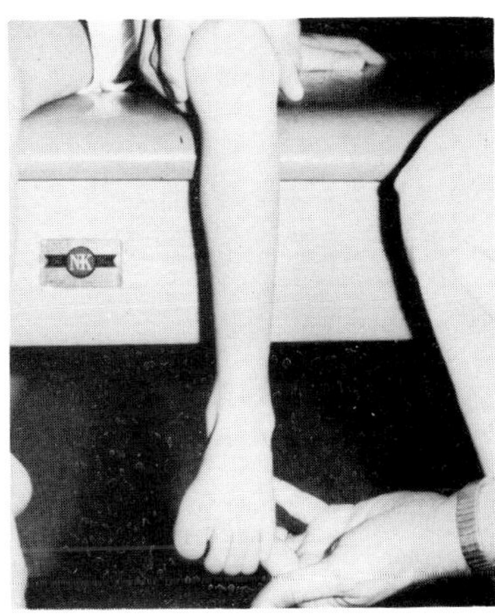

Fig. 36. Dorsiflexion confusion test.

Ankle Tests—Laboratory

X-ray evaluation should be made in the standing position, with the knee extended. A standing antero-posterior ankle view will demonstrate any talar tilt in the ankle mortise (Fig. 37). Failure to recognize valgus tilt of the talus in a standing antero-posterior view will lead to over-correction at the subtalar joint, if a Grice procedure is performed. A standing lateral view will reveal the position of the os calcis. In the presence of fixed equinus (heel cord contracture), the os calcis will be in equinus position, with the point of heel cord insertion displaced relatively superiorly (Fig. 38). Persistence of this in an ambulatory patient may lead to rocker-bottom foot. Where dorsiflexors are strong and plantar flexors weak, the os calcis will assume a calcaneus position, with the point of heel cord insertion displaced relatively inferiorly (Fig. 39).

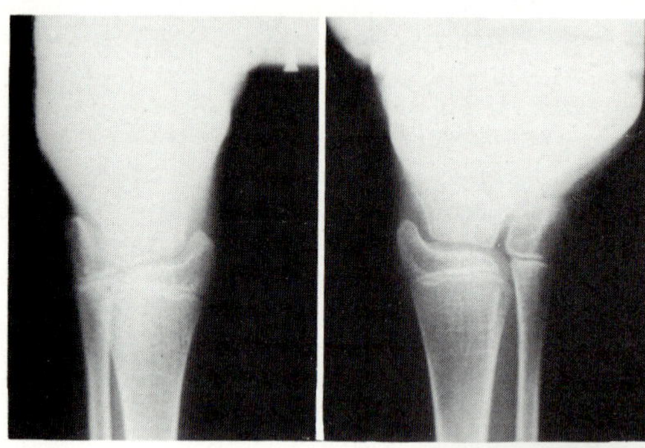

Fig. 37. Standing A-P view of ankles. Note valgus tilt in ankle mortise (from Samilson 1973).

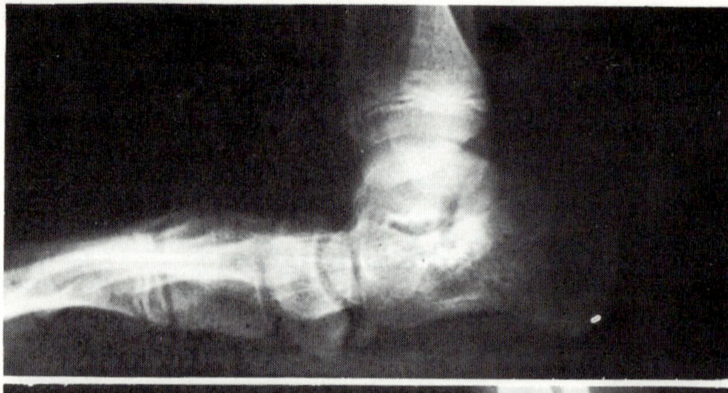

Fig. 38. Standing lateral of foot. Heel cord is tight and os calcis is in horizontal position.

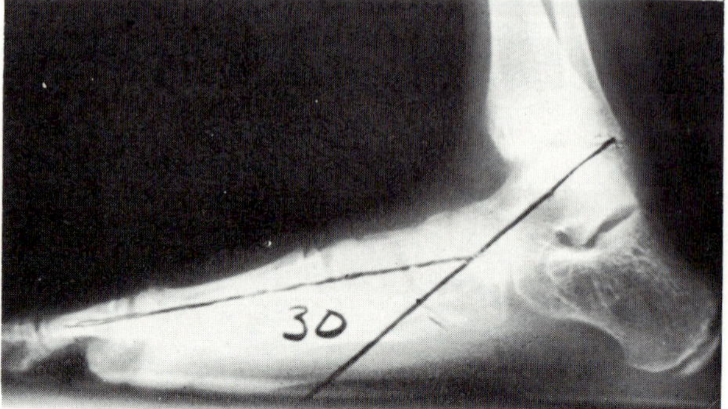

Fig. 39. Standing lateral of foot. Heel cord is not tight and os calcis is tilted upwards.

Electrical stimulation of dorsiflexors will assist in determining the muscle power in this group, electromyography will demonstrate the presence or absence of phasic activity in the muscles about the ankle.

Local procaine block may obviate reflexogenic areas on the plantar surfaces of the foot, obliterating equinus temporarily. Ethyl chloride is relatively ineffectual for such purposes.

Foot Tests — Clinical

Much that has been said already applies to the foot. For ease of understanding, it is wise to consider the hind-foot, mid-tarsus, and fore-foot separately, recognizing the functional impositions one places on the other.

The *position of the os calcis* has been discussed, but the influence this has on the remainder of the foot is of paramount importance. For example, calcaneus is almost always accompanied by cavus deformity and eventual claw toes, whilst equinus frequently imposes rocker-bottom deformity at the mid-tarsus if the equinus is fixed and the child continues to bear weight. Varus and valgus tilt of the os calcis usually results in the mid-foot and fore-foot following suit (Fig. 40). Consequently, *passive calcaneal* shift in the weight-bearing position, with observation of the effects of such shift on forefoot position, can assist in determining the outcome of calcaneal osteotomies.

Frequently, long toe flexors play a significant rôle in persistent equinus deformity. They should be evaluated in this regard. Often, clawing of the toes will occur, long after heel cord lengthening or gastrocnemius aponeurotomy, as a consequence of over-active toe flexors (Fig. 41).

Whether or not the *plantar fascia* is tight should be tested with the toes extended. In the presence of calcaneus position of the os calcis, tightness of the plantar fascia is not infrequent.

Position of the talar head is determined by observation and palpation. Normally the talar head rests on the sustentaculum tali of the os calcis. With valgus deformity and increased talo-calcaneal divergence, the talar head slips medially and plantarwards off the sustentaculum, and is observed and felt in its new position (Fig. 42a).

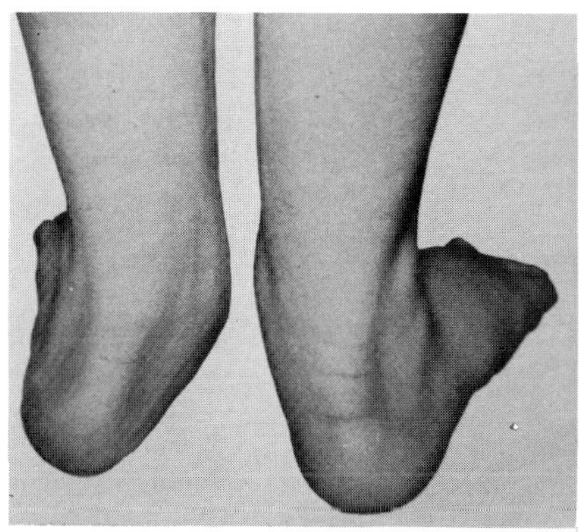

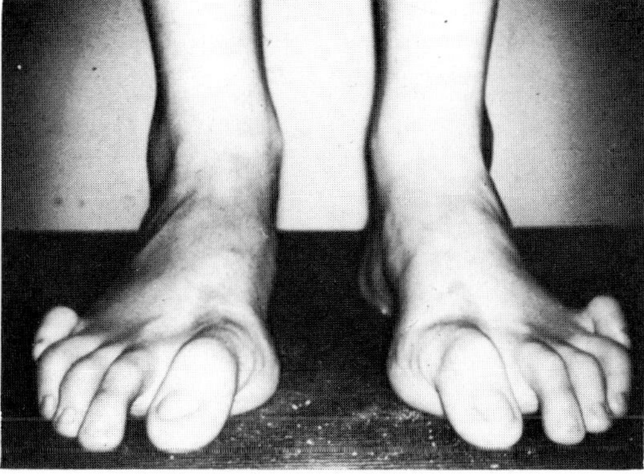

Fig. 40 (*left*). Valgus feet (from Samilson 1973).

Fig. 41 (*right*). Toe flexor spasticity following heel cord lengthening.

Persistent ankle clonus may be an indication for selective soleus and/or gastro-cnemius neurectomy, using a neurostimulator to identify those motor branches which contribute to the clonus.

Having the child stand on a lucent glass or plastic surface, and observing the foot print from below is quite revealing. Any callosities should be noted, and the *plantar print* recorded photographically.

Foot Tests—Laboratory

Standing X-rays of the foot are evaluated for os calcis position, talar head position, talo-calcaneal divergence, naviculo-cuneiform sag, cavus, and metatarsal position. A special *Anthonsen view* (Anthonsen, W., personal communication) will reveal the axial position of the os calcis as regards valgus or varus, and the axis of the subtalar joint posteriorly. It is of help in pre-operative evaluation of children who undergo calcaneal osteotomy. Shoe inserts, particularly the University of California os calcis insert (Henderson and Campbell 1967) (Fig. 42*b*), are of value in determining the effect of passive correction of os calcis position on the rest of the foot.

Electrical stimulation and *electromyography* may indicate the status of foot intrinsics.

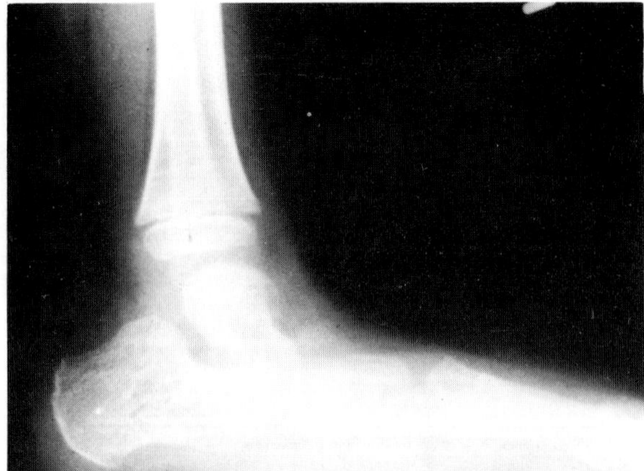

Fig. 42*a*. Talus is plantar flexed and talar head is medial to sustena-culum.

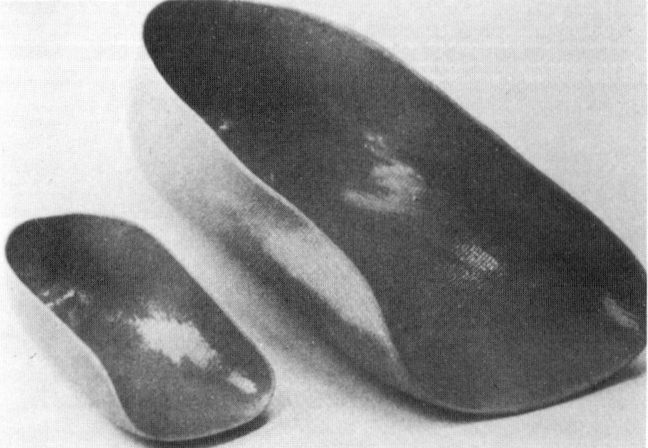

Fig. 42*b*. University of California Biomechanics Laboratory Insert (from Samilson 1973).

Pelvic obliquity in cerebral palsy may be due to suprapelvic factors, infrapelvic factors, or both (Fig. 43) (Crome 1971). The obliquity may be correctable or fixed. Persistent neonatal reflexes (*e.g.* incurvatum or Galant reflex) may result in tonic postural attitudes conducive to muscle contracture which results in eventual fixed pelvic obliquity.

Infrapelvic factors leading to pelvic obliquity are related to increase or decrease of effective valgus (femoral neck-shaft angle). An increased effective valgus may be due to true coxa valga (probably from iliopsoas over-activity), femoral anteversion and/or adduction contracture.

Decreased effective valgus results from abduction contracture or, rarely, associated congenital and/or developmental coxa vara. A short leg in hemiplegia is rarely a cause of pelvic obliquity.

Suprapelvic factors leading to pelvic obliquity are poorly understood. Lordosis occurs first, followed by rotary imbalance, often associated with persistence of neonatal reflexes (such as obligate asymmetrical tonic neck reflex, or incurvatum or Galant reflex). In addition, asymmetrical righting reflexes lead to rotary spinal instability.

The management of pelvic obliquity and spinal deformities associated with cerebral palsy is outlined in Chapter 8.

Kyphosis in cerebral palsy (Garrett 1971) is often associated with hamstring spasticity and/or a 'collapsing spine due to major weakness of spinal extensors'. Again, a failure of righting reactions and equilibrium reactions to occur probably plays a rôle as well.

Lordosis is most frequently associated with hip flexion contracture in cerebral palsy, but is also seen with marked spinal extensor spasticity (Garrett 1971).

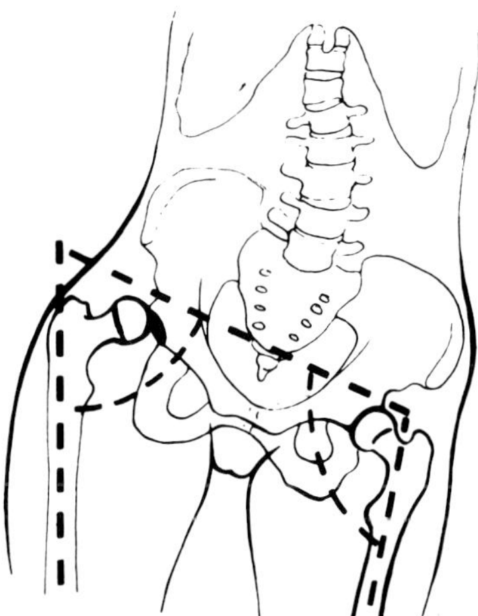

Fig. 43. Pelvic obliquity.

Spasmodic torticollis and cervical arthritis are sometimes seen in athetoid patients, and are most difficult to manage (Garrett 1971).

Scoliosis (Fig. 44) in cerebral palsy is most common in severly involved, neurologically immature quadriplegics (Samilson and Bechard 1973). Approximately 7 per cent of ambulatory patients, 25 per cent of sitters, and 39 per cent of total bed care patients have scoliosis. The over-all prevalence varies according to the relative numbers of the above categories one sees.

The commonest type of curvature is thoraco-lumbar (Fig. 45), followed by lumbar, thoracic, and double primary curves, in that order.

Again, persistence of an asymmetrical incurvatum reflex and/or failure of symmetrical righting reactions to occur are possible etiological factors. There is a high incidence of associated hip dislocations.

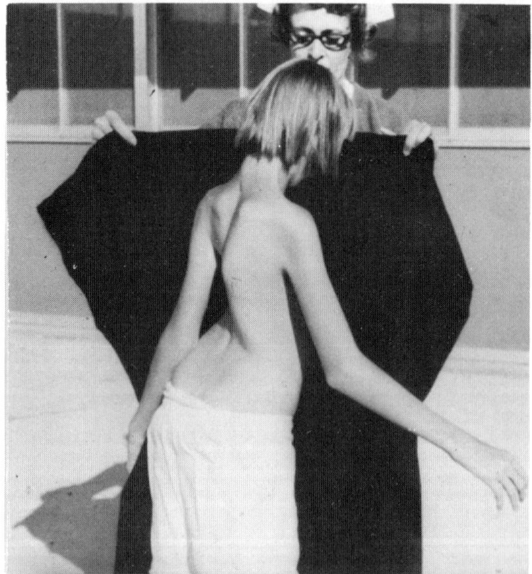

Fig. 44 (*left*). Scoliosis and lordosis.

Fig. 45 (*below*). Thoraco-lumbar scoliosis with windblown hips towards concavity of spinal curve.

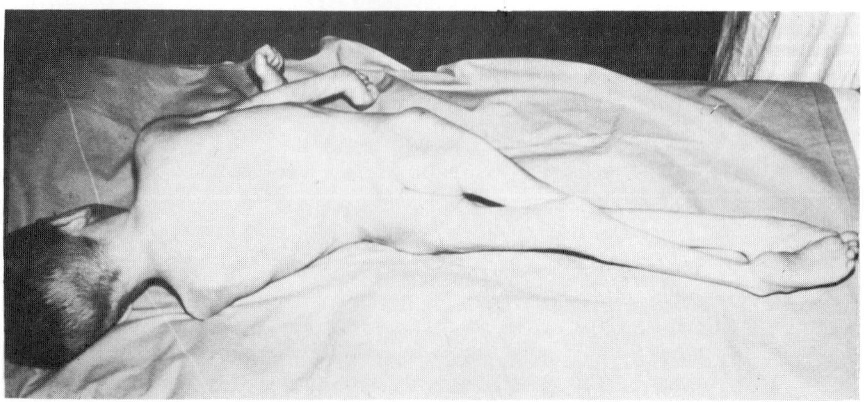

Influence of the Type of Cerebral Palsy on End Results

Spasticity differs from rigidity, in that the former is velocity sensitive, and is manifest only during a small arc of the range of motion of the joint over which the tested muscles pass. Rigidity is not velocity sensitive and is present during most of the range of passive motion, and often prevents motion. The *poorest prognosis is in those children manifesting rigidity.* Surgical procedures in the upper limb or those designed to permit ambulation are contra-indicated in the patient manifesting true rigidity.

We must *differentiate spasticity from contracture* as well. Contracture denotes actual physical shortening of the muscle. The latter can be corrected only by surgical lengthening of the musculo-tendinous unit, or by removal of bone over which the contracted muscle passes, resulting in relative lengthening. Spasticity, on the other hand, may be amenable to physical therapy, bracing, local nerve blocks, and sometimes, temporarily, to neurectomy. A continuing spasticity of a muscle group is likely to eventuate in a myostatic contracture, but when and how this occurs is poorly understood. Sometimes it is necessary to examine a child under general anesthesia to differentiate severe rigidity from myostatic contracture.

Rarely do we see a pure neurological state of spasticity, athetosis, rigidity, or ataxia in cerebral palsy. Most patients have mixed manifestations, with one type predominating. Athetosis, itself, is not a contra-indication to surgery, but problems are far more frequent in this group than in spastics. For example, it is more difficult to achieve an arthrodesis is an athetoid patient, because of the constant involuntary movement occurring during the healing phase. Similarly, the so-called 'athetoid shifts' occurs occasionally, but less frequently than has been purported. This 'athetoid shift' may result in a reverse deformity to the one corrected by a tendon transfer.

For a discussion of the effects of 'patterns' of involvement on potential surgical procedures, please see Chapter 12.

Timing of Surgery in Cerebral Palsy

Growing children have certain peculiarities, for which neither the orthopaedic surgeon nor the physical or occupational therapist should take credit. In the first few years of life, the normal child goes through an amazingly complex process of neurological maturation which normally occurs in a reasonably sequential manner. This maturation is *always* delayed in the cerebral palsied child, but its propensity to resume and advance is a fact which we must never forget. A therapist who relates that she 'worked out a Babinski' on a child is just as ridiculous as an orthopaedic surgeon who tells the family, 'your child would never have walked unless I had done that Achilles tendon lengthening!'

It is because of the ever-changing neurological state of the growing child, that we must be very careful in the planning of potential operations. In a non-ambulatory child of seven or eight years, for example, the likelihood of eventual ambulation is dim indeed. In such an instance, surgical procedures to facilitate ambulation (*e.g.* achievement of a plantigrade foot) should be delayed and abandoned altogether, once the child reaches age eight years. Similarly, operations to improve nursing care (*e.g.* adductor tenotomy and obturator neurectomy) or to prevent dislocated hips (*e.g.* soft tissue releases and varus-derotation femoral osteotomy) may be done early on, whether or not the patient will become ambulatory eventually.

Bony growth must be considered in potential surgery. Interference with epiphyseal growth, for example, will delay arthrodesis of the foot until age ten to eleven years and of the wrist until age twelve to thirteen years. Similarly, bone growth may necessitate repetition of soft tissue surgery early on (*e.g.* Achilles tendon lengthening). In a hemiplegic child, particularly a female, with relative shortening on the affected side, it would be wise to avoid correction of equinus on that side, since it compensates for the shortening, and will be masked later on when the young lady wears shoes with moderate heels.

Neither braces nor physical therapy can correct true myostatic contracture, and, in fact, attempts to do so sometimes results in additional deformity (*e.g.* development of rocker-bottom foot from bracing a myostatic contracture of the triceps surae in an ambulatory child). Most soft tissue surgery should be delayed until age three to four years, since oftentimes non-operative management during the early years obviates the necessity for surgery. Once myostatic contracture occurs, surgery is indicated. In and about the hips, knees and wrists, myostatic contracture can often be prevented by splinting, physical therapy, and proper positioning, and/or by tendon transfer (*e.g.* flexor carpi ulnaris to radial wrist extensors, provided that other indications for this procedure are present).

No operative procedure is a 'cure-all', and all surgery must be followed by appropriate post-operative splinting and physical therapy, to retain the gains achieved. Similarly, teachers should understand proper positioning of the children in the classroom, post-operatively.

Ambulation and Gait in Cerebral Palsy

To evaluate the prognosis for ambulation in the cerebral palsied child, Beals (1966) measured the severity of lower extremity motor involvement, severity of upper extremity motor involvement, birth weight, intelligence, seizures, hip stability and surgical treatment. By assessment of motor skills, he determined a motor age (or neurological age). 'Severity index' was defined as the motor age, in months, at a chronological age of three years. This severity index had a possible range of 0 to 36. All children with a severity index of 12 or more achieved ambulation by seven years of age, and no child ever ambulated freely with a severity index less than 10. An index of 4 to 9 was consistent with crutch-walking. Seizures and hip dislocation adversely affected the ability to ambulate. He outlined the principles of orthopaedic management, relating this to the severity index. In the 0 to 9 severity index group, maintenance of the integrity of the hip joint is most important. In the severity index 10 to 11 group, hamstring transfers should be delayed until age six or seven years. In addition, triceps surae release in this group, in the presence of knee flexion, tended to increase the latter and jeopardize free ambulation. In those children with a severity index of 12 to 18, surgery was utilized only to improve gait, once free ambulation was obtained.

Bleck (1965) relates locomotor prognosis to neurological development, and, with 90 per cent predictability at age four years, indicated that any two of the following signs were considered to give a zero prognosis for ambulation: symmetrical tonic neck reflex, asymmetrical tonic neck reflex, absence of parachute reaction, positive supporting reaction (extensor thrust), absence of the foot placement reaction, neck righting reflex, and Moro reflex.

REFERENCES

Anthonsen, W. *Personal communication.*

Baker, L. D., Dodelin, R., Bassett, F. H. (1962) 'Pathological changes in the hip in cerebral palsy.' *Journal of Bone and Joint Surgery,* **44A**, 1331.

Banks, H., Green, W. T. (1958) 'The correction of equinus deformity in cerebral palsy.' *Journal of Bone and Joint Surgery,* **40A**, 1359.

Bassett, F. H., Baker, L. D. (1966) 'Equinus Deformity in Cerebral Palsy.' *In* Adams, J. P. (Ed.) *Current Practice in Orthopaedic Surgery,* Vol. 3. St. Louis, Mo: C. V. Mosby Co.

Beals, R. K. (1966) 'Spastic paraplegia and diplegia: an evaluation of non-surgical and surgical factors influencing the prognosis for ambulation.' *Journal of Bone and Joint Surgery,* **48A**, 827.

Bleck, E. E. (1965) 'Locomotor prognosis in cerebral palsy.' *Paper presented at the Annual Meeting of the American Academy for Cerebral Palsy, Cleveland.*

Bobath, K. (1959) 'The neuropathology of cerebral palsy and its importance in treatment and diagnosis.' *Cerebral Palsy Bulletin,* **1**, (8), 13.

—— (1965) 'The motor deficit in patients with cerebral paresis.' *Paper presented at the Study Group on Orthopaedics and Physical Medicine in Cerebral Palsy, Bristol.*

—— Finnie, N. (1958) 'Re-education of movement patterns in everyday life in the treatment of cerebral palsy.' *Occupational Therapy,* **21**, (6), 23.

Boyes, J. H. (1962) 'Selection of a donor muscle for tendon transfers.' *Journal of the Hospital for Joint Diseases,* **23**, (1), 1.

Bunnell, S. (1964) *Surgery of the Hand,* 4th edn, (revised by Boyes, J.) Philadelphia: Lippincott. p. 24.

Carroll, R. E. (1958) 'The treatment of cerebral palsy of the upper extremity.' *Bulletin, New York Orthopedic Hospital,* (December).

Chapchal, G. (1972) *Reconstructive Surgery and Traumatoly,* Vol. XIII Basel: S. Karger Ag.

Cooper, W. (1952) 'Surgery of the upper extremity in spastic paralysis.' *Quarterly Review of Pediatrics,* **7**, 139.

Crome, W. (1971) 'Pelvic obliquity in cerebral palsy.' *Instructional Course Volume, 25th Annual Meeting of the American Academy for Cerebral Palsy, New York.*

Crothers, B., Paine, R. S. (1959) *The Natural History of Cerebral Palsy.* Cambridge, Mass.: Harvard University Press.

Denhoff, E., Robinault, I. (1960) *Cerebral Palsy and Related Disorders.* New York: McGraw-Hill.

Duncan, W. *Personal communication.*

—— (1960) 'Tonic reflexes of the foot: their orthopedic significance in normal children and in children with cerebral palsy.' *Journal of Bone and Joint Surgery,* **42A**, 859.

Eggers, G. W. N., Evans, E. B. (1963) 'Surgery in cerebral palsy.' *Journal of Bone and Joint Surgery,* **45A**, 1275.

Fiorentino, M. R. (1973) *Reflex Testing Methods for Evaluating C.N.S. Development.* Springfield, Ill.: C. C. Thomas.

Garrett, A. L. (1971) 'The spine in cerebral palsy.' *Instructional Course Volume, 25th Annual Meeting of the American Academy for Cerebral Palsy, New York.*

Gesell, A. L., Amatruda, C. S. (1947) *Developmental Diagnosis, 2nd edn.* New York: Harper.

Goldner, J. L. (1955) 'Reconstructive surgery of the hand in cerebral palsy and spastic paralysis resulting from injury to the spinal cord.' *Journal of Bone and Joint Surgery,* **37A**, 1141.

—— (1961) 'Upper extremity orthopedic surgery in cerebral palsy or similar conditions.' *A.A.O.S., Instructional Course Lectures,* **18**, 169.

Green, W. T., Banks, H. H. (1962) 'The flexor carpi ulnaris transplant and its use in cerebral palsy.' *Journal of Bone and Joint Surgery,* **44A**, 1343.

Henderson, W. H., Campbell, J. W. (1967) *UC-BL Insert-casting and Fabrication Biomechanics Laboratory, Technical Report, 53.* San Francisco: University of California.

Holt, K. S. (1965) *Assessment of Cerebral Palsy.* London: Lloyd-Luke.
—— Reynell, J. K. (1967) *Assessment of Cerebral Palsy—II.* London: Lloyd-luke.
Illingworth, R. S., (1962) *An Introduction to Developmental Assessment in the First Year.* London: Spastics Society—Heinemann Medical.
Jensen, G. D. Alderman, M. E. (1963) 'The prehensile grasp of spastic deplegia. *Pediatrics*, **31**, 470.
Keats, S. (1965) 'Surgical treatment of the hand in cerebral palsy: correction of thumb-in-palm and other deformities. Report of 19 cases.' *Journal of Bone and Joint Surgery,* **47A**, 274.
Lewis, F. R., Samilson, R. L., Lucas, D. B. (1964) 'Femoral torsion and coxa vara in cerebral palsy—a preliminary report.' *Developmental Medicine and Child Neurology,* **6**, 591.
Martz, C. D. (1960) 'Talipes equinus correction in cerebral palsy.' *Journal of Bone and Joint Surgery,* **42A,** 769.
Paine, R. S. (1965) 'Early recognition of cerebral palsy and prognostic signs.' *Instructional Course Lecture, American Academy of Cerebral Palsy, Cleveland.*
—— Oppé, T. E. (1966) *Neurological Examination of Children. Clinics in Developmental Medicine, Nos. 21/22.* London: Spastics Society with Heinemann.
Peiper, A. (1963) *Cerebral Function in Infancy and Childhood.* New York: Consultants Bureau.
Pollock, G. A. (1962) 'Surgical treatment of cerebral palsy.' *Journal of Bone and Joint Surgery,* **44B,** 68.
Ralston, H. *Personal communication.*
Rushworth, G. (1960) 'Spasticity and rigidity—an experimental study and review.' *Journal of Neurology, Neurosurgery and Psychiatry,* **23**, 99.
Ryder, C. T., Crane, L. (1953) 'Measuring femoral anteversion: the problem and the method.' *Journal of Bone and Joint Surgery,* **35**, 321.
Samilson, R. L. (1973) 'Neuromuscular diseases affecting the foot.' *In* Inman, V. T. (Ed.) *Du Vries' Surgery of the Foot.* St. Louis, Mo.: C. V. Mosby Co.
—— (1966) 'Principles of assessment of the upper limb in cerebral palsy.' *Clinical Orthopedics and Related Research.* **47**, 105.
—— Bechard, R. (1973) 'Scoliosis in cerebral palsy.' in *Current Practice in Orthopedic Surgery.* St. Louis, Mo.: C. V. Mosby Co. 183.
—— Morris, J. M. (1963) 'Surgical improvement of the cerebral palsied upper limb—electromyographic studies and results of 128 operations.' *Journal of Bone and Joint Surgery,* **46A**, 1203.
—— Carson, J., James, P., Raney, F. L. (1967) 'Results and complications of adductor tenotomy and obturator neurectomy in cerebral palsy.' *Clinical Orthopedics and Related Research,* **54**, 61.
—— Tsou, P., Aamoth, G., Green, W. (1972) 'Dislocation and subluxation of the hip in cerebral palsy.' *Journal of Bone and Joint Surgery,* **54A**, 863.
Stack, H. G. (1962) 'Muscle function in the fingers.' *Journal of Bone and Joint Surgery,* **44B**, 899.
Stamp, W. G. (1963) 'Bracing in cerebral palsy.' *Orthopaedic and Prosthetic Appliance Journal,* (*December*).
Steindler, A. (1952) 'Pathokinetics of cerebral palsy.' *A.A.O.S., Instructional Course Lectures,* **9**, 118.
Stelling, F. H., Meyer, L. C. (1959) 'Cerebral palsy: the upper extremity.' Clinical Orthopedics and Related Research, **14**, 70.
Swanson, A. B. (1960) 'Surgery of the hand in cerebral palsy and the swan-neck deformity.' *Journal of Bone and Joint Surgery,* **42A**, 951.
Tachdjian, M. O., Minear, W. L. (1958) 'Sensory disturbances in the hands of children with cerebral palsy.' *Journal of Bone and Joint Surgery,* **40A**, 85.
Zuh, T. (1961) 'Indications and check-out of results of treatment for spastic palsies on the basis of electro-diagnostic studies.' *Chirurgja Narzedów Ruchu i Ortopedja Polska,* **26**, 157.

Cerebral Palsy Gait

JACQUELIN PERRY

Introduction

Among the many definitions of walking, one useful for the analysis of gait is to consider it as a sequence of standing postures which advance the body while continuously retaining balance and security (Fig. 1). The two basic requirements are a stable standing posture and the ability to accomplish an effective stride. Even a slight abnormality of posture or stride will lead to less efficient walking, but only in the presence of quite considerable deformity will walking be totally impossible. Thus one need not be physically perfect to walk effectively, although the basic requirements must be met. By relating errors in a patient's gait to his clinical abnormalities, appropriate corrective measures can be selected for both functional and cosmetic improvement.

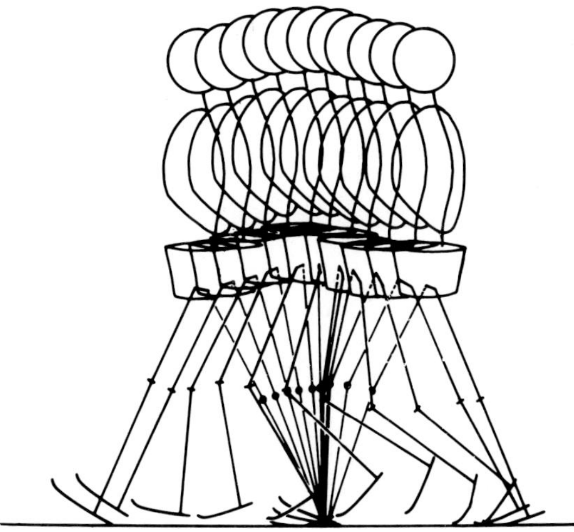

Fig. 1. Double gait: recorded with interrupted light (strobe) photography. Note that as the left leg swings forward the stance limb, while supporting the body, also constantly alters its posture to allow the trunk to move forward with the swinging limb.

With most types of disability, there is a close correlation between the physical findings and the observed gait. The effects of local joint trauma or arthritis can be forecast quite accurately. So too with many types of paralysis, such as poliomyelitis, muscular dystrophy and peripheral nerve injuries, the functional consequences of the muscle loss are predictable.

Such predictions are not possible with cerebral palsy. The reasons for this are multiple: (1) the lesions causing the motor dysfunction are hidden within the control centres of the brain and spinal cord; (2) motion is controlled through a hierarchy of numerous sensory-motor exchange centers; and (3) disruption of this hierarchy through brain damage has diverse effects.

Neurological Control Mechanisms

The definable types of motor activity are voluntary selective motor patterns, primitive locomotor patterns, mass limb reflexes, erect postural responses and spasticity. They represent five levels of sensory-motor exchange within the neurological system (Table I). As no motion occurs without a stimulus, the nature of the sensory functions at each particular level determines the type of motor action that will ensue.

TABLE I

Neurological levels of control

Clinical sign	*Stimulus*	*Neurological level*
Spasticity (rigidity)	Quick stretch (slow stretch)	Reflex arc from muscle spindle
Mass limb reflex extension flexion	Hip and knee extension (or flexion)	Spinal cord multisegmental interaction
Erect postural tone	Trunk upright	Vestibular system in brain stem
Primitive locomotor patterns	Desire to stand or step	Midbrain/subthalamus area
Selective control	Normal volition	Cerebrum

Spasticity is an unmoderated display of the simplest form of motion. The muscle responds directly to the stretch stimulus. This action, requiring only the reflex arc of a single spinal segment, represents the lowest level of the motor control hierarchy. Electromyographic analysis has shown two types of response: sustained action and clonus. The sustained response is recorded only with a slow stretch or as a continuation of an earlier clonic reaction. The pattern of distribution of spasticity represents an exaggeration of the ordinary bipedal posture.

The *mass limb reflexes* of the lower extremity represent a postural relationship between the hip, knee and foot. Through intrasegmental connections within the spinal cord, the position of one of these joints influences that of the others (Krieg 1945). In their most primitive form (*e.g.* in patients with a spinal cord injury) the mass limb reflexes are manifested as the flexor withdrawal to a noxious stimulus and the extensor thrust response to firm plantar pressure. The cerebral palsied patient displays a more subtle relationship between joint posture and muscle action. Grossly the 45 degree position of hip and knee divides the flexion and extension synergistic responses.

Either the hip or knee, but more particularly the knee, may influence activity in the ankle and foot muscles, and hence, joint posture. With flexion at the hip or knee, the ankle plantar flexors are relaxed and the foot is easily dorsiflexed (Fig. 2a); with

72

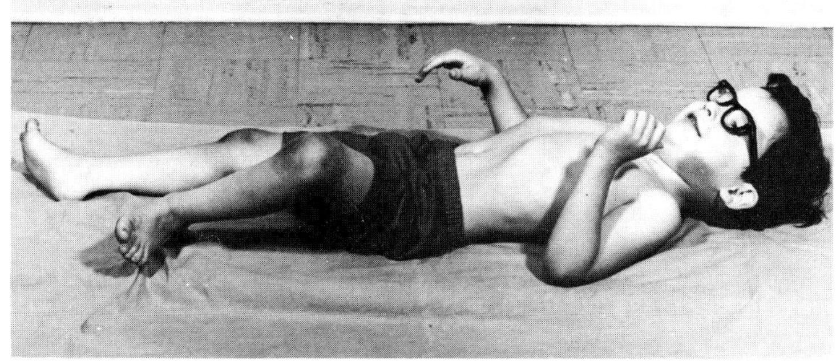

Fig. 2*a*. Mass limb reflex: mass flexion. Note prominent ankle dorsiflexion accompanying flexion of hip and knee.

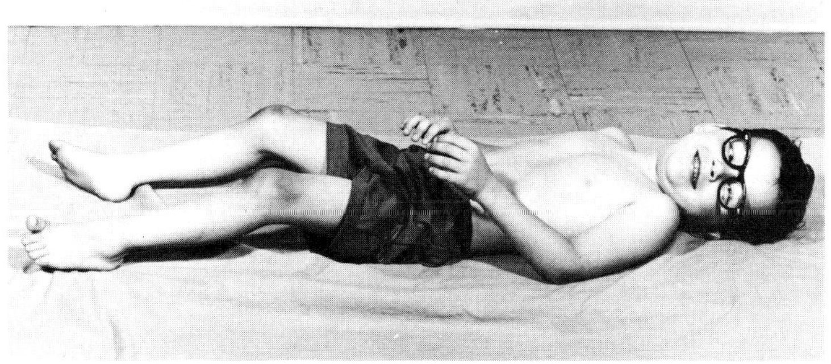

Fig. 2*b*. Mass limb reflex: mass extension. Note marked ankle plantar flexion accompanying hip and knee extension.

the hip or knee in extension, the ankle plantar flexors are tense and hold the foot in plantar flexion (Fig. 2*b*). Using stretch as a test of muscle tension, the change in muscle tone between the two positions may be displayed by the difference in the duration of clonus. To the clinician this means that the Silfverskiöld test, commonly employed to differentiate contracture in the gastrocnemius from that of the soleus, is invalid (Giovan *et al.* 1974), if the patient's neurological lesion has exposed his mass limb reflexes. It also means there will be active ankle plantar flexion due to contraction of both the soleus and gastrocnemius muscles whenever the child extends his knee. This is clearly demonstrated in the hemiplegic cerebral palsied child. Similar mass limb reflexes occur in the upper extremity.

Erect Postural Tone is mediated through the vestibular system within the lower brain stem. In response to vestibular stimulation (there are tracts extending from the brain stem to the spinal cord segments), extensor tone in the lower extremities is

73

increased when the patient is erect (Elliot 1969) (Fig. 3). (In the upper extremities it is the flexors which become hypertonic.) The induced tone also increases the spastic response. Thus examination of a patient supine will not reveal the function one will observe when he is standing.

In *primitive locomotor patterns* the mass limb reflexes are used for locomotion. Stimulated by the patient's desire to walk, this control center in the mid-brain subthalamic area initiates the flexor synergy (to take a step) and the extensor pattern (to provide limb support) (Figs. 4a and b). The three joints respond in a stereotyped fashion, which the patient cannot modify. There are, however, variations among patients as to the strength and completeness of the patterns.

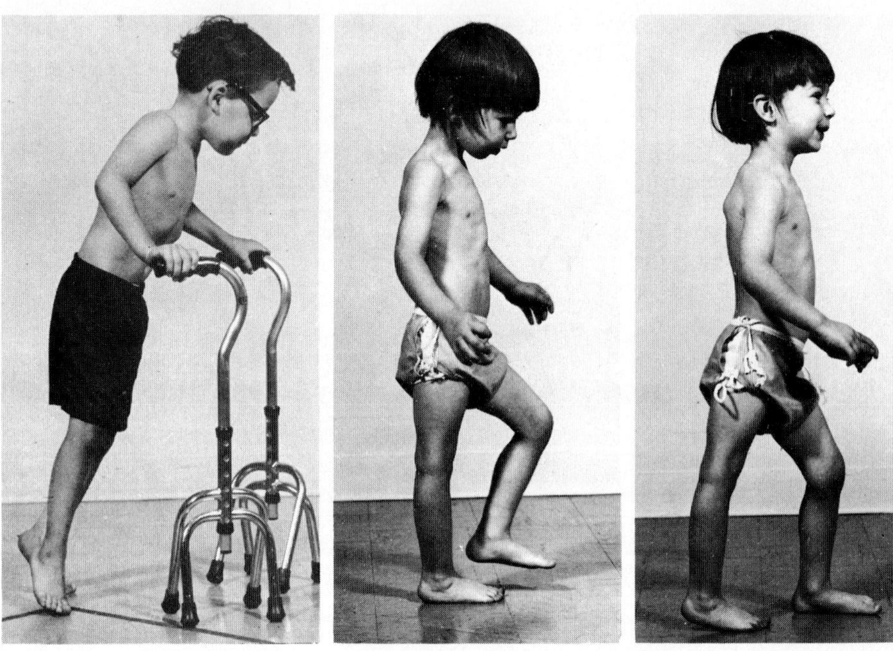

Fig. 3. Erect postural tone. Note increased plantar flexion with patient erect.

Figs. 4a and 4b. Primitive locomotor patterns. (a) (*left*): flexion pattern. Note simultaneous hip flexion, knee flexion and ankle dorsiflexion as the patient takes at step. The ankle dorsiflexion is more pronounced than that which occurs during normal gait. (b) (*right*): extensor pattern. Note combined hip extension, knee extension and ankle plantar flexion.

Selective control is the normal way to move. Emanating from the cerebral cortex, selective control permits one to move any one joint (or muscle) independently, or to combine various actions as desired, either sequentially or simultaneously. Strength and velocity also are modified at will. All these characteristics are used to attain the smoothness and efficiency of normal walking that makes this complex task seem so easy (Close 1964).

Selective motor control is essential for manual muscle testing, as careful isolation of an action is a prime requisite for an accurate assessment of its strength. Manual muscle testing is appropriate in patients with paralysis from poliomyelitis, muscular dystrophy, peripheral neuritis and nerve injury, or in persons with localized joint pathology. As such patients are able to control their muscles accurately, failure to perform as instructed, or a display of weakness, is direct evidence that the peripheral structures being tested are deficient. For the cerebral palsied patient, the situation is just the reverse. His peripheral system is intact, but he cannot control it accurately. Consequently his responses to a manual muscle test will tend to be inconclusive, incomplete, and highly misleading when ever joint and body postures are active influences, though this is not true in all cases (Sutherland *et al.* 1969).

The typical cerebral palsied patient presents a mixture of these many forms of motion as he walks. Spasticity is induced by limb or body weight stretching the muscles. Major changes of joint position alter muscle tone through the mass limb reflexes. The general character of the gait is determined by the relative amounts of patterned and selective control available to initiate the walking act; both standing and stride characteristics are influenced by the level of control.

STANCE STABILITY

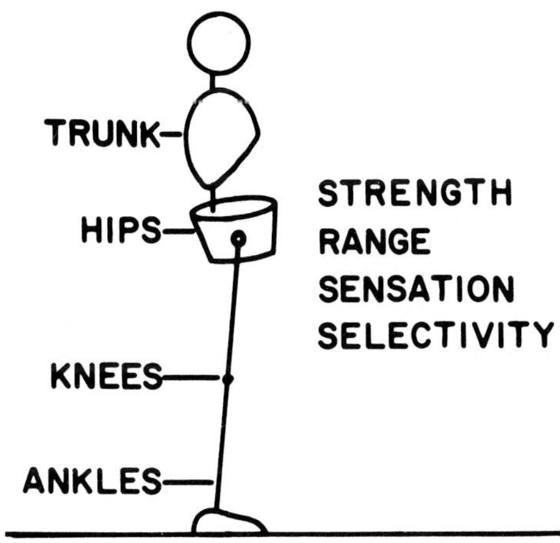

Fig. 5.

Stationary Standing Posture

The posture assumed during quiet standing will give an idea of the alignment available to the patient during walking. Stability is automatic when the feet are flat on the floor, the knees and hips are slightly hyperextended, and the trunk is erect and centered over the feet (Fig. 5). Deviations from this alignment, due to deformity or muscle imbalance, indicate a need for active support of the mal-aligned joints. In addition, there must be compensatory adaptations of the adjacent segments if the patient is to stand independently. Regardless of individual joint postures, the trunk must be 'centered' over the supporting base offered by the feet contacting the floor. Denervation-type weakness is not a characteristic of cerebral palsy, so the stabilization of mal-aligned joints is seldom a problem, although the attainment of compensatory alignment frequently is. When this alignment cannot be accomplished spontaneously, crutches or other types of external support are needed.

The apparent weakness one observes in cerebral palsy most commonly represents failure of the central control mechanism to initiate action at the proper time or to an adequate extent. This failure also leads to strength loss as a result of disuse. An additional cause of weakness is mechanical impairment of the muscle through chronic overstretching by hyperactive antagonists.

Because mal-alignment of one segment influences the stability of the next, the examiner must check each anatomical part individually.

The trunk. The trunk is a large, influential mass, representing 50 per cent of the body's weight. The head and arms each represent another 10 per cent, so a total load of 70 per cent of body weight has to be balanced by the lower extremities (Fig. 6). Normally, movements of the head and trunk are slight, and are directed towards counteracting those at the pelvis. Deformities such as scoliosis transform the erect, well-balanced trunk into an asymmetrical mass and tend to pull the patient off balance (Figs. 7a and b). With 70 per cent of the body's weight involved, this can be an overwhelming problem to extremities which are already under poor control. Loss of alignment also lessens the patient's ability to use his trunk in maneuvers to counterbalance hip, knee, or ankle alignment difficulties.

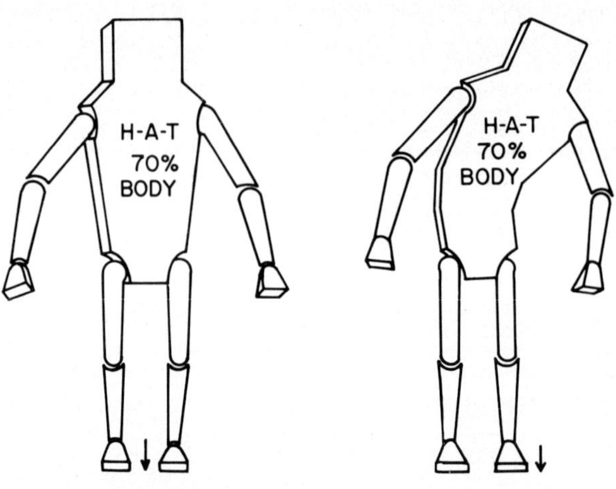

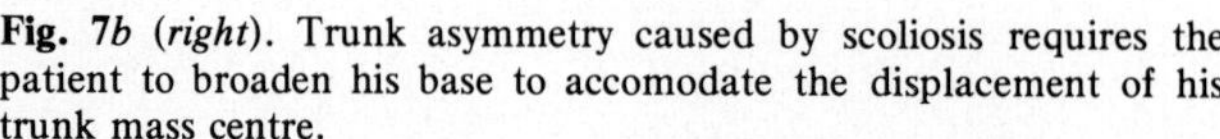

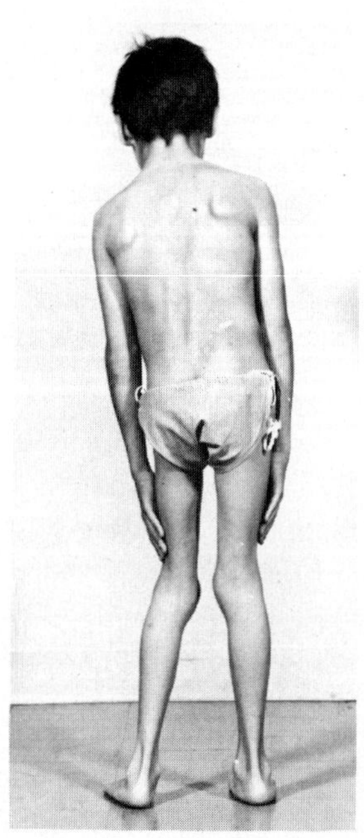

Fig. 6. (*above left*). The head, arms and trunk (H.A.T.) comprise a heavy mass to be carried by the lower extremities.

Fig. 7a (*above right*). Asymmetrical trunk. The body mass now falls outside the base, and cannot be supported unless the patient can adapt his base.

Fig. 7b (*right*). Trunk asymmetry caused by scoliosis requires the patient to broaden his base to accomodate the displacement of his trunk mass centre.

The hips. Spastic or contractural hip flexion deformity prevents the patient aligning his trunk over his feet, unless there is adequate lordosis or the knees are flexed (Fig. 8). As hypermobility of the lumbar spine is not a characteristic of the cerebral palsied child, lordotic substitution, though it occurs, is usually limited. Hence, if by operation one corrects a patient's excessive knee flexion without also lessening his hip flexion, the trunk will lie anterior to its support, and crutches will be needed post-operatively, even though the child was independent before (Fig. 9). Fixed adduction and abduction at the hip create similar lateral alignment problems.

The knees both reflect and dictate the posture of the hips and ankles during stance. In the erect posture, flexion at the knee so tilts the femur that the hip will also be flexed. The converse also occurs if the hip moves freely into extension, but spasticity of the hip flexors reflects the postural change to the trunk. As the hip and knee represent the two ends of a common bone (the femur) one must treat these two joints as a functional couple, always planning for them together. This relationship is enhanced by the demand of the erect posture (Fig. 10).

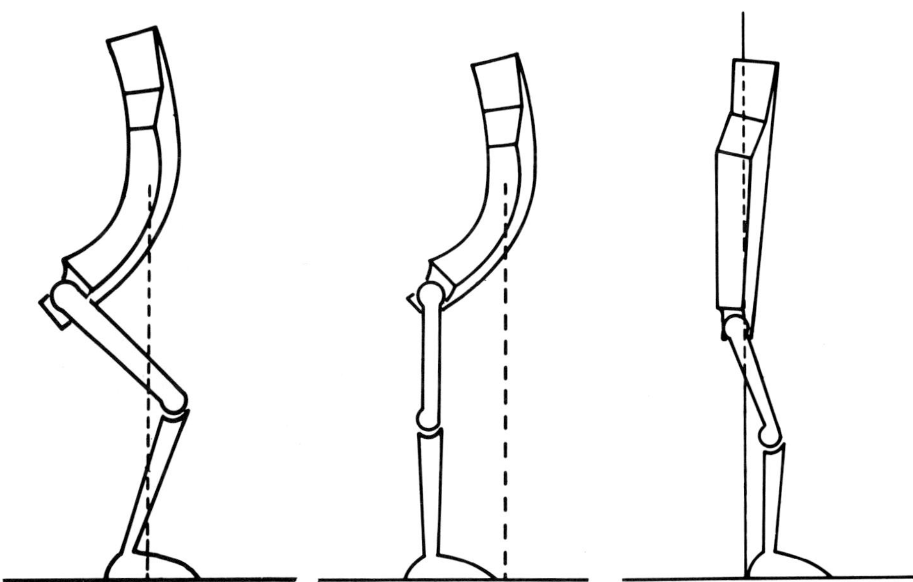

Fig. 8 (*left*). Postural balance achieved with fixed hip flexion by lordosis and knee flexion. (From Perry 1974.)

Fig. 9 (*centre*). The patient with fixed hip flexion loses postural balance when the knees are independently extended.

Fig. 10 (*right*). Inter-related postures adopted by hip and knee in order to maintain erect posture. To maintain balance, the hip and knee must flex the same amount, as they represent opposite ends of the same bone.

A second functional couple is formed by the knee and ankle (Saunders *et al.* 1953). If the knee is flexed, either the ankle must dorsiflex a comparable amount or the patient is obliged to stand on his 'toes' (Fig. 11). In the latter situation, attempts to correct toe-stance without paying attention to the knee can lead to surgical over-lengthening of the Achilles tendon (Fig. 12). A significant cause of complications following Achilles tendon lengthening is the nature of the ankle joint. There is great intrinsic stability when the ankle is in plantar flexion. The weight of the patient's body mass directed through a posteriorly angled tibia is an added restraint to ankle movement, so no extrinsic force is needed to lock the joint when the patient is standing with his ankles plantar flexed. However, once travel is initiated, the ankle passes through its full range of motion with utmost ease (Klevin 1970). As the tibia advances across the ankle, the locking mechanism of body weight is quickly lost. Considerable muscle force is now required to restrain the tibia from falling forwards (Fig. 12). In the absence of stability at the ankle, the knee also becomes more difficult to lock, as its inferior segment (the tibia) is mobile (Fig. 13).

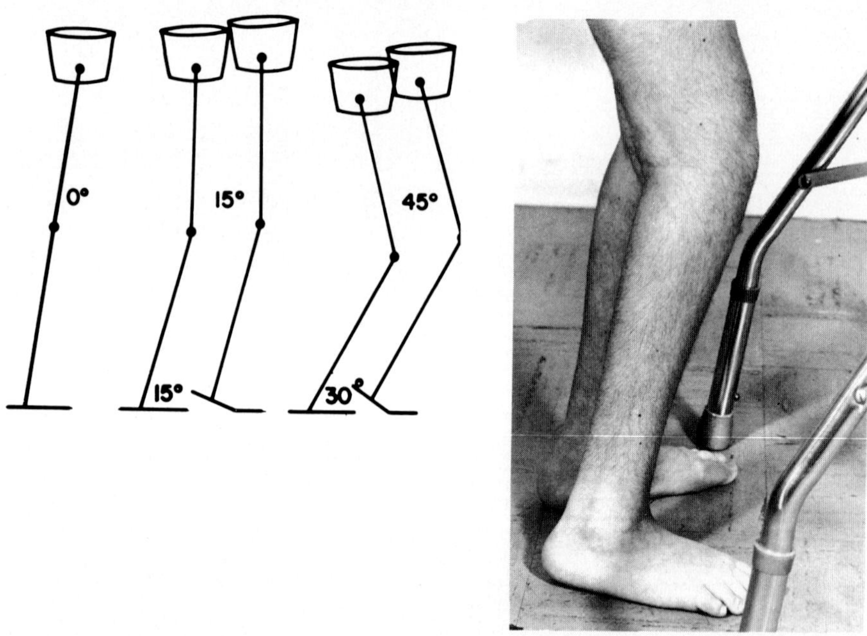

Fig. 11. (*left*). Inter-related postures of knee and ankle, necessary if the trunk is to be balanced over the flat foot. When the ankle cannot dorsiflex sufficiently to compensate for the knee flexion, the patient is obliged to adapt by raising the heel and standing on his 'toes' (from Perry 1974).

Fig. 12. (*right*). Operation to get the foot flat on the floor has resulted in over-lengthening of the tendo achillis, because the influence of knee flexion was not appreciated.

With dependence on primitive patterning for locomotion, the cerebral palsied patient cannot modify his plantar flexor force according to the situation. A response that is adequate in slight plantar flexion will be insufficient to control the tibia as it moves forward over the highly mobile ankle joint. The resulting posture is dorsiflexion of the foot at the ankle, with the tendo achillis stretched to its maximum length and a corresponding degree of knee flexion to keep the patient erect.

Functional coupling between ankle plantar flexion and knee hyperextension is well known, but the need for it is seldom appreciated. Just 15 degrees of plantar flexion of the ankle places the trunk behind the supporting foot (Fig. 14a), unless there is hyperextension at the knee (Fig. 14b), flexion at the hip (Fig. 14c), or a two-inch heel on the shoe. Only with an appropriate mixture of these compensatory measures can the patient stand erect. A co-existing knee flexion of a mere 15 degrees so exaggerates the posterior position of the trunk, that not even 45 degrees of hip flexion or a three-inch heel will restore trunk-foot alignment. Independent standing balance is therefore lost.

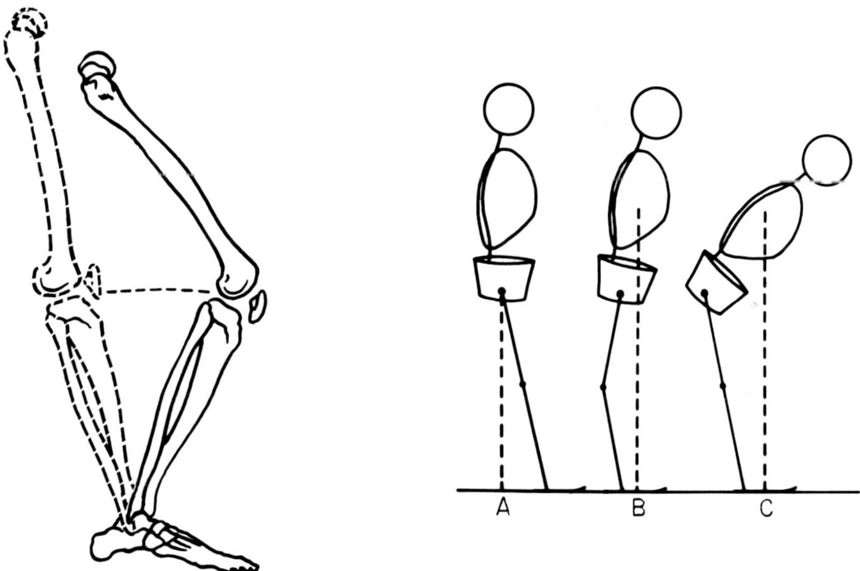

Fig. 13 (*left*). Ankle postures found with a weak soleus or an over-lengthened tendo achillis. With the body weight behind the ankle axis, the ankle is plantar flexed (*left*), but when the body mass is anterior to the ankle axis (*right*), the tibia falls forwards due to the lack of direct muscular control at the ankle. The consequent ankle dorsiflexion causes the knee to flex and leads to gait instability.

Fig. 14 (*right*). The influence on stance of fixed ankle plantar flexion. (A) Without accommodation by the other limb joints, the body mass will be aligned behind the supporting foot. (B) Knee hyper-extension makes it possible for the body mass to lie over the foot. (C) Alignment of the body over the foot can also be achieved by hip flexion, but only if the patient has strong hip extensors; otherwise the patient must support his trunk weight with crutches (from Perry 1974).

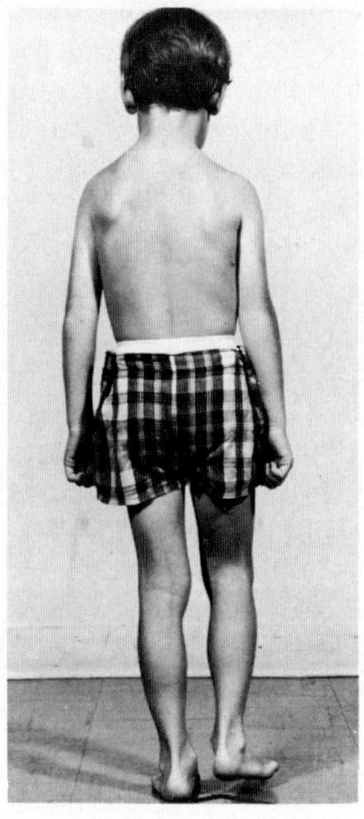 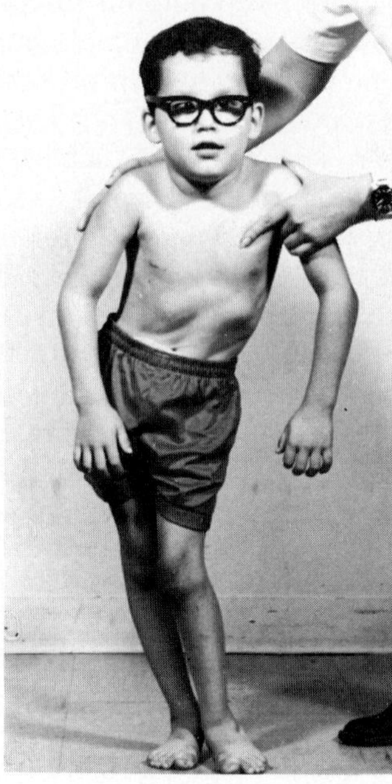

Fig. 15 (*left*). Normal single limb stance. Note that the trunk has shifted to align over the supporting foot. The hip abductors are locking the pelvis at neutral.

Fig. 16 (*right*). Diplegic child with inadequate hip abductors. The trunk falls away from the supporting limb, and the child is unable to compensate for this by adapting his trunk posture.

Standing Stability During Walking

The dynamics of walking present two further challenges to the patient's standing stability. He must be able to support the trunk over only one limb, and the abrupt motion changes which follow floor contact must be controlled.

Supporting the body's weight on one limb requires lateral balance (Perry and Hislop 1967) in addition to the sagittal alignment just discussed. To balance over one foot, the body is shifted about 2 cm towards the supporting limb (Saunders *et al.* 1953), and the hip abductors contract strongly to maintain a level pelvis (Fig. 15). Timely shifting of the body is a function of one's body schema. This is often disturbed with brain damage. The patient lacks an awareness of his body segments, and hence does not account for their weight. If, when attempting to balance over one leg, the patient falls *in toto* towards the unsupported side without trying to catch himself, body image is impaired. This *in toto* falling must be distinguished from a positive Trendelenberg test, which is indicative of weak hip abductor muscles. In the latter case, the unsupported pelvis drops and the trunk falls to that side, but the body as a whole does not. Also the patient promptly moves to catch himself. He is aware of his unsafe plight.

Hip abductors are not a part of the primitive locomotor pattern, and therefore the support they provide is lacking in pattern-dependent patients (Fig. 16). Such patients will exhibit a Trendelenberg drop during single limb support, unless they have sufficient proprioceptive awareness and selective control to compensate by leaning over the supporting limb.

During gait, when the swinging limb makes contact with the floor, its momentum is abruptly interrupted. When contact is made with the heel, the foot acts as a rocker, efficiently perpetuating the forward motion. The tibia continues to advance rapidly, and if this advance is not controlled, it leads to excessive knee flexion and a sense of instability. In patients dependent on primitive locomotor patterns, the advance of the tibia is checked by the patterned activation of the ankle plantar flexors that accompanies knee extension during late swing. However, the advance of the tibia will not be controlled if surgical attempts to provide a 'good' range of dorsiflexion have resulted in over-lengthening of the tendo achillis, as the patient who is dependent upon primitive locomotor patterns cannot selectively increase the action of his plantar flexors to meet this increased demand. If the quadriceps are spastic, they will react and provide the necessary stability. The observed action in this case will be a brief knee flexion thrust and a quick retraction. Attention will be focused on the knee, but the seat of undesired function at the moment of floor contact is the ankle, with its plantar flexors providing insufficient restraint.

Knee stability is no problem when the ankle is held in plantar flexion by strong triceps surae, though advancement of the body is seriously curtailed. This latter problem will be covered in the discussion on stride length. When muscle action is stereotyped, correction of equinus must be a compromise between the need for stance stability and the need for adequate stride length.

Gait Characteristics

Because the requirements for postural stability and stepping ahead vary during the course of a stride, investigators have defined several phases of action. The basic ones are 'stance' and 'swing'. These terms are used to distinguish between the limb's weight-bearing period and its interval of free advancement. Further sub-divisions have been introduced to specify the different events occurring within these broad categories. The terminology customarily used to describe normal function has been modified to accommodate the variation seen in paralytic gait. The sub-phases are as follows: floor contact (heel-strike), contact response, mid-stance, terminal stance ('push-off'), pre-swing (follow-up of 'push-off'), 'pick-up' (early swing) and 'reach' (late swing).

Floor contact describes the phase during which a previously freely swinging limb becomes a stable weight-bearing member. Mid-stance is that interval during which the trunk advances over a stationary foot. Terminal stance refers to the subsequent period when the foot alters its position on the floor. Pre-swing refers to the moment when the knee flexes in preparation for 'pick-up'. 'Pick-up' describes the initial mechanics of advancing the unloaded limb, while 'reach' identifies the motion complex of gaining the final length of stride.

Stride Length

The distance one spans with each stride is generally attributed solely to the efficiency of the swinging limb. Such is not the case. Sixty per cent of the stride length is achieved only as a result of postural modifications by the stance limb. Thus the actions of both limbs must be considered when assessing this aspect of gait.

Floor Contact and Contact Response (Fig. 17)

Trunk advancement is uninterrupted when floor contact is made with the heel, as the forward motion is perpetuated by a rocker-like response in the foot and knee. The normal response to heel contact is a rapid but controlled drop to a flat foot position accompanied by moderate advancement of the tibia.

Normal heel strike is dependent, not only on the ankle being at 90 degrees, but also on full knee extension and on hip flexion of 30 degrees. Failure to achieve any of these three positions causes the toe to approach the floor. The result is either a flat foot or toe contact, depending on the degree of position loss.

In cerebral palsy, a flexed knee and equinus ankle are commonly seen. When the two occur together, the floor contact is made with the toe. Bracing of the ankle to restore the 90 degree posture converts this contact to a flat foot alignment, but does not give heel strike. Only by also restoring full knee extension will the latter be accomplished.

When the toe contact is due to sustained ankle plantar flexion (active or contractural) the effect of weight-bearing is to produce a backwards thrust of the tibia as body weight pushes the whole foot to the floor. This prevents the limb from advancing—in fact, its course of motion is reversed. Trunk advancement is correspondingly halted momentarily. Toe contact also creates a rapid stretch on the tense plantar flexor causing increased spasticity.

If the foot is in such severe equinus that weight is borne only on the most anterior area of the metatarsal heads, the foot serves as a small rocker and forward momentum is not interrupted.

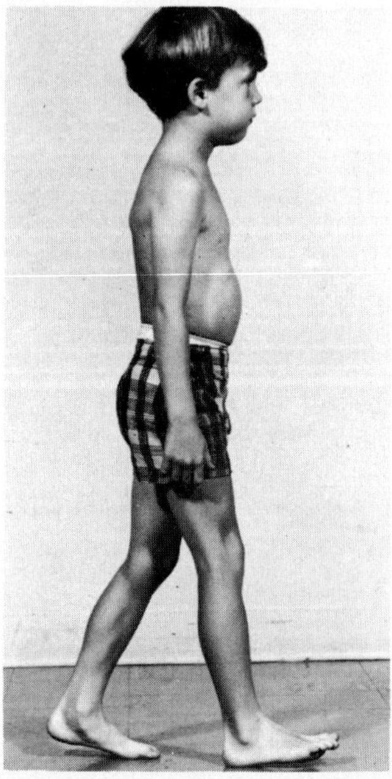

Fig. 17. Initial contact and contact response. Note heel strike and partial drop of foot to flat foot posture.

Mid-stance (Fig. 18)

During this single support period, the foot is stationary and is normally flat on the floor. Advancement of the trunk over this stationary foot is continued by momentum and as a result the ankle is dorsiflexed. Progression from an original 15 degrees of plantar flexion to about 10 degrees of dorsiflexion (at which point the heel rises) is gradual and is under the control of the soleus. Both this muscle and the gastrocnemius which joins it a bit later, undergo a yielding contraction, as they restrain the tibia from advancing too fast, yet do not restrain it completely (Sutherland 1966).

Such graduated muscle action is not available to the patient dependent on primitive locomotor patterns and subject to vestibular extensor tone and spasticity. Instead, the plantar flexor muscles remain strongly contracted at one position, thereby excessively restraining the tibia and perpetuating the plantar flexion posture at the ankle. The momentum that continues to carry the trunk forward creates a hyper-extension thrust on the knee. If the knee does not yield, the force is reflected upwards to the hip, causing it to flex. Stride length at this moment is limited to the amount of advancement permitted at the ankle, knee and hip. The effect is visualized as a short swing by the other limb. If the hip and knee yield sufficiently to place body weight over the most anterior portions of the forefoot, a rocker is created that lets the trunk advance smoothly. However, lack of terminal stance, hip extension or knee flexion severely limits advancement of the trunk, and the contralateral swing is shortened. If the mechanism causing sustained plantar flexion is spasticity superimposed on selective control, tendo achillis lengthening is an effective way of gaining ankle mobility during mid-stance. The stretch response is thereby avoided. If patterned muscle action is prominent, however, the post-surgical gain will be less evident, as the patient will still lack the ability to graduate his muscle action.

In patients with soleus overactivity (patterned or spastic), the need to place the trunk ahead of the supporting foot as one walks leads to progressive genu recurvatum. The young child with his rapidly growing tissues is, of course, most susceptible.

A weak soleus leads to a flexed knee stance and a reduction in stride length. The cause may be either poor spontaneous activity or excessive surgical tendo achillis lengthening. Lacking soleus restraint the tibia falls forward in response to the foot contacting the floor. As the femur and trunk are advancing less rapidly, knee flexion results. The loss in stride length corresponds to the failure of the trunk to advance beyond the flexed knee.

Terminal Stance (Fig. 19)

This phase of gait is the final period of single support. In normal gait, the onset of 'terminal stance' is when the heel rises from the floor as the trunk passes over the toe. With strong triceps surae action stabilizing the ankle at neutral, body weight is progressively transferred to more anterior parts of the forefoot. By the end of this phase, the trunk has moved well ahead of the foot, so increasing the length of the stride by about 20 per cent. Because during terminal stance there is increased pressure against the floor followed by rapid plantar flexion of the ankle, this was initially called 'push-off'. More recent analysis denies any actual push. Instead, the foot action during this final period of single support should be considered as a rocker action to further advance the trunk.

The cerebral palsied patient is denied this rocker action by his fixed plantar flexion. The posteriorly aligned tibia and the foot become one lever, which is too long to roll over unless forward momentum is sufficient to produce the necessary marked elevation of the trunk. Trunk advancement is therefore curtailed. In this situation, the knee tends to lock and the foot is prevented from being lifted until weight has been transferred to the other foot (Fig. 20).

Weak plantar flexor muscles deny the patinet sufficient ankle stability for heel rise. Hence a position characteristic of terminal stance is lacking. Instead the limb is lifted *in toto* after weight is on the other foot, with a corresponding loss in stride length and momentum.

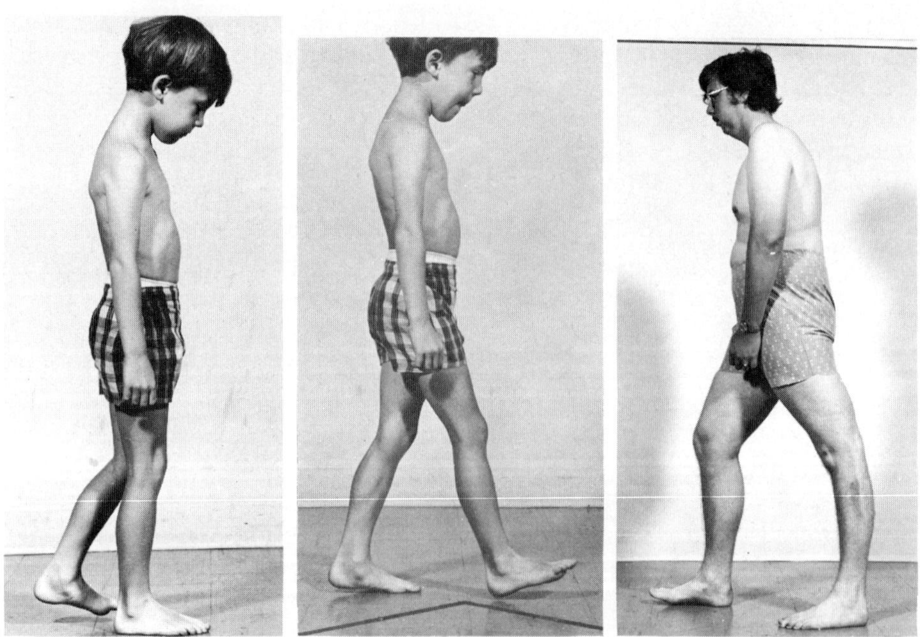

Fig. 18 (*left*). Mid stance. The body is balanced over the supporting foot. The ankle is in slight dorsiflexion (5 to 10 degrees).

Fig. 19 (*centre*). Terminal stance or 'push off' (more appropriately called 'roll-off'). The heel rises (left foot) and the body weight moves forward onto the forefoot. Note that the other foot is not yet on the ground.

Fig. 20 (*right*). Head injury patient with a spastic hemiplegia lacking the roll off (push off) of terminal stance. His hyperextended ankle prevents weight transfer of the forefoot.

Pre-Swing (Fig. 21)

This is an interval of double support during which the trailing limb maintains floor contact while the leading limb is accepting body weight. Of prime importance is the 35 to 40 degrees of knee flexion that occurs during the final moments of toe contact. It prepares the limb for the further knee flexion needed for easy toe clearance during early swing. The mechanism for the rapid knee flexion seems to be the considerable forward alignment of the trunk mass unlocking the previous extensor alignment. An additional factor may by abrupt unloading of the previously taut gastrocnemius, as there is an associated ankle plantar flexion and virtual cessation of weight-bearing, and continued floor contact and knee stability are maintained by slight quadriceps activity.

Like the terminal stance, the pre-swing phase is denied to the cerebral palsied patient. Slight rather than full tension of the quadriceps is not available with patterned action. Also the approach into flexion creates a stretch on tense muscle, inducing a spastic response that adds further tension. Hence an extended, rather than flexed knee is the final posture. This does not occur if knee flexion and ankle plantar flexion are so severe that weight is borne only on the more anterior part of the forefoot.

Swing

With body weight entirely on the other limb, the trailing extremity is free to swing forward for the next stride. Differences in knee motion divide the swing phase into two separate tasks: 'pick-up' and 'reach'.

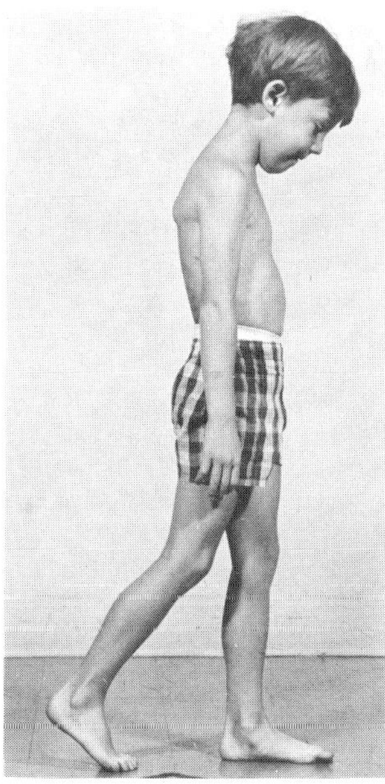

Fig. 21. Pre-swing. The knee is abruptly flexed approximately 35 degrees in preparation for swing.

Initial Swing ('pick-up') (Fig. 22)

'Toe-off' is the common designation for the onset of the swing phase of the gait. The dominant action at this time is knee flexion. The postural relationship between the limb and the trunk at the end of stance places the limb behind the body with the toe pointing down, *i.e.* there is a natural equinus. The knee is in about 35 degrees of flexion as a result of the pre-swing stance action. To avoid dragging the toe while the limb advances, the knee must flex an additional 35 degrees (Murray 1964). The hip need flex only half this amount. Following a brief continuation of the plantar flexion rebound seen during the last moments of stance, the ankle progressively dorsiflexes. By the time the foot passes the supporting limb, the previous position of 20 degrees plantar flexion has been recovered (Fig. 23).

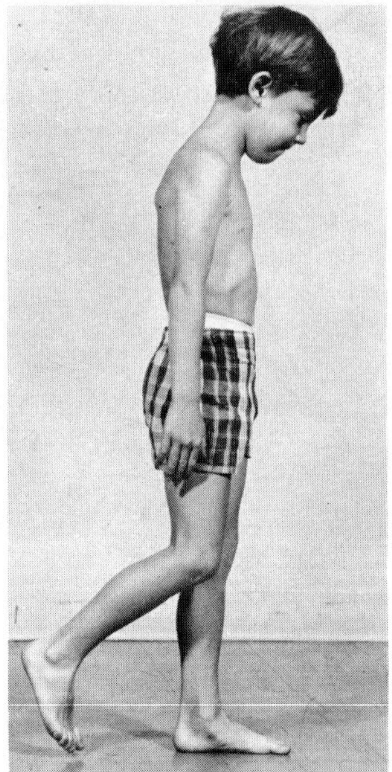 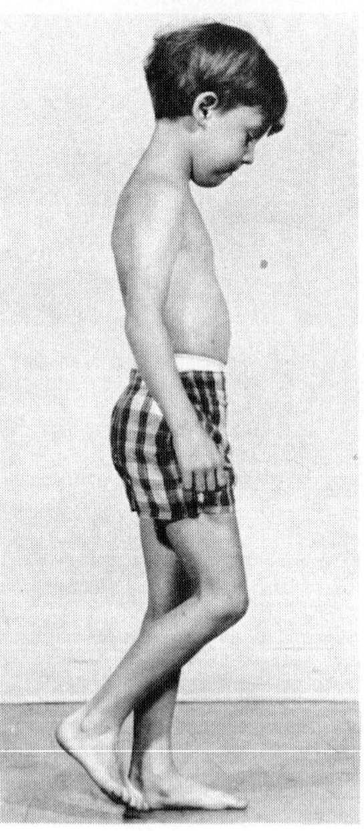

Fig. 22 (*left*). Initial swing. The key action during this phase is knee flexion to keep the toes clear of the ground. The ankle is in approximately 15 degrees of plantar flexion, so knee rather than ankle motion is the key action at this time.

Fig. 23 (*right*). End of initial swing. Knee flexion is maintained, and the foot has recovered its dorsiflexed posture.

In cerebral palsy, toe clearance is difficult to achieve, and the limb appears stiff. The pre-swing knee flexion of terminal stance is lacking. In fact, because at the end of 'stance' the hip is in extension, knee flexion at this time is likely to provoke a spastic re-action of the quadriceps and, in particular, of the rectus femoris (Fig. 24). In patterned gait, dependence on the flexor withdrawal reflex means that flexion of the knee is always accompanied by roughly an equal amount of hip flexion. Yet for normal gait the knee should proceed twice as fast. One advantage of the patterned gait is that knee flexion is accompanied by simultaneous dorsiflexion of the foot. A second advantage is the relative shortness of the stride, which lessens the obstacles created by the trailing position. The advantages thus partly balance the disadvantages, and permit minimal toe clearance, but with a stiff-looking limb.

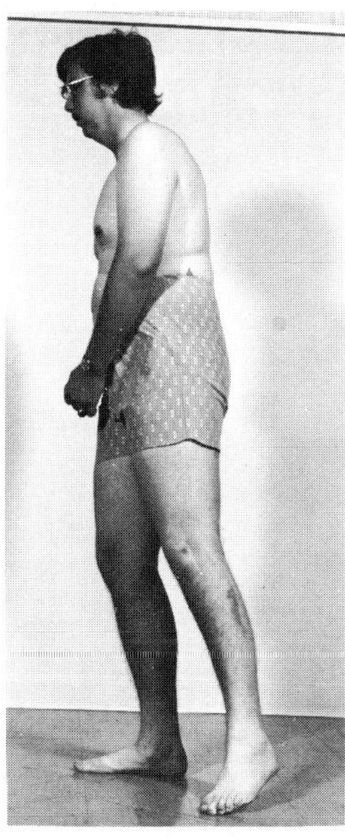

Fig. 24. This patient with traumatic hemiplegia lacks knee flexion. As a result he drags his toe during initial swing.

Terminal Swing (Reach) (Fig. 19)

With the foot now ahead of the body, the need for knee flexion to avoid a dragging toe no longer exists. Now the objective is to extend the knee for maximum stride length. During the first part of this knee extension period, the hip and ankle continue to flex, until hip flexion of 30 degrees and neutral ankle alignment are attained. These positions are then maintained, while the knee continues to extend during the rest of the reach phase.

Knee extension is primarily a passive pendulum-like motion. After 'pick-up' the knee flexors (short biceps and gracilis) relax and the limb swings forward (Inman 1953).

The functional requirements for an effective 'reach' seem simple, but have proved to be neurologically complex. Only the patient with unfettered selective control can fully accomplish the necessary mixture of motions—the cerebral palsied patient with his spasticity and dependence on primitive locomotor patterns cannot.

Poor reach due to incomplete knee extension may be caused by hamstring spasticity. Delay in the relaxation of the knee flexors following 'pick-up' subjects them to the pendulum-like swing of the shank (tibia). These hypersensitive muscles are stretched, leading to a spastic restraint of knee extension.

Dependence on patterned locomotor control permits use of the flexor or extensor limb synergies, but not a mixture of the two. Thus, while the hip is held in flexion, the knee automatically flexes an equal amount. The result is a vertical shank (tibia), with foot parallel to the floor and a short stride. Efforts to extend the knee initiate the extensor synergy, and hip flexion is lost. This causes general retraction of the limb. Many cerebral palsied patients have some degree of selective control and are able to partially escape the restraints of purely patterned gait.

Foot posture is similarly influenced by patterned action. As the knee is extended to reach forward, the triceps surae is also activated, causing a plantar flexion at the ankle. A combination of increasing ankle flexion, a loss of hip flexion and incomplete knee extension, results in a 'toe-down' foot position. The anterior tibialis commonly exhibits a spastic response which is detectable on electromyography but is too weak to hold up the foot. It must be recalled that the gastrosoleus muscle mass is five times greater than that of the anterior tibialis, so the odds favor an equinus posture.

Because of the cerebral palsied patient's limited ability to modify his responses, correction of postural irregularities must be planned so as not to deprive him of his ability to move. The basic requirements during standing are a stable base, centering of the trunk over this base (the feet), and sufficient latitude in alignment for the patient to be able to move without falling. To take a step he must be able to pick up the limb sufficiently to clear his toe and to advance it a useful amount.

Management of cerebral palsy gait is a compromise between the need for standing stability and the need to be able to take a step. The more a patient is dependent on patterned control for walking, the less opportunity therapists and surgeons have to improve his gait.

REFERENCES

Close, J. R. (1964) *Motor Function in the Lower Extremity.* Springfield, Ill.: C. C. Thomas.

Elliot, H. C. (1969). *Textbook of Neuroanatomy, 2nd edn.* Philadelphia: J. B. Lippincott.

Giovan, P., Perry, J., Hoffer, N. (1974) 'EMG analysis of the triceps surae action in cerebral palsy hemiplegia.' (*in Preparation.*)

Inman, V. T. (1953) *The Patterns of Muscular Activity in the Lower Extremity During Walking. Prosthetic Devices Report. Series II, Issue 25.* University of California.

Klevin, D. K. (1970) *The Ankle Joint; An Anatomical and Mechanical Study Using Amputated Specimens.* Thesis.

Krieg, W. J. S. (1945) *Functional Neuroanatomy.* Philadelphia: Blakiston.

Murray, M. P. (1964) 'Walking patterns of normal men.' *Journal of Bone and Joint Surgery, 46A,* 335.

Perry, J., Hislop, H. (1967) *Principles of Lower Extremity Bracing.* New York: American Physical Therapy Association.

Saunders, J. B. de C. M., Inman, V. T., Eberhart, H. D. (1953) 'The major determinants in normal and pathological gait.' *Journal of Bone and Joint Surgery, 35A,* 543.

Sutherland, D. H. (1966) 'An electromyographic study of the plantar flexors of the ankle in normal walking on the level.' *Journal of Bone and Joint Surgery, 48A,* 66.

—— Schottstaedt, E. R., Larsen, L. I. (1969) 'Clinical and electromyographic study of seven spastic children with internal rotation gait.' *Journal of Bone and Joint Surgery, 51A,* 1070.

The Non-operative Aspects of Orthopaedic Management of Cerebral Palsy

SAMUEL B.THOMPSON

The rôle of the orthopaedic surgeon in the non-operative management of the cerebral palsied child varies greatly in different communities. In the British Isles and urban areas of the United States and Canada, some other member of the management team is likely to have the rôle of primary physician; on the other hand, in more sparsely populated areas of the United States, the orthopaedic surgeon may very well assume the primary rôle, with the other members of the management team functioning as consultants. The author's rôle has been that of an orthopaedic surgeon functioning as the primary physician in the management of the cerebral palsied in an area where treatment centers are few and far between, and where difficulties of transportation make the direct application of treatment through treatment centers impracticable in many instances. It is understandable that this chapter will be colored by this experience.

During infancy and the pre-school years, the developmental program of going through the stages of changing lying postures, crawling, knee standing, sitting, assisted walking, ambulation using aids and devices, inhibition of persistent primitive reflexes and facilitation of the development of righting reflexes is the policy followed if a center is available (Bobath and Bobath 1957). The implementation of this program may be carried out by the various members of the management team, as described in other sections of this book (Deaver 1953, Knott and Voss 1956, Bobath and Bobath 1957).

If, as has been the case with most of the patients the author has treated over the past 25 years, such a center is not available, some variant of this management program must be developed. The alternative that the author has followed has been to have the child and parent attend for sessions with the physical therapist, the occupational therapist, and, as the child gets a little older, the speech therapist. At these meetings, the parent, usually the mother, is taught the specific techniques of handling the child in the home, in such a manner as to bring about the desired progress of the child through the various developmental stages.

This instruction is reinforced by visits to the home by a public health nurse, by return visits to outpatient clinics held in or near the individual's community, or by the child being brought to the doctor's office. Such return visits to the orthopaedist will usually take place once every three to four months. At these visits, the orthopaedist will normally consult directly with the other members of the team, but in the absence of a centrally located team, this consultation may be conducted over the telephone and by written correspondence. Particular attention is given to analysis of the functional state attained by the child, and to the range of motion of the joints affected by the spasticity or excessive tone. Physical and X-ray examinations are carried out, to detect early joint contractures and such complications as subluxation or dislocation of the hips.

One of the pitfalls of having the cerebral palsied patient and his parent seen by each member of the team separately is that, after receiving separate detailed instructions in a number of different aspects of the child's care, the mother (or mother substitute) may find herself faced with a program which is too demanding and time-consuming for her to carry out satisfactorily. It would seem, therefore, that an important aspect of the non-operative management of these children is the co-ordination of the various prescribed procedures in such a manner as to allow the mother to carry out her physical therapy, occupational therapy and speech therapy techniques simultaneously, and to make the routine one which can be somewhat akin to play for the child. If this is done, it is to be hoped that neither the mother nor the child will become so fatigued that the program is abandonded.

Day or night bracing, if used, is rarely begun until the infancy stage is passed. Attempts should be made to free a patient from bracing before school age is reached. The author's own thinking as regards the use of braces has gradually changed over the past 25 years. With greater experience he has found it necessary to prescribe fewer and fewer braces, and those that have been prescribed have been kept on for shorter and shorter periods of time.

Where the attainment of some functional self-sufficiency can reasonably be expected, every effort is made to remove a child's braces by the time he starts school. To achieve this aim, particular emphasis is placed on physical and occupational therapy, and care is taken to ensure that surgical intervention is early enough to have the child free of encumbering devices by the time he reaches school age.

The setting of realistic goals for each child is of paramount importance and becomes progressively even more important as the child goes through the pre-school program.

In general, it is anticipated that the hemiplegic, whose mental abilities are good and who has either no seizures or controlled seizures, will go to into the public school system rather than into classes for the orthopaedically handicapped or into special education classes. Every effort is concentrated on teaching him the activities of daily living (Deaver 1953), so that, in spite of the involved upper and lower extremities, he will be able to compete in the non-handicapped environment in a satisfactory manner. This brings the orthopaedist, if he is the primary physician, into close collaboration with the regular classroom teachers in the public school system, and, particularly, with those in the school departments of physical education.

The diplegic patient who becomes ambulatory without the use of external devices may make it into the regular classroom, but may have to be placed in a class for the orthopaedically handicapped. Every effort is made to integrate these classes with the school system as a whole, so the child can acquire experience of functioning with the non-handicapped. As with the hemiplegic, emphasis is placed on the activities of daily living (Deaver 1953).

Totally involved patients, including those with spastic quadriplegia, athetosis and other types of dyskinesia, will usually be educated in classes for the orthopaedically handicapped, or, if their mental ability is sufficiently poor, in special education classes. Again, if the orthopaedist is functioning as the primary physician, he must liase with those who are responsible for the child's education. Physical, occupational and speech therapy will be continued, with the emphasis placed on functional activities. These programs should not, in the author's opinion, be so time-consuming that they interfere with the child's academic education. The emphasis should be on his schooling, with his physical rehabilitation being scheduled in such a manner as not to interfere with such schooling.

The adolescent patient presents additional problems of management. Careful psychological and vocational counselling are necessary to guide the patient through the stormy period of transition from childhood to adult life. Again it is essential to establish realistic goals. Particularly careful scrutiny from the orthopaedic standpoint is necessary at this time, as some patients lose range of motion and functional ability. It may be necessary to decide that continued attempts at independent ambulation are impractical, and that the individual's best interests will be served by making him more mobile by the use of a wheelchair.

Surgical procedures may be considered during adolescence (a) for correction of recurrent deformities, (b) as the last of a series of procedures for establishing optimal function of an extremity, or (c) as an aid to those patients who have, for various reasons, been neglected during the earlier stages of their development.

Bracing

The prescription of bracing, and the management of the child while wearing and using braces, traditionally come into the sphere of the orthopaedic surgeon. As mentioned above, the author has tended to use braces less and less frequently, but has not abandoned their use completely, and still finds them quite useful in many instances on an empirical basis. This empiricism is practised primarily in the ordering of specific braces, orthoses or other aids to meet the specific needs of an individual patient. It is not the author's feeling that a specific diagnosis warrants a specific brace; rather, he feels that a brace may be indicated in an individual case, where, after a period of observation and functional analysis, the orthopaedic surgeon, in collaboration with other members of the team (including the physical and occupational therapist), decides that it may be beneficial.

Day Braces

The full control brace (Fig. 1) (Phelps 1953)—consisting of double upright long-leg braces attached to a pelvic band with back uprights and a high thoracic band, and including 90 degree stop ankles, slip lock knees with finger springs, knee caps and slip lock hip joints which lock both in the straight position and in 90 degrees of flexion—was a rather common prescription 25 years ago. Developmental measures of inhibition of primitive reflexes, facilitation of righting reflexes, development of synergistic activity (Rood 1954, Knott and Voss 1956, Bobath and Bobath 1957), and the early use of surgery in and about the hips, knees and ankles, have eliminated the need for such braces in a number of patients, and freed others earlier than in the past.

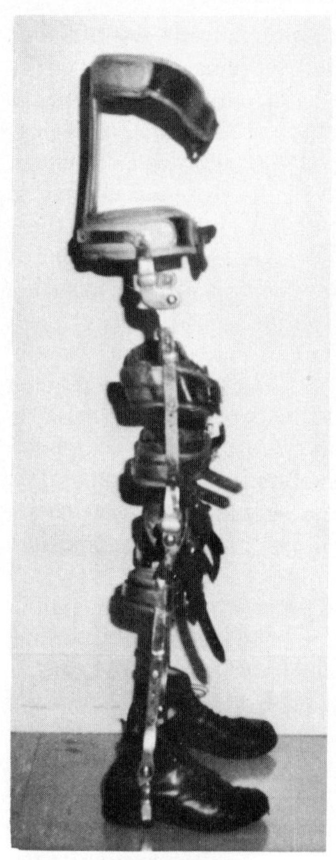
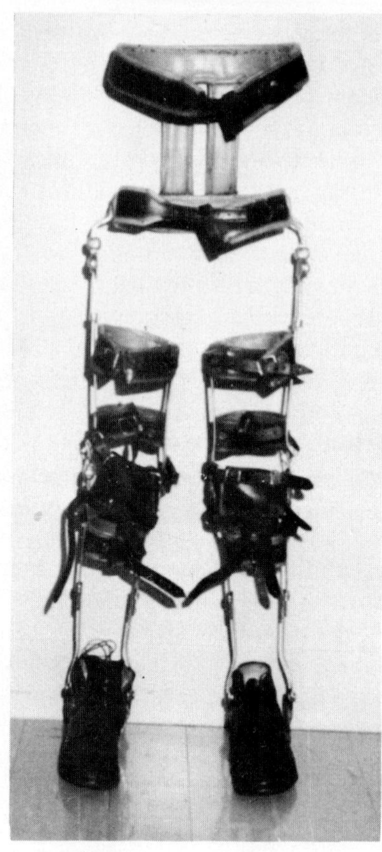

Figs. 1*a* **and** *b*. Full control brace. Anterior and lateral views.

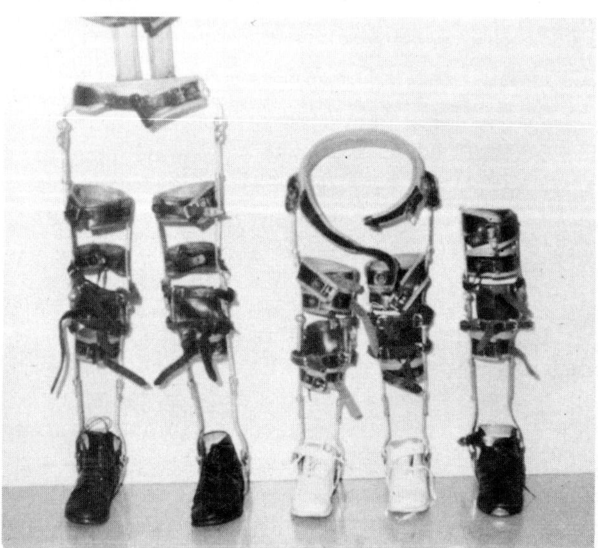

Fig. 2. Progressive removal of parts of the brace, following the Deaver technique.

The Deaver (1953) technique of starting with the full control brace and pulling it off, piece by piece, from the top downwards, as the child's function improves at each level, may be helpful in some patients who are not responding to the more commonly employed techniques; it may also be useful in the post-operative rehabilitation of muscles whose strength and direction of pull have been altered (Fig. 2).

If the aim of the brace is to control flexion and extension of the hips, it seems reasonable that the upright bars and thoracic bands should be added to the pelvic band, in order to provide a longer lever arm. If the pelvic band is being used for control of rotation and adduction at the hip joints, the upright bars are not necessary. Garrett *et al.* (1966) have used the pelvic band and thigh cuffs alone to prevent hip adduction, while allowing free abduction and free flexion and extension.

Some totally involved patients develop an abduction deformity of one hip and an adduction deformity of the other (the 'windblown' hip), but still have enough balance control to be ambulatory with assistance and devices. These deformities may be controlled by using a trolley device placed on the inside upright thigh pieces of the braces, so that rolling friction is applied against each abnormal thrust (Thompson 1957) (Fig. 3). This trolley device is necessary only if the forces are so great that the bars of the braces are bent, or the hip rivets will not hold against the force.

It is felt that in most instances, particularly in patients with spastic involvement, the need for pelvic bands and hip locks may be eliminated surgically by the time school-age is reached. Occasionally, such a brace may still by used as an adjunct to the activities of daily living. There are patients who, with the use of such a brace, can be moved from bed to chair and from chair to desk, and ambulated with assistance across the room, whereas without it they would require to be lifted. In such instances, the brace may be prescribed for the child, in order to avoid having to prescribe a brace for the mother's back later.

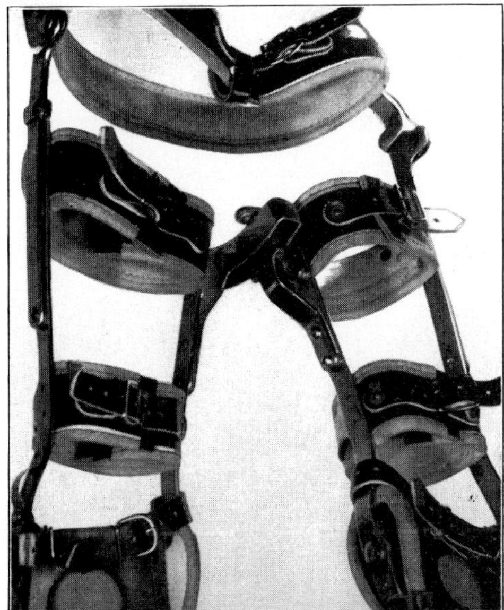
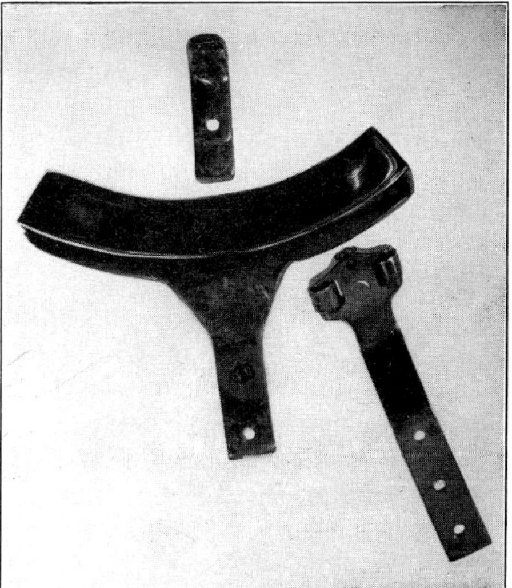

Fig. 3. The trolley device added to control braces for adduction of one hip and abduction of the other.

The use of locked knees to overcome the crouch position assumed by some diplegics is not always effective, but will be used occasionally, largely at the express request of the physical therapist, as an adjunct to training.

The short leg brace to control equinus, complete with appropriately placed T-straps to control varus or valgus, has been a useful functional aid to many patients, and has allowed the therapist to concentrate more attention on the control of knee and hip function. It may be that a total contact orthosis will prove to be a better device for this purpose in the future, since it is lighter, cleaner, easier to apply, and meets less psychological objection on the part of both patient and parent. Such an orthosis may well prove useful in overcoming genu recurvatum (Rosenthal *et al.* 1973). The brace the author uses consists of a double upright brace with a 90 degree stop, an outside T-strap for correcting a varus tendency of the foot, and an inside T-strap for correcting a valgus tendency (Fig. 4).

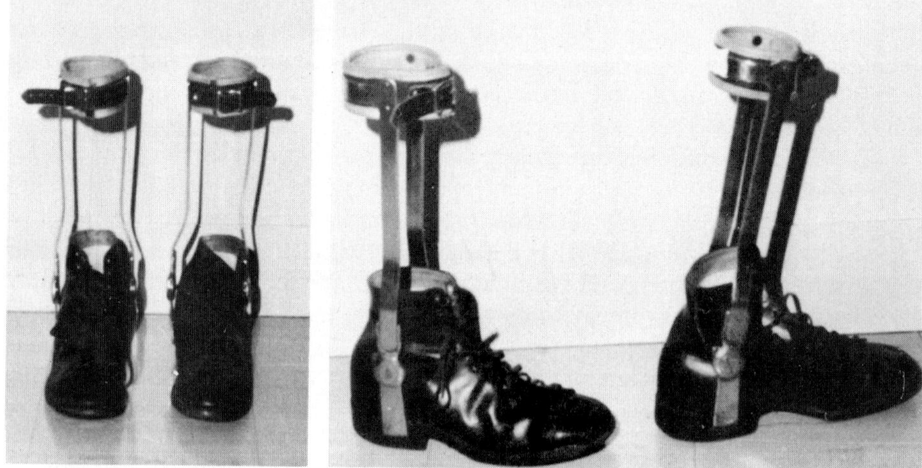

Fig. 4. Short leg, double upright, 90 degree stop brace.

In the smaller child, the simple round bar brace, fixed in caliper fashion into the heel of the shoe, with the motion occurring at the heel rather than at the ankle joint, has been used. There are of course, valid biomechanical objections to the use of this device if the patient is to do much walking.

Night Bracing

The brace used most frequently by the author is the short leg night brace for the spastic hemiplegic (Fig. 5). This is a single round bar brace with a calf cuff and a caliper insertion at the outside or the inside of the heel, according to whether the tendency is to equinovalgus or to equinovarus; a metal plate is attached to the sole of the shoe and extends to the tips of the toes. As long as the bar is straight, the foot is held at a right angle, and the T-strap on the opposite side from the bar can be adjusted to control the valgus or varus deformity. With the use of bending irons, the bar can be bent, as desired, into more dorsiflexion or plantar flexion, or into more varus or valgus, which makes this a simple tool for holding desired positions at night. The author has, even in varus feet, put the bar on the outside of the leg rather than the inside, to prevent discomfort caused by the bar hitting the other leg in bed. In such cases, the use of bending irons makes it possible for the foot to be held in valgus even though the bar is on the outside, and the need for the T-strap is eliminated.

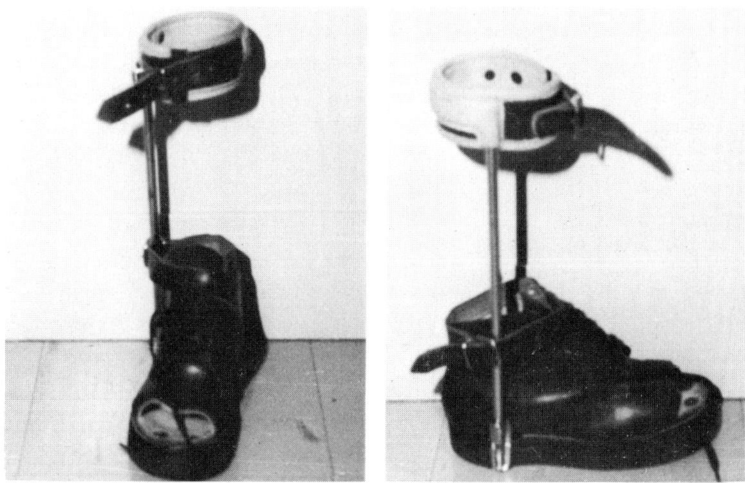

Figs. 5a and b. The single short upright round bar caliper brace for night use.

The use of plaster of paris moulds bandaged in place at night is reported as being highly effective. The total contact orthosis is a development which may be an improvement over the standard night brace.

A bar from one shoe to the other has been added to bilateral night braces of the type described above, in an effort to control adduction and excessive internal or external rotation of the hips. It may be that this device derives such success as has been claimed for it from the fact that the patient is simply prevented from sleeping in an undesirable posture, with the result that the normal processes of growth prevent the development of bony alterations. If so, they would appear to have some usefulness. Many patients do not tolerate braces with bars as well as they tolerate those without bars.

The long leg night brace has been used following gastrocnemius surgery and hamstring surgery about the knee, but has been less readily accepted by patients and parents than the short leg night brace, and a night brace that is not worn is of no value. The use of plaster moulds at night has been somewhat better tolerated, and it may be that a total contact orthosis may be useful for this purpose.

Apart from plaster of paris moulds and plastic splints used for a few months following surgical intervention, the author has abandoned the use of night braces for the upper extremity.

The Management of the Child with a Brace

The orthopaedist's responsibility does not end with the prescription of a brace and the selection of a competent orthotist. The brace should be checked after its application and before its use. The parent and, if he is old enough, the child should be carefully instructed in the reason for its being used, the expected result, the method of application, and the problems that may arise.

Of prime importance is the need to keep the heel down in the shoe, so that the foot itself rather than just the shoe is held at the desired position in relation to the leg. To accomplish this, it is important to use a high-top shoe, which should be carefully laced, with the greatest tension being on the bottom lace, and the tension evenly distributed to the top, so that the force is applied equally throughout the length of the tongue of the shoe. A padded tongue may be a useful adjunct, but by far the most important need is to teach the mother, and/or the child if old enough, to lace the shoe properly. The practice that some fall into if not instructed is simply to leave the lace loose, and pull tightly from the top lace, so producing a tourniquet-like effect. Elastic laces are not adequate for this purpose.

The shoe must be checked, and if necessary changed, at frequent intervals, to ensure a proper fit. If the shoe is too big, the heel will ride up in the shoe; a shoe that is too small is painful to wear.

When night braces are applied, it is important that the shoe should not be set to the maximum dorsiflexion that the foot will tolerate, but that some ten degrees or so of leeway should be left so there will not be a constant force applied to the sole of the foot throughout the night. With the aid of a physical therapy program and normal use of the foot during the day, there will be instances in which, if bending irons are used, the bar of the brace may be bent slightly every six to twelve weeks, so as to gradually increase the angle of dorsiflexion of the foot until the foot is held at a right angle—or at even more than a right angle—to the leg. Appropriate bends can also be made to change a varus or valgus deformity gradually in the opposite direction.

The cutting out of the toecap of the shoe to allow ventilation of the toes at night will help obviate the excessive sweating and maceration of the skin which can result from both day and night use of the shoes.

It is alleged that the total contact orthosis is more effective in keeping the heel down in the shoe at night, and is better tolerated by the child. However, a disadvantage of the total contact orthosis would seem to be that to bring about a slight change in the posture of the foot involves changing the whole device rather than simply bending a bar. The total contact orthosis would appear to be a particularly useful device after the best possible correction had been obtained surgically.

When the child outgrows the shoe on his night brace, the expense of buying another can be deferred by making a simple cut along the join between the upper and the sole on each side where the toecap has been removed, and another one on each side of the tongue. This will increase the room for the forefoot, and allow the foot to come further forward in the shoe. It will also take pressure off the heel, which is the usual source of complaint when a child, having previously tolerated the night brace, ceases to do so.

One objection to a night brace is that it interferes with toilet training. This problem may be overcome by putting a sole over the metallic devices on the bottom of the shoe, in such a manner as to allow the child to walk to the bathroom.

Conclusion

Orthopaedic management amounts to attention to details. The orthopaedist must always be ready to listen to the mother; he must regularly follow the progress of the patient, both in and out of braces, and be quick to make appropriate recommendations to alleviate the multitude of mechanical problems which may arise.

REFERENCES

Bobath, K., Bobath, B. (1957) 'Control of motor function in the treatment of cerebral palsy.' *Physiotherapy,* **43,** 295.

Deaver, G. G. (1953) *Braces, Crutches and Wheelchairs.* Rehabilitation Monograph, No. 5. New York: University of New York, Bellevue Medical Center.

Garrett, A. L., Lister, M., Dresnan, J. (1966) 'New concept in bracing for cerebral palsy.' *Journal of the American Physical Therapy Association,* **46,** 728.

Knott, M., Voss, D. S. (1956) *Proprioceptive Neuromuscular Facilitation, Patterns and Techniques.* New York: Hoeber.

Phelps, W. M. (1953) 'Braces—lower extremity—cerebral palsy.' *Instructional Course Lectures, American Academy of Orthopedic Surgeons,* **10,** 303.

—— (1958) 'The role of physical therapy in cerebral palsy.' *in* Illingworth, R. S. (Ed.) *Recent Advances in Cerebral Palsy.* London: Churchill. p. 251.

Rood, M. S. (1954) 'Neurophysiological reactions as a basis for physical therapy.' *Physical Therapy Review,* **34,** 444.

Rosenthal, R. K., Deutsch, S., Miller, W. (1973) *Unpublished material presented at the American Academy for Cerebral Palsy Meeting, December.*

Thompson, S. B. (1957) 'An anti-scissoring device for patients with cerebral palsy.' *Journal of Bone and Joint Surgery,* **39A,** 218.

The Physiotherapist's Rôle in the Treatment of Cerebral Palsy

DAVID SCRUTTON and MOYNA GILBERTSON

It is not possible in this chapter to give a great deal of detail about the work of the physiotherapist, not least because, as we shall indicate later, there are many varying approaches to cerebral palsy treatment by physiotherapists. We hope, however, to give some indication of the rationale behind the physiotherapist's work to help the doctor to understand and co-operate with the therapist in managing movement disorders in children.

CLASSIFICATION

The traditional diagnostic methods of classification of cerebral palsy on the basis of the clinical signs (spasticity, rigidity, *etc.*) and the distribution in the body (quadriplegia, hemiplegia, *etc.*) are useful and give diagnostic information, but they do not provide enough information for the therapist. The therapist has two additional methods of classification which make it easier to appreciate these disorders. The first is based on the *primary functional difficulty,* the second on the *age of onset.* The various categories in these systems of classification are set out in Table I.

TABLE I

Classification of cerebral palsy for physical management

(A) Classification according to the primary functional difficulty	(1) Difficulty in producing movement	hypertonia hypotonia hyper- + hypotonia
	(2) Difficulty in preventing (involuntary movement)	Type of involuntary movement How it disrupts voluntary movement Degree of hypertonia Emotional influence
	(3) Difficulty in controlling movement	Type of movement involved Additional motor difficulties
(B) Classification according to the age of onset	Congenital	
	Acquired	before 1 year between 1 and 5 years after 5 years

A. The Primary Functional Difficulty

The primary functional difficulty may be classified as (1) a difficulty in producing movement; (2) a difficulty in preventing involuntary movement; or (3) a difficulty in controlling a movement. Within these three main categories the physiotherapist will look for sub-groups.

Difficulty in Producing Movement

Patients with difficulty in producing movement are sub-divided according to whether they have hypertonia, hypotonia or a combination of the two. Because difficulties in producing movement are clearly related to, if not caused by, these disorders of tone, the subdivision of patients into these three categories on the basis of classical diagnostic criteria provides useful information for the therapist.

When assessing a patient for hypertonia, it is important to realise that the extent and severity (degree) of hypertonia will vary according to a number of immediate factors, not least of which are the confidence with which the child is handled and his emotional state.

The distribution of hypertonia is constant, in the sense that it is confined to certain areas of the body in a particular child, but variable in that it may shift from one muscle group to another within those areas; these shifts are very much related to the child's preferred posture.

Difficulties in Preventing (Involuntary) Movement

While disorders of tone (hyper- or hypotonia) have an obvious direct relationship with difficulty in producing movement, difficulty in preventing (involuntary) movement cannot be related so readily to any physical finding. Phelps (1950) divided cerebral palsies with involuntary movements into eleven groups, which he considered relevant to his treatment methods. However, in our experience, once a classification of this sort is started the possibilities are infinite for, as Crothers and Paine (1959) observed, it is partly aetiological, partly topographical and partly descriptive. For our purpose, therefore, we find it more suitable to sub-divide patients with involuntary movements in relation to four variables: (1) the type of involuntary movement; (2) the manner in which the involuntary movement disrupts voluntary movement; (3) the degree of background hypertonia; and (4) the extent to which emotional state influences movement.

The Type of Involuntary Movement. The type of involuntary movement is mentioned only to emphasise that it is almost irrelevant to physical treatment, which cannot directly reduce involuntary movement.

The Manner in which Involuntary Movement Affects Voluntary Movement. Involuntary movements can disrupt movement ability in two ways, acting separately or together: (a) the involuntary movement supersedes (superimposes itself on) the willed activity, which is distorted; (b) the involuntary movement disrupts the proximal fixation of a limb performing a willed movement—a willed movement cannot be performed adequately without a stable background posture.

The Degree of Background Hypertonia. Although involuntary movements alone sometimes comprise the disorder, there is often associated hypertonia, which implies activity of tonic postural responses. If the patient has proximal hypertonia (of the trunk and proximal limb joint muscles) this may mask some of the involuntary movements for a part of the time.

The Extent to which Emotional State Influences Movement. Labile abnormal postures are associated with a lack of emotional stability, and disturbance of the emotions can release massive outbursts of involuntary movement activity. In some patients this activity is so marked that their involuntary movements appear to be caused almost solely by a failure to suppress this emotional influence.

It is appreciated that a classification of involuntary movement on the basis of the above criteria may have no fundamental relevance for the physician, but it is important for the physiotherapist because it describes the various elements which she can or cannot treat, and makes clear what she is treating.

Difficulty in Controlling a Movement

It is obvious that a child with any of the movement disorders described above will have difficulty in controlling movements, but in this third group we are concerned only with those patients whose difficulty in control is primary, *i.e.* those with ataxia.

The term ataxia is used to cover a very wide range of disorders, from ineptitude at games, untidy writing, clumsiness and repeated falling, to incoordination so severe that the child can hardly perform any purposeful movement. This wide variety of disorders can be subdivided by the physiotherapist in two ways (1) according to the type of movement involved (*e.g.* gross postural movements, fine movements or both) and (2) according to the additional locomotor difficulties (*e.g.* hypotonus, hypertonus, involuntary movements, or none).

B. The Age of Onset

The second important means of classification used by the physiotherapist is the age of onset (see Table I). The selection of age groups is somewhat arbitrary, but the cut-off points do represent ages at which the prospects for rehabilitation using physiotherapy are generally considered to change. It is clear that, according to the age of onset, a child either will or will not have had experience of normal movement and normal sensation. Thus, for children under one, the outlook is much as it is for the child with a congenital (*i.e.* present from birth) lesion, whereas the child aged between one and five years at the time of onset has the advantage of having had previous sensory and motor experience, and may well re-learn old skills with comparative ease. In our experience, in cases where the onset is after the age of five years, physiotherapy seems to have less to offer than it does in younger children. Spontaneous recovery in a large number of school-age children may foster extravagant claims for specific types of treatment, but despite such claims the authors consider that specialised treatment techniques have yet to prove their worth in this field. This is not to say that the physiotherapist has no part to play; her attitude of enlightened common sense towards rehabilitation is of the greatest need during the two years following the onset of a motor disorder in a school child.

A RATIONALE FOR EARLY TREATMENT OF MOVEMENT DISORDERS

The case against the treatment of many movement disorders caused by dis-

100

organisation of the higher centres of control can be summed up by three statements:
(1) a deficiency of the central nervous system is responsible for the disorder;
(2) physical treatment cannot reduce this deficit;
(3) therefore physical treatment cannot alter the disorder.

This argument is as unassailable as it is irrelevant. Physiotherapists need not refute it, because their case can be put another way:
(1) a deficiency of the central nervous system is responsible for the disorder;
(2) this will inevitably prevent the patient from functioning above a certain level of competence;
(3) but, without help, will he *inevitably* function up to that level?

We contend that, unless he receives help, a cerebral palsied patient is unlikely to function at the highest level possible for him; in fact, we would go further and suggest that in many disorders and circumstances he certainly will not. The movement limitation and deformity which is often taken to be the inevitable outcome of brain damage is inevitable only if the child is subjected to a normal environment. To have a movement or postural deficit is (by implication) to be unable to cope with the normal environment; the activity of a patient with such deficits is restricted, his opportunities for practising pathological movement responses are greatly increased and his opportunities for experiencing the environment are decreased. Having accepted that a patient will inevitably have some motor disability, the physiotherapist aims to ensure that it is no greater than that directly attributable to the neural deficit.

The paths from a child's minimum potential disability to his maximum disability as a result of a brain lesion are set out in Figure 1. The limited movement potential inevitably leads to some sensory deprivation, incorrect movement habits and frequent movement failure. There is probably poor child-parent feedback and usually

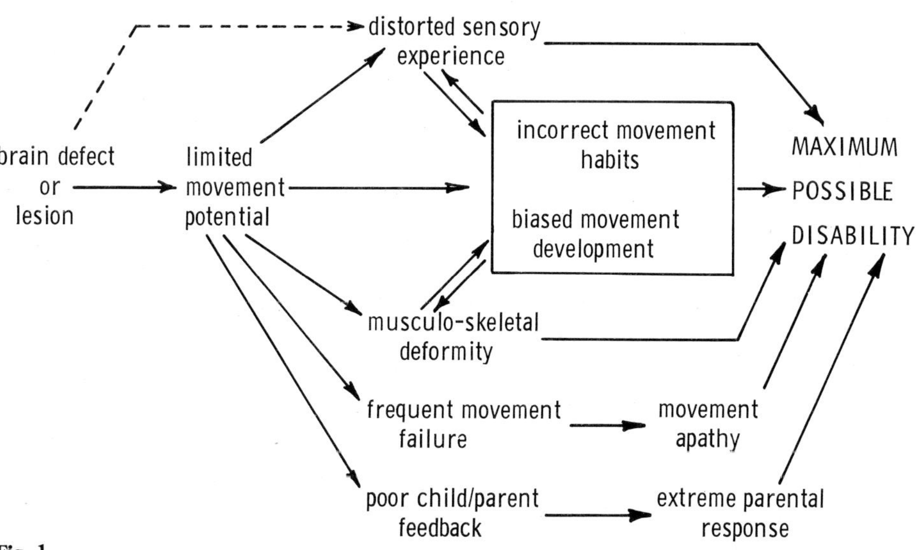

Fig. 1.

musculo-skeletal deformity. The incorrect movement habits, while reinforcing the inevitable limited movement potential, also tend to increase both the sensory deprivation and musculo-skeletal deformity. Each of these in its turn makes correct movement more difficult and so reinforces the incorrect habit. All these factors together make movements difficult to achieve and frequent failure reduces the motivation to move. Figure 1 highlights the basic aims of treatment, without putting them in any order of importance, as this is likely to vary from physiotherapist to physiotherapist and from treatment method to treatment method.

TREATMENT

Physical treatment can be started from the first days of life but the earliest practical age for treatment is likely to be between the ages of six and twelve months for children with congenital disorders, and immediately following the acute episode for those with acquired disorders. Although ideally infants are initially referred at these ages, in practice they are often not referred until the early period of movement development is over, by which stage they may already have some deformity. These late referrals present many different problems, but the following general points should be appreciated.

(1) Because a child has not been having treatment in the past, it may be possible to get some immediate rapid improvement in function, but it is unlikely that this rate of improvement will be maintained.

(2) There is an element of *fait accompli* about these children's disabilities, and the neurodevelopmental treatment suitable at a younger age may not be so effective when the early period of movement development is over, although it may (like any other approach) produce some marked immediate benefits.

Treatment will be discussed under four headings:

(1) musculo-skeletal deformity;

(2) management of posture and movement;

(3) sensory stimulation;

(4) advice to parents.

Musculo-Skeletal Deformity

Soft Tissue Deformity

Sharrard (1971) has pointed out that children's muscles/tendons lengthen as a consequence of bone growth, which, by thrusting apart the muscles' origins and insertions, applies a force to them; a fixed deformity results when the forces applied to antagonistic muscle groups are unequal, as occurs for example, in a locomotor disorder having differential muscle weakening. However, in the normal body, in spite of a marked disparity of available muscle strength across many joints, no deformities occur. It seems unlikely, therefore, that unequal muscle strength by itself can be the cause.

It would appear that muscle/tendon growth (or rather hypertrophy in response to bone growth) operates on a fundamental physical principle, *i.e.* le Chatelier-Braun principle that 'if any change of conditions is imposed on a system at equilibrium, then the system will alter in such a way as to counteract the imposed change'. In this

102

instance, the system is the whole of the locomotor system required to maintain a normal posture at that joint, and the constraint is bone growth. The cerebral palsied infant is not born with contractures or bony deformity, but with a tendency to develop abnormal postures. These preferred postures imply *an abnormal ratio of muscle lengths* between opposing muscle groups. Since the same physical principle operates, muscle hypertrophy occurs *so as to maintain the disorder of posture.* Thus a deformity which was postural gradually becomes fixed.

Any attempt to prevent fixed deformity by applying a 'constraint' upon the system is bound to fail, since the system will respond so as to retain its previous state. Therefore, traditional splinting and passive stretching are self-defeating. Success can be achieved only by altering the system itself, and there are three lines of approach.

(1) Exercises designed to inhibit pathological postural activity *and* substitute more normal activity. Such a treatment needs to be started early in the child's locomotor development (certainly by 6 to 9 months of age). It cannot be emphasised too strongly that the aim is not to strengthen muscles but to increase the likelihood of certain, previously unfavoured, movements occurring. In these disorders, any muscle weakness is secondary to the disorder of posture.

(2) Splinting, which in this context is part of the child's movement re-education and not, as often stated, to stretch a fixed deformity. The new posture alters the proprioceptive input and so changes the output: this effectively alters the system. The method has limited application, but is nonetheless of use. An example is in *postural* equinus: if the foot can be held at about ten degrees of dorsiflexion, not only does the plantar flexor spasm cease but the dorsiflexors are activated. Thus a below-knee caliper with back stops on a well-fitted boot can be very effective when worn by a child just learning to stand and walk. The authors have never found night splints to be very effective, but consider that day splints do have an important rôle in the management of some children. Reluctance to prescribe splinting constitutes a contra-indication in itself, as it is then used only as a last resort (which is too late) and by those who lack the experience to apply it to the correct patient. Splinting in cerebral palsy causes a strong division of opinion amongst physiotherapists, partly due to a sharp division in treatment methods: the mechanical versus the neuro-developmental approach. The splint (whether a caliper, moulded support or plaster of paris) being the archetype of the mechanical approach is often abhorrent beyond reason to those favouring a neuro-developmental treatment. Both sides have sound arguments, but they usually relate to differing circumstances, and are more complementary than antagonistic.

(3) Surgery is obviously the most direct method of altering the system. It is usually claimed that the purpose of surgery is to eliminate the fixed deformity and at the same time produce a balance of muscle strength across the joint, so as to maintain the correction. However, in cerebral palsy, the significant fact in maintaining correction appears more likely to be the alteration of proprioception.

Bone and Joint Changes

The shape of bones and joints is determined in part by the use to which they are put, *i.e.* the forces applied to them. Nowhere in the body is this more apparent than in the formation of the acetabulum and femoral head and neck. Hypertonia may lead to gradual subluxation/dislocation of the hips, usually accompanied by femoral neck anteversion and a failure of the femoral shaft/neck angle to decrease; both these accompanying deficits usually present as a marked increase in the range of internal, at the expense of external, rotation of the hip, when tested with the hip in extension. There is sometimes little change in the ranges of external and internal rotation when the hip is tested in flexion, a difference which is relevant to physical treatment.

Children who sit between their heels (see Fig. 2) usually show the altered joint ranges both with the hip in flexion and extension. However, it is standing rather than sitting which appears to hold the key to combatting the problem of the hip joint deformity, insofar as what is needed is the encouragement of correct and early weight bearing. Bouncers (which stimulate the extensor thrust response) are to be avoided at all costs, since they combine all the disadvantages—they do not allow full weight bearing, they encourage the deforming posture and they teach the child that, as in sitting, his trunk is his base (from which his legs hang), whereas the very essence of standing is that the feet form the fixed point. Whether the infant is developmentally ready to stand or not, weight bearing through extended hips should be started at about age one year. The feet should be plantigrade and the hips slightly abducted and rotated away from the position of deformity of that child. This exercise, together with measures mentioned later, will usually avoid severe hip joint deformity.

Limb Shortening

Limb shortening is significant only if it is in the legs, if it is asymmetrical, and if the patient is standing and walking. Its effects are varied. For a child with asymmetrical diplegia, shortening may lead to some alteration of spinal posture, but more typically it has no spinal effect, as it is compensated by an increased equinus of the short leg or an increased hip/knee flexion of the other. The hemiplegic patient may also compensate in this way, but more typically the pelvis drops on the affected side, causing a postural scoliosis concave to the unaffected side. A lightweight heel (and perhaps sole) raise is needed if the shortening is greater than half an inch, but it need not correct the full amount.

Management of Posture and Movement

The means of treatment will vary with the child's primary movement difficulty, his age at onset, intelligence and circumstances, but although the emphasis will change the underlying aims will remain the same. These aims are:
(1) to ensure that the child experiences a large choice of movement possibilities in a wide range of circumstances;
(2) to prevent the dominance of any postures or movements;
(3) to give experience of stable posture, from which movements can be performed;
(4) to give the child the opportunity to experience movement of his body as a whole to achieve an objective, *i.e.* to show him that coordinated movement is purposeful;
(5) to ensure he appreciates that he has responsibility for his body, *e.g.* that his head is *his* and not something which is propped up by his mother's shoulder.

There are many methods of treatment, and the difficulties in describing the techniques have led to the use of eponyms. A discussion on treatment becomes a roll-call: Bobath, Brunnstrom, Collis, Doman, Kabat, Phelps, Petö, Rood, Fay, Vojta . . . . All of these methods 'work', some perhaps better than others all of the time, and some better than others with certain patients and therapists. Lip service is given to an eclectic treatment, and to a certain extent all but the most rigid disciples of a method do treat eclectically. We consider that true eclectic treatment (however desirable it may be) is not really possible for two reasons:

(1) it takes a long time to become proficient at even one method;
(2) the treatment must suit the physiotherapist as well as the patient; and to do all treatments equally well is probably to do them all equally badly.

It is difficult to appreciate the value of a particular treatment method unless it has been practised for a time, for none should be judged from the rationale put forward by its proponents. The majority of the methods grew out of empirical observations, and the rationale was added later. As a general rule, the more 'scientific' the explanation appears, the less the likelihood of its withstanding criticism, for explanations often fail to take account of how crude our treatment methods must be in relation to the physiological mechanisms expounded!

It may seem reasonable to ask which system has the best results over-all. It is difficult to judge for several reasons. The aims of treatment are somewhat different. Those who advocate one method might prefer to be judged on their ability to prevent deformity, whilst those who advocate another might consider the prevention of deformity to be secondary to the achievement of a more normal pattern of movement. One method may be directed towards the early achievement of walking, while another may deliberately delay walking until it can be performed better. It is impossible to match children of equal handicap, for the handicap is not an isolated and direct result of the brain insult. It is a combination of the direct results of the insult with all that has happened since. Hence, if two children, one treated and one untreated, have the same degree of handicap, it does not follow that the former has not been helped by treatment. Just as plausible an explanation is that the treated child would have been worse without treatment. Until a means of making a more accurate early diagnosis (and therefore prognosis) has been devised, the influence of early treatment will remain unsettled. In older patients, once the handicap has become established, the effects of different techniques can be more accurately judged, but it does not follow that treaments more (or less) successful at this age are also more (or less) effective in infancy. In fact this would seem unlikely, as the problems are different.

However, one approach to the treatment of these disorders is in a category by itself, and not to single it out would be to present an unbalanced picture. The work of Dr. and Mrs. Bobath challenged the established treatments and influenced physiotherapy more than is often appreciated. Perhaps the highest compliment that can be paid to them is that much which was previously considered controversial is now unanimously accepted.

The essence of any treatment for managing or preventing a posture or movement disorder is the creation of circumstances in which the patient can experience more natural movement (or posture). To begin with this may require that the movement be done for the child, to give him the sensation of it. This assistance will be withdrawn as quickly as possible, so that he can carry out the movement on his own, though still in a very circumscribed set of physical conditions. Once a movement is achieved, the child is gradually given more and more difficult circumstances in which to achieve it, until (ideally) the movement can be performed in everyday situations. In point of fact, this final stage will be accompanied by a falling off of the quality of the movement, and part of the skill in treating these patients is the achievement of a balance between the quality of the movement and the difficulty of the situation in which it is performed.

Much of the treatment frequently utilizes the balance and protective responses. Balance and protective responses involve patterns of movement which are nearly always opposed to those preferred by the damaged brain, yet they can often be elicited without the voluntary assistance of the child. Consequently, they are a particularly convenient method of widening the infant's and the young child's movement experience.

As the child grows older, the emphasis of treatment should gradually shift away from the teaching of different patterns of movement to the achievement of the most economic and advantageous use of those he already has. Much more of the available treatment time will be needed for training in activities of daily living which will allow him greater independence. This change of emphasis does not mean that the previous treatment would not continue to give some benefit, but that the benefit would probably be small in proportion to the time required to produce it, and less relevant to the child's needs.

After any orthopaedic surgery, an intensive treatment regime is well worthwhile, as the operation should have altered the child's potential and opened up new avenues of movement.

Involuntary Movements and Ataxia

The early treatment of these disorders ensures that the children get the maximum opportunity to experience normal movement and posture. This appears to be important, and the authors consider it very desirable. However, ignoring those patients with any hypertonic element, there is, in our experience, little to recommend intensive treatment of older children with involuntary movements and ataxia. Such children continue to improve gradually until they are well into their teens, through what may be a combination of late maturation, increased experience and greater determination and purpose. What these older children need is the opportunity to explore the limits of their ability in their everyday life. Learning new skills at a late age is not extraordinary in these children, it is natural, but it demands great persistence and courage on the part of the child. It is for all those concerned with him to appreciate this, and to sustain persistent encouragement as well as providing the necessary movement opportunities.

Sensory Stimulation

It has already been pointed out that the disorder is sensory/motor, and that proprioceptive experience is the key to motor ability. In this section, the sensory stimulation referred to is mainly exteroceptive, although for an understanding of the environment, proprioception (*e.g.* appreciation of weight and shape) may sometimes be of equal or greater importance.

From the earliest age, a baby with cerebral palsy should be helped to feel his body: to play with his feet and legs, and to put his hands in his mouth, on his face and through his hair. If two-handed play is difficult, he should be encouraged, with only as much help as is necessary, to clasp and clap his hands and to play with toys and transfer them from one hand to the other. Toys should be of different colours, textures, sizes and weights, as well as having a built-in noise (like a bell or rattle). In this way, an association between vision, hearing, touch and proprioception may be built up.

Experience of reaching out towards a face or toy is needed to help the child appreciate distance. An understanding of distance, particularly as regards near-to (personal) space, is important not only to preclude secondary dysmetria but also for an appreciation of speed (which would seem to require knowledge of a time-distance ratio). In this context, it is interesting how often severely handicapped children with an over-active startle response shy away from a hand brushing hair out of their eyes or a spoon taking food to their mouths. Bearing in mind that a child may get a better understanding of distance and speed from watching and moving his own limbs, it is better to put the spoon in the child's hand and guide it to his mouth, even if he is unlikely ever to be able to feed himself. In this way his proprioceptive experience can supplement his inadequate visual appreciation of the speed at which the object is approaching.

Experience of differing temperature, textures, weights, colours, sounds and distances is important. Concepts such as above/below, inside/outside and behind/in front can be introduced earlier than might be thought as part of dressing and bathing.

Advice to Parents

Those readers who are interested in how to help parents to understand and manage their children's movement disorders can refer to the book 'Handling the Young Cerebral Palsied Child at Home' by Finnie (1974). It is to be emphasized that, wherever possible, the treatment involves the training of parents in their child's every-day care. It is this all-day, every-day management, far more than the specific treatment given by the physiotherapist, which will influence the child's sensory/motor development. However, the advice given to the parents must be specific for the child and his particular circumstances.

SITTING AND CHAIRS

The question of sitting and chairs is given particular attention here, as frequently the doctor is responsible for ordering such equipment, and very often inadequate attention is paid to the design and planning of sitting and the provision of ordinary chairs and wheelchairs for the cerebral palsied child.

Sitting is the most commonly used intermediate position between the relaxation of lying and the active postures of crawling and standing. It is the best position for many activities, and the one in which many handicapped children are expected to live. There are six basic sitting positions: long sitting, cross-legged sitting, between-heel sitting , side sitting (left and right) and chair sitting (Fig. 2). Their common factor is that a large proportion of the body weight is taken through one or both the ischial tuberosities. Providing comfortable and desirable sitting positions for handicapped children becomes very much easier when this is borne in mind.

Long Sitting

Long sitting is the natural first sitting position for the majority of infants. By leaning forwards, they keep their centre of gravity well inside a large triangular base. Infants are usually propped up in this position a couple of months before they can get up into it by themselves. Long sitting gives infants good opportunities for seeing what is going on around them and for play, and allows them to practise their rapidly emerging gross motor skills (*e.g.* trunk equilibrium, arm propping and protective extension). However, it presents them with problems in remaining upright without over-extending the trunk and so falling backwards. Poor motor control exaggerates this problem. Short spastic hamstrings tend to throw the body weight onto the sacrum rather than the ischial tuberosities. As a result, the lower vertebrae are incorrectly aligned and compound the problems of trunk control; it is better for these children to flex their knees slightly and so allow more hip flexion.

Trunk control cannot be learnt without a secure base, so the infant needs his buttocks firmly supported. A corner seat may help, but should be made for the particular child and be measured for height of back-rest, distance from crutch support to corner, and height and size of tray. Unless the back-rest is also a head support, it rarely needs padding: an infant is well padded by his napkins and his clothes.

Cross-Legged Sitting

Cross-legged sitting is not a very useful position. The combination of a smaller base, together with total flexion of the lower limbs, makes this a difficult position for most movement-handicapped children. It is misused by some physiotherapists for children who perpetually sit between their heels, as a means of getting their hips away from an internally rotated position. Unfortunately, it is these very children who find it hardest to do anything when placed cross-legged.

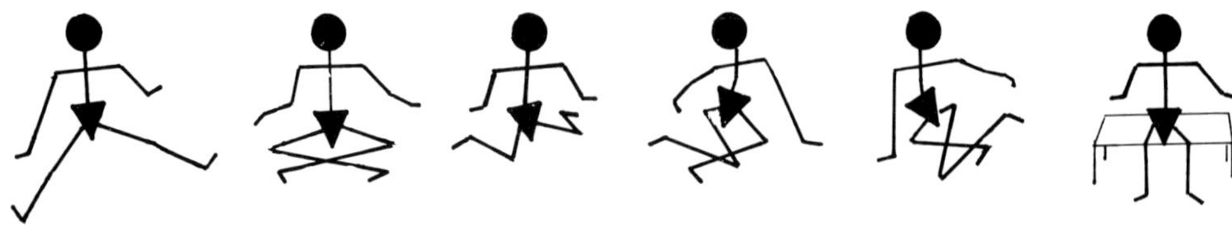

Fig. 2 (*left to right*). Long sitting, cross-legged sitting, between-heel sitting, side sitting (left), side sitting (right), chair sitting.

Between-Heel Sitting

Between-heel sitting is perhaps the *easiest* floor sitting position, particularly for a child (normal or abnormal) who has good prone development. It is their natural resting posture from crawling, and leads easily into upright kneeling and standing. The vertebral column is in the middle of a large base: the hamstrings are relaxed, and so the pelvis is not tipped back upsetting the trunk alignment. It is the classic sitting position of the spastic diplegic patient, and is blamed by many for their typical femoral neck deformities. In its favour, it is probably the best position for many children to learn correct trunk control, and the relaxed hamstrings allow the development of the secondary lumbar curve.

Side Sitting (Left and Right)

Side sitting is a natural playing position for many normal children. It gives a good base, and allows the child to be right on top of what he is doing. For the handicapped child it has the disadvantage that it requires two good arms, one for support and the other for play. Consequently, it is of little significance *as a posture* in handicapped children apart from those with spastic hemiplegia, amongst whom it is a favourite sitting and shuffling position. Side sitting to the unaffected side is comfortable for these patients because it gives full reign to all their abnormal postural tendencies (*e.g.* hip adduction/internal rotation, shortened hamstrings, and side flexion to the trunk to the hemiplegic side) and requires no effort by the hemiplegic arm.

Therapy for these spastic hemiplegic patients includes side sitting to the affected side. In this position, the child can use his good hand for play, while learning (with help) an extension position of his hemiplegic arm, trunk side flexion away from the involved side, and hip external rotation.

Chair Sitting

From the design of most children's chairs, it might be thought that sitting means no more than being in a chair, regardless of the position adopted on it. Whereas for a normal child sitting is easier if the chair is designed so as to fit him reasonably well, for the handicapped child the fit of the chair can make all the difference between his being able or unable to sit.

But what do we mean by 'fit'? Basically, a chair which fits is one which is of the right size and provides the right support.

Chair Size

Length. If the seat is too long, the child will lean back and his buttocks will probably slide forwards; if it is too short he will lack adequate support for his thighs.

Height. If the seat is too high the child will be unable to get support through his feet; too low, and he will lack full-length thigh support. The height of the seat can be measured not to the ground but to a foot rest if this is more convenient.

There is a division of opinion about foot rests. Those in favour maintain that they give a constant floor surface, allow the feet to be fixed (if necessary), prevent thrusting with the feet from tipping the chair over backwards, and prevent the child from pushing himself around backwards. Those against foot-rests maintain that it is easier to get on and off a chair without one, and they *like* children to push themselves around backwards.

Back Rest

Height of Back rest. The back rest should not support the head unless the child cannot control it well enough by himself, or unless for some other reason the chair has to be tipped backwards.

Slope or Angle. As a general rule, the back rest should be at an angle of approximately 100 degrees to the seat.

Chairs which Offer Additional Support

Pelvis. Having a chair which fits for size may not be enough. The child may be too floppy, stiff, or lacking in the necessary balance to sit on it. The cardinal rule when it comes to supporting a child on a chair is to fix his pelvis in the correct position, *i.e.* with his body weight taken equally on both ischial tuberosities. If this position is not achieved, all other measures to improve sitting will be in vain. It is surprising how often efforts are made to support a child with a strap around his chest without first controlling his pelvis.

Most infants' chairs are unsuitable for children who cannot maintain a correct sitting position unaided, because the restraining straps are fixed at the front of the seat and allow the child to slide too far forward. In such cases, it is necessary to find some means of holding the pelvis back, or all thoughts of correct sitting will have to be abandoned. Three methods, each of which has its advantages and disadvantages, are a backward-sloping seat, groin straps, and a crutch block.

Trunk. With the pelvis secure, the child has the opportunity to learn trunk control. Trunk support may still be needed, but it is important to remember that the purpose of this support may vary from patient to patient. Support is needed in the following situations.

(1) If the patient has insufficient head control, then the trunk support will be designed to supply a firm enough base for head control to be learnt.

(2) If the patient has fair or good head control, then the trunk support must be sufficient to give him the opportunity to learn trunk control, *i.e.* there must be opportunity for free movement within and just beyond his range of ability.

(3) If the patient has little or no chance of learning better control, then trunk support may still be needed (a) to give him the best opportunity to function to his maximum ability, and (b) to prevent deformity.

Feet. It is sometimes necessary to help the child who is chair sitting to hold his feet in the correct position. Correctly placed feet can give good support to the rest of the body. At the same time, the child has the opportunity to appreciate postural control through his feet to his body, which may help his understanding of the function of the feet in standing.

Wheelchairs

It is hard to over-state how difficult it is to design a good wheelchair, because so many of the requirements are mutually exclusive. When considering a wheelchair

for a particular child, it may be pertinent to ask the following questions.
(1) Is it needed as a push chair or a self-propelled chair?
(2) Will it be used indoors, outdoors, or both?
(3) Will the child be travelling in it to and from school, and will he be using it at school?
(4) Will it have to be taken by car, or on a bus or train?
(5) Where will it be kept at home?

All too often, wheelchairs are issued without thought for the other user—the parent. A chair which suits the child may be far from what is needed by the parent, who may not realise what his or her own real needs are until closely questioned and shown the various alternatives available. Very often, one chair alone cannot fulfil all the needs of both the patient and his parents. For instance, one chair could give good support, provide a useful sized tray and be self-propelled indoors, whilst another altogether lighter chair may be needed for going out shopping or for walks. The solution may not be cheap, but it is no less correct for that.

Acknowledgement. This article is based on material from the book 'Paediatric Physiotherapy' by David Scrutton and Moyna Gilbertson (Butterworth 1975).

REFERENCES

Crothers, B., Paine, R. S. (1959) *The Natural History of Cerebral Palsy.* Cambridge, Mass.: Harvard University Press.

Phelps, W. M. (1950) 'Etiology and diagnostic classification of cerebral palsy.' *in Proceedings of the Cerebral Palsy Institute.* New York: Association for the Aid of Crippled Children.

Finnie, N. R. (1974) *The Handling of the Young Cerebral Palsied Child at Home. 2nd Edn.* London: Heinemann.

CHAPTER 6

Pre- and Post-operative Medical Management of the Cerebral Palsied

ERIC DENHOFF
(Prepared with the assistance of NATHAN RAKATANSKY, CARROL SILVER, HENRY LITCHMAN, NANCY CASTRO and NANCY D'WOLF)

The medical management of the cerebral palsied child given orthopedic surgical treatment focuses on getting the child into the best possible physical and emotional condition for surgery, and maintaining him in this condition during the entire period related to surgery, *i.e.* during the pre-admission build-up, the hospital stay and the convalescence. If, throughout this time, proper attention is paid to the following seven aspects of the child's care, the chances of successful surgery are increased substantially.

(1) Nutritional balance.
(2) Emotional stability.
(3) Seizure and/or behavior control.
(4) Fluid and metabolic balance.
(5) Anesthesia.
(6) Nursing care.
(7) Post-operative rehabilitation.

When their particular requirements are met, cerebral palsied children respond to surgery like normal children. In my own experience with the cerebral palsied, orthopedic surgery has caused no deaths, and the morbidity has been negligible—being generally limited to discomfort or irritability immediately after surgery.

PRE-ADMISSION BUILD-UP

Nutrition

A requirement for elective surgery is an acceptable nutritional balance. Some cerebral palsied children are chronically undernourished, and it may require an eight- to twelve-week period to achieve a good nutritional state. The major problems encountered are anemia and hypoproteinemia. These require early evaluation and prompt intervention, since responsiveness to diet may be sluggish.

Poor nutrition (iron deficiency) is the most common cause of anemia, although anticonvulsant drugs such as phenytoin ('Dilantin'), oxazoladine ('Tridione') and mephenytoin ('Mesantoin') may also be responsible. Occasionally, intestinal parasites, hemolytic syndromes, sickling, and chronic blood loss are to blame. Laboratory studies are a pre-requisite to anticipated surgery, and should at the very least include the following: a blood count and hemoglobin or hematocrit, a differential blood smear (white blood cell count if indicated), with special attention paid to the morphological appearance of the cells, platelets, and eosinophils, a routine urine analysis, and a total protein with albumen-globulin ratio if moderate to severe protein deficiency is suspected. The use of other tests depends upon the clinical situation.

Oral treatment for anemia is usually satisfactory (*e.g.* 5 mg/kg body weight/24 hours of ferrous sulphate), but if a child cannot tolerate oral medication, parenteral iron administration is acceptable. Transfusions are never indicated, unless the hemoglobin is below 7.0 grams and an emergency surgical procedure is required.

When the patient has anemia due to drug intoxication, apart from anticonvulsant substitution, it is necessary to prescribe folic acid, 5 mg three times a day, along with vitamin B complex. When intestinal parasites are found, prompt anthelmintic therapy is required.

A well-balanced high protein diet is essential during the pre-operative period. A menu for handicapped children can be developed which is both nutritious and encourages better chewing habits. If the child can gain a few pounds of weight prior to hospitalization, it will be helpful, but this may be hard to accomplish. Generally, cerebral palsied children have high caloric requirements and poor energy conservation.

The handicapped child may need 10 to 25 per cent more calories than his normal peers. Growth requirements for normal children are listed in Table I.

TABLE I

Normal daily requirements of calories, protein and water for children at various ages

Age	*Calories* (*No. per kg body weight*)	*Protein* (*g/kg body weight*)	*Water* (*cc/kg body weight*)
Infancy	110	4.0	150
1 to 3 years	100	3.5	125
4 to 6 years	90	3.0	100
7 to 9 years	80	2.5	75
10 to 12 years	70	2.0	75
13 to 15 years	60	1.5	50
over 15 years	50	1.0	50

In developed countries, hypoproteinemia is generally of a mild degree, but in certain sections of the underdeveloped countries it is not unusual to find clinical signs such as edema of the trunk and abdomen. Generally, a high protein, high vitamin diet is sufficient to correct protein imbalance. To get a cerebral palsied child to eat such a diet often requires ingenuity, as cerebral palsied children are notoriously poor eaters. Since some children insist on continuing to eat infant or infant-type foods, protein supplementation is often achieved by adding one to two tablespoonfuls of instant, vitamin-fortified dried milk or some flavored or unflavored gelatin to milk, jello, custards or juices. Mixed, strained baby meat can be added to soup, vegetables or a favorite food. The new fortified breakfast or diet liquid foods are generally popular. Constipation may be an annoying complication of a high protein diet, but can be modified by forcing fluids, vitamin B complex compounds ('Lederplex'), or stool softeners such as dioctyl sodium sulfosuccinate ('Colace').

113

Emotional Stability

Serious consideration must be given to the emotional needs of the cerebral palsied child who is being prepared for or convalescing from surgery. Emotional turmoil resulting from insensitive handling can defeat the best surgical efforts, and the emotional effects can last for many months.

Those involved in the rehabilitation process need to be aware of the processes of emotional development in normal children. Cerebral palsied children generally have more exaggerated behaviour responses than non-handicapped children, and many characteristics are slow to mature.

A child's personality will often echo his parents' hopes, fears, and anxieties. The handicapped child with uneven personality development will often react unpredictably to stress. Limited contact with a normal peer group, added to an excessive involvement with a medically oriented world, fosters such reactions. Complications which further interfere with behavior and emotional reactions are mental retardation or normal intelligence which cannot be demonstrated because of serious physical limitations.

Many cerebral palsied children never completely emerge from the self-centred infantile dependent stage. Normal ego development is often impeded. Ego development*, which starts in a rudimentary fashion at birth and normally is well-established by the second or third year of life, depends upon the intactness of central nervous system, particularly of the perceptual apparatus. Inadequate ego development almost invariably leads to distortions of self-image, which are a common complication in patients with cerebral palsy.

By three years of age, the normal child is developing unconscious self-protective and survival mechanisms. Shortly after this age, he develops a conscience, which ultimately leads to self-control and an ability to make ethical and moral decisions. Cerebral palsied children often lag in this area of emotional growth. The cerebral palsied child fears punishment and loss of parental love, and feels completely helpless when exposed to a threatening environment. His fears are mainly parent-directed.

It is easy to understand why hospitalization during this developmentally critical period can leave long-lasting emotional scars, unless the child's reactions are anticipated and his needs met meticulously. The occurrence of destructive, episodic rages generally reflects a conscious or subconscious attempt to survive. The hospital staff must be able to transmit a feeling of warmth and understanding to the child. This is an essential requirement of successful surgery. The physicians, parents, nurses, laboratory technicians, therapists, and child care workers, all of whom are involved directly or indirectly in the surgical procedure, must accept that there is a very close relationship between emotional stability and successful rehabilitation.

Before the child enters the hospital, it is the surgeon's responsibility to interrelate the feelings of the child and his family with the hospitalization and the surgical procedure. He should seek the aid of the pediatrician, anesthetist and the nursing

---

*Ego development concerns that part of the mind which perceives, thinks, remembers, recalls, and conceptualizes about self as opposed to non-self.

staff, and ask them to take every precaution to minimize emotional trauma. In general, if the child's intellectual level is adequate (a mental age of 7 or 8), this is done by explaining and discussing everything that is to happen as carefully and fully as possible. The surgeon should meet with the child and his parents in his office about a month before surgery. He should outline a plan to help make separation from the family a non-traumatic experience. The age of the child, and his ability to communicate and reason, will affect this planning.

Since surgery is indicated only after multiple evaluations by the surgeon to assess fully the mechanical physiological disabilities of the child, the surgeon has the opportunity to develop more than a superficial relationship with the child and family. Although some of the diagnostic studies are carried out by para-medical personnel, the surgeon should participate in muscle and sensory testing and in gait analysis. Such participation increases his contact with the child, as well as providing a better understanding of the nature of the problem.

Generally, younger cerebral palsied children do not grasp the implications of surgery as quickly as normal children. Bright cerebral palsied teenagers may be extremely apprehensive or overly cheerful about surgery which they hope may help make them walk better or use their hands better. With the younger child and the child who cannot talk or relate to adults, serious thought must be given to parent 'rooming-in' during the hospital stay. With the older child (and adult) fear of pain is often a very real worry, and reassurance that adequate 'pain-killers' will be given is important. Adolescents will often exhibit more anxieties than younger children. They may require much reassurance during the preparation phase as well as during hospitalization. It is reasonable to use tranquilizers for a short period if the patient is over-anxious.

Seizure and/or Behavior Control

Many cerebral palsied patients who undergo surgery are taking anticonvulsant medication. Every effort must be made to have the child seizure-free before he enters the hospital. Usually, full control of seizures is not difficult to attain. However, apprehension associated with a hospital admission can precipitate an unexpected convulsion, even in a child previously well-controlled or believed to be clinically free of seizures. If there is any question that seizures may occur, investigations (such as electroencephalograms) should be completed before hospitalization. If after these investigations there remains a suspicion that seizures may occur, it is wise to start anticonvulsant medication. Prophylactic medication may prevent a seizure on admission. However, if a seizure does occur, it can usually be aborted by the intravenous or intramuscular injection of 1.0 or 2.0 cc (5 or 10 mg) of diazepam ('Valium'). If a seizure occurs in a child who has never previously had one, it is wise to defer surgery until seizure control is reasonably certain.

In cases where seizures are a prominent feature, it is a wise precaution to admit the child to the hospital 48 hours before elective surgery to make necessary medication adjustments. Hospital anticonvulsant drug schedules are patterned after home schedules. Medications are given orally until four hours before operation, when the 'nothing by mouth' order is instituted. A double dose at night will make up for

TABLE II

Common anticonvulsant medication

Medication	Dosage (mg/kg/24 hrs)	Average dosage (mg/24 hrs)	Therapeutic blood level (mg/ml)	Side effects
Generalized, focal or psychomotor attacks				
primidone ('Myosline')	5-20	125-1000 once nightly	1.0-3.0	Initial headache and vomiting possible. Use 25-50 mg as a starting dose, and increase by 50 mg every four days until proper dosage is attained.
phenytoin ('Dilantin')	5-10	32-300 once nightly	1.0-2.0	Morbilliform rash; ataxia; gingival hyperplasia is common; multiple systemic side effects are possible with long-term usage.
phenobarbital	3-6	32-200 three times per day	1.0-3.0	Over-sedation interferes with cognitive function. Paradoxical agitation effect not uncommon in hyperkinetic children.
Petit mal triad ethosuximide ('Zarontin')	20-60	250-500 three times per day	2.5-3.5	Morbilliform eruption; blood dyscrasias occur, but are rare.
trimethadione ('Tridione')	20-60	150-600 three times per day		Nephritis; platelet and red blood count deficiency not uncommon.
acetazolamide ('Diamox')	12-25	125-250 three times per day		Rash, drowsiness, parathesia of face and extremities.

missed morning tablets. If the child cannot tolerate the medication, sodium phenobarbital, intramuscularly, is a good substitute. Oral medication is re-instituted as promptly as possible after surgery (Table II).

Behavior Ameliorators

Medications designed to modify undesirable behavior and attitudes can play a beneficial rôle in obtaining perfect surgical results. The Hyperkinetic Impulse Syndrome often creates a considerable barrier to the cerebral palsied child's ability to cope with stress. Hyperactivity, short attention span, variability, impulsivity, inability to delay gratification, irritability and explosiveness with tantrums are particularly difficult to deal with in the convalescent period. Psychostimulant drugs such as dexamphetamine ('Dexedrine') or methylphenidate ('Ritalin') can be used to provide the child with some internal controls, and so make the home environment tolerable during the time the child is in the cast or receiving post-operative therapy.

There are other children who become extremely anxious during the hospitalisation

116

and during the early weeks of convalescence. In such cases tranquillizers such as chlorpromazine ('Thorazine') can serve a useful purpose for a limited period.

The muscle relaxant drugs play an extremely important rôle. Diazepam ('Valium') is used to combat hypertonia. If lethargy occurs, the dosage is reduced. Diazepam is omitted the day before surgery. It is resumed as soon after the operation as possible, and is continued until at least a month after the cast is removed. This drug has reduced post-surgical complications to a minimum. It may, however, produce irritability and hyperkinetic behavior when used over a long period, in which case it is omitted and generally dexamphetamine sulfate or thioridazine ('Mellaril') is substituted.

In the post-surgical period, diazepam ('Valium') has lessened the need for medication for pain, as post-operative pain is most often related to spasm in the operated muscles. Table III summarizes important features in the use of these medications.

TABLE III

Useful medications related to orthopaedic surgery for cerebral palsied children

Drug	Dosage (mg/kg/ 24 hours)	Average Dosage (mg)	Side effects
Psychostimulants dexamphetamine ('Dexedrine')	0.2-1.0	5-10 three times per day	Loss of appetite, sleep and weight, possible hypertension.
l-amphetamine ('Benzedrine')	0.4-2.0	10-20 three times per day	Loss of appetite, sleep and weight; possible hypertension.
methylphenidate ('Ritalin')		5-10 three times per day	same as above, but less intense.
Tranquillizers (major) chlorpromazine ('Thorazine')	1-2	10-25 three times per day	Sedation, hypotension, and possible extrapyramidal effects: photosensitivity.
thioridazine ('Mellaril')	1-5	10-25 three times per day	Excessive weight gain and abdominal stria; drowsiness; other side effects similar to those of chlorpromazine.
Tranquillizers (minor) chlordiazepoxide ('Librium')	0.5	5-10 three times per day	Drowsiness, syncope and, rarely, ataxia.
Skeletal muscle relaxants diazepam ('Valium')	0.12-0.8	2-10 three times per day	Over-sedation and hypotonia.

Most children find the hospital a strange and awesome place. It generally provokes feelings of fear when parents discuss it. Thus every effort must be made to make the hospital environment friendly. A warm, well-organized staff helps to produce a feeling of confidence in the parents and the child. By contrast, a hospital staff unable or unwilling to meet the needs of a handicapped child and his family can nullify surgical preparation and prejudice the outcome.

Admission Procedure

When a handicapped child arrives for hospital admission, it is important that the administrative procedures should be brief and to the point. The family should be sped promptly to the pediatric ward. Here they are met by the head nurse and the nurse assigned to the case. To instil immediate confidence, the head nurse explains the reasons for the various hospital precautions, such as crib restraints and laboratory tests, and suggests the parents ask questions. The nurse then explains the possible complications which could arise to delay surgery, such as hypersensitivity, or an idiosyncratic response to antibiotics or certain foods. Recent exposure to contagious disease is explored, dietary preferences or dislikes are recorded, and prescribed medications listed. Parent sleeping-in arrangements are discussed in detail.

By now the resident physician assigned to the case has arrived, and he is alerted to possible problems. He explores, specifically, blood-coagulation or bleeding problems, family history of adverse anesthetic reactions, previous systemic steroid therapy, and need for a tetanus booster. He examines the child, and pays special attention to the presence of contagious disease, signs of respiratory infection and loose teeth. Later that evening, the anesthetist re-examines the child to assess the anesthetic risk.

Routine laboratory tests will normally have been done during the pre-hospital period, but a final haemoglobin check and any other necessary investigations can be done at this time.

Parents' 'Rooming-in'

The parents have a definite rôle to play during the hospital period. While it may be impracticable for all parents to be allowed to 'sleep-in' during the hospital stay, it is highly desirable that the hospital should have some facility to permit this when emotional turmoil is at a high level. Rooming-in privileges are especially to be recommended for the parents of infants and toddlers.

When the parent is not to 'sleep-in', the mother is encouraged to provide a favorite toy, dressing garment or blanket to comfort the child during the hospital period. Parents are encouraged to relate to other children in the ward, to minimize a concentration of attention on their own child. The mother's presence is expected at meal times, as with her help it is easier to ensure that adequate nutrition is maintained.

On ward rounds, loose medical talk and discussion of the case in front of the parent or the child is prohibited. Check lists are reviewed daily for special diet requirements, and for food or drug idiosyncracies.

Generous parent visiting hours are a necessity, but limits may have to be set for other visitors. Even when parents are visibly disturbed, visits must be encouraged. While the consequences of separation due to hospitalization are unclear in most children, there is sufficient accumulated evidence to show that the effects of the hospital stay may demonstrate themselves in a variety of subtle and bizarre ways during the months or years that follow. Highly susceptible to emotional stress are children aged between six months and three years, and their mothers in particular should be encouraged to 'sleep in'.

The hospital pediatric ward must be child-oriented and comfortable, with a minimum of hustle and bustle of adult activity. The hospital stay should not exceed a week (generally it can be reduced to three days), if post-operative rehabilitation is to be successful.

Nursing Care

After the nursing staff has established a basic rapport with the child, preparations for surgery begin. The field of surgery is shaved and scrubbed for ten minutes with 'Phisohex', and then wrapped in sterile towels. The patient is then readied for bed. Sedation is rarely needed, but if the child is extremely agitated chlorpromazine ('Thorazine') (5 to 25 mg in 5 cc distilled water) is injected intramuscularly.

In the morning, the scrubbing and wrapping of the surgical area is repeated. The nurse describes the surgical 'trip', including the manner of transportation to and from the operating room, the type of clothes worn by the hospital personnel, and the receiving of anesthesia—which starts by 'blowing up a balloon'. The child is told he will return to his room wearing a cast, which may be stained with blood, but that this is all part of a routine operation.

Diet

Routinely, the night before surgery, a normal evening meal is permitted. Subsequently, clear fluids are given until four hours before surgery. The last feeding consists of a mixture of sweetened water and orange juice to avoid glycogen depletion. After surgery, clear liquids are reinstated for 24 hours or until the effects of anesthesia and sedation have worn off; then a routine hospital diet, supplemented by a multivitamin with a high vitamin C content, is given orally. Tube feedings are generally avoided if possible. Occasionally, a gastrostomy is recommended for a marasmic child whose intake is insufficient for nutritional balance.

Fluid Requirements

Some cerebral palsied children are in a state of chronic dehydration as well as undernourishment. While every effort should be made during the pre-admission build-up to achieve as close to normal hydration as possible by the oral route, it is often difficult to attain acceptable hydration prior to and immediately following surgery. Although the majority of children require little special care if certain nutritional principles are followed, as in all patients submitted to surgery, adequate management of electrolyte or fluid imbalance is essential in the cerebral palsied.

Anesthesia

Preparation for Anesthesia

A good rapport between the child and the anesthetist is a pre-requisite for successful anesthetic results. With understanding, the need for sedatives before anesthetization can be minimized. Reassurance from the anesthetist, plus a carry-over of the effects of medications prescribed to calm the child on hospital admission, will usually be sufficient to ensure a smooth transfer to the operating room.

If, after examining the child the night before surgery, the anesthetist decides that any pre-operative sedation is necessary, this is given an hour before the call to surgery. Atropine and meperidine ('Demerol'), in approximately half the dose prescribed for a normal child, is a favored choice*. Barbiturates are avoided, since they often stimulate these children rather than quiet them. Scopolamine may have a similar but less striking action.

The most popular inhalent anesthetic is halothane ('Fluothane'). It has virtually replaced ether in recent years, because it is non-explosive and provides a high safety factor in surgical procedures where motorized instruments are used; it is reasonably pleasant to inhale, and does not leave the patient with undesirable side-effects when he or she awakes. It can be combined with a relatively high level of oxygen in a non-re-breathing system which provides minimal resistance to breathing. Usually halothane is combined with oxygen and nitrous oxide in a 50/50 mixture.

The child is kept in as light a plane of anesthesia as the surgical procedure permits. With halothane ('Fluothane'), it is possible to slowly decrease the ratio of the gas so that, by the end of the surgery, the level of unconsciousness is minimal. A small anesthetic bag (1 to 2 liter size) is used, and breathing is assisted by giving the bag a light squeeze with each breath. It is best to maintain a constant flow of fresh gas to lessen the chances of depressed respiration.

In an orthopedic surgical procedure, intubation is rarely needed, and should be avoided unless absolutely necessary. If it is needed, however, there should be no hesitation to use it. Relaxant drugs are rarely needed during the operation. In a very disturbed child a pre-medication combination of 'Demerol' (50 mg), 'Phenergan' (25 mg) and 'Thorazine' (25 mg), made up in a 2.0 cc dose, is helpful. It is used in 1.0 cc amounts for each 20 pounds of body weight.

If a child has a seizure during the induction of anesthesia or during the operation, intravenous diazepam ('Valium') has replaced intravenous barbiturates and phenytoin sodium ('Dilantin') as the most effective form of medication. It is used in amounts of 1.0 cc (5 mg) per 40 pounds body weight.

Coinciding with the start of anaesthetization, an intravenous drip consisting of 2.5 per cent dextrose in 0.45 normal saline solution is set up; this is maintained during the entire operation as a safety factor in case emergency resuscitative drugs are required. Precordial stethoscope monitoring is used from start to finish, to provide a very early indication of possible cardiac or vagal reflex complication.

If a seizure occurs during surgery, it is considered to be a reaction to anesthesia and a prompt change is made to another gas. Surgical complications virtually never

*Normal child dose: meperidine 0.5 mg/lb body weight; atropine sulphate 0.01 mg/lb body weight.

occur, because the surgical team, each working on a limb, will complete a procedure in no longer than 45 minutes. Pneumatic tourniquets and controlled bleeding techniques minimize post-surgical bleeding.

Recovery Room

When surgery is completed, the patient is moved to the recovery room, where he is watched carefully until the full effects of anesthesia have dissipated. Since restlessness is short-lived, narcotics are never ordered. Constant turning, always keeping the head to one side, prevents asphyxiation from vomiting or excess thickened mucus. By keeping the patient as lightly anesthetized as possible, post-operative complications are generally avoided. If a child's breathing does become over-depressed, an oxygen mask or tent can be used. Other predicaments which may occur are atelectasis or aspiration pneumonitis, post-surgical bleeding and blood incompatibility reactions. These are all handled in the standard manner.

Post-operative Phase

As soon as the effects of anesthesia have worn off and the vital signs and reflexes are stable, the child is returned to his room in the pediatric ward where, especially if he is young, his parents await him.

For protection, he is placed in a body harness, and the side rails of the bed are elevated. His assigned nurse pays special attention to the limb(s) in the cast for changes in temperature, circulation or color and for bleeding or swelling. If an area of bleeding is noted on the cast it is outlined. If it increases in size, it is reported promptly to the surgeon. One should remember that wet plaster may act as a sponge, and a substantial amount of bleeding may occur before it will show on the cast.

The nurse pays special attention to body care at this stage, and elevates the limbs on pillows, rolled blankets or towels. Exposed toes or an exposed heel are not allowed to touch the bed, and frequent changes in body positions are in order to allay anxiety and fear. 'Valium' is generally started as soon as the child can swallow and retain food. Intramuscular 'Valium' can be used earlier if there is a need.

Aspirin and, occasionally, codeine will be used as pain-killers during the first 24 hours. Fluids are encouraged early, and it is standard to keep a record of voiding and bowel movements. A careful watch is made during this early post-operative phase for dehydration, renal complications, and respiratory distress.

Post-operative fever is a common complication. Temperature regulation mechanisms in cerebral palsied children are frequently disturbed, and thus great fluctuations can result from relatively minor triggering mechanisms. After surgery, temperature elevations may start immediately and may last for several days. Since the fever most often starts on the day of surgery, it tends to camouflage post-operative infections, but these must be considered in the differential diagnosis. The fever generally responds favorably to salicylates and fluid.

Parents are alerted to the child's needs, and are encouraged to help. The anesthetist and the surgeon visit the child on the ward as soon as they can, and the surgeon reviews with the parents in simple terms what was done and what he hopes to accomplish.

As soon as the cast is dry, the edges are lined with Saran Wrap and tape, and, after a final trim by the surgeon, several coats of shellac are applied. Where pressure phenomena are likely to occur, for example at the heel in a patient with a leg cast, the offending portions of the cast are removed in the immediate post-operative period. Where sensory impairment is present, painless ulcers often develop insidiously. This complication can be avoided by prophylactic care of pressure areas. Where ulcers do develop, they must be treated promptly. This can be done without loss of the cast, stability, or immobilization.

If there are no unexpected after-effects, the child is discharged within three days. During the hospitalization period the parents are taught how to turn the child over and position him, how to dress him, how to care for the cast, the bladder and the bowels, and feeding techniques. On the morning of discharge they are given prescriptions for medication, and a set of instructions, with dates for suture removal or cast change.

The physical therapy department of the hospital works conjointly with nursing staff, the parents, and the cerebral palsy center to make the transition from hospital to home as smooth as possible.

CONVALESCENCE

Seven to fourteen days after discharge, the child, still in a cast, is brought back to the cerebral palsy center and resumes a program of limited group participation. When the cast is removed approximately six to eight weeks later, he returns to full activity.

When the casts are removed, the physical therapist outlines specific exercise procedures that can be supervised by the parents. Warm baths are recommended three or four times a day. When in the tub, the child should be encouraged to bend his operated limb(s) and splash about. A skin softener should be added to the water. This helps get rid of the dry skin which has developed under the cast, and makes skin care easier. Following the bath, the parent should dry the child briskly with a towel, and gently but firmly stroke or massage the entire limb(s) for five minutes. This improves circulation, removes dry skin, and helps to build up a tolerance of handling which will have been lost, because the limb(s) have been overprotected by the plaster cast(s). Further massage helps to speedily restore in a natural way the sensory-kinesthetic intake-integration motor (output) pathways so necessary for learning.

When the therapist feels that the time is appropriate, the mother is shown how to move the limb(s) through normal ranges of motion with the child lying supine. She is shown how to support the child while he performs weight-bearing exercises. The therapist stresses that the child should be gently encouraged and never forced to co-operate in these exercises. During this phase, crawling or other forms of propulsion around the house are encouraged, as complete bed or chair rest is to be avoided. Slowly but firmly, the child is permitted to advance to the desired level of gross motor development.

In severely impaired children, where surgery has been performed to improve nursing care rather than ambulation, bathing, massage and movement of the limb(s) through ranges of motion are regularly scheduled. In these cases, there is no need for weight-bearing exercises.

In the child where ambulation is anticipated following surgery, the child is encouraged to proceed at an even pace through the normal stages of gross motor development starting with standing and progressing to independent walking and improved gait function. These methods have been outlined in detail previously (Denhoff and Langdon 1966).

To review, first the child is encouraged to stand unsupported in the corner of a room, using magazine splints if necessary to maintain knee extension. The splints are eliminated as quickly as possible, and the child is encouraged to shift weight from one hip to the other, while the parents hold him firmly about the hips in an upright position. Hand walking is quickly eliminated, and walking with the child's trunk supported by a harness or folded towel is encouraged. Then the parent stands behind the child, and provides additional support by pushing the buttocks forward to help establish a more erect position. A kitchen chair with metal buttons under the legs to reduce friction is then substituted for parent support and sequential walking patterns are encouraged until independence is established. When the child has gained independent walking, constant exposure to and stimulation of gross motor activities that fall within the sequential pattern of development should be encouraged.

Diet

The pre-hospital diet is resumed, but the continuing use of iron or fortified foods depends upon the hemoglobin level at discharge.

Some children are so upset by the hospitalization that they refuse to eat after they go home. In some, cyproheptadine ('Periactin'), an antihistamine with appetite stimulating qualities, is prescribed in doses of 4 mg three times a day. In others, thioridazine ('Mellaril'), a mild tranquillizer, given in doses of 5 to 10 mg three times a day, appears to stimulate appetite. Anabolic agents are not recommended, but have been used for four to eight weeks in severely handicapped marasmic children.

Sleep

Sleep resistance often presents a real problem in the convalescent care of these children. Phenobarbital is contra-indicated because it may cause irritability or excitement. 'Temaril', a phenothiazine derivative, in doses of 5 to 10 mg at bedtime, or 'Phenergan Forte' syrup (25 mg per teaspoonful) are helpful in inducing sleep.

Respect for the inherent weaknesses of cerebral palsied children and their families, meticulous attention to detail, and team work, will provide the orthopedic surgeon with a superior supportive base for the surgical approach to cerebral palsy.

REFERENCES

Denhoff, E., Langdon, M. (1966) 'Cerebral dysfunction: a treatment program for young children. *Clinical Pediatrics*, **5,** 1332.

CHAPTER 7

Deformities of the Spine and Pelvis in Cerebral Palsy

EUGENE E. BLECK

Because orthopedists have concentrated on locomotion and the limbs in cerebral palsy, spinal and pelvic deformities have been neglected. Exposition demands subdivision, but it is important that one should also be able to view these different facets of cerebral palsy as an integral whole. Spinal and pelvic deformities can be classified as follows:

Spinal deformities: (1) Scoliosis
(2) Thoracic kyphosis
(3) Lumbar lordosis
(4) Degenerative disc disease

Pelvic deformities: (1) Increased posterior inclination
(2) Increased anterior inclination
(3) Rotation
(4) Obliquity

Scoliosis

Prevalence

Recent studies (MacEwen 1968*a*, Robson 1968, Samilson 1969, Balmer and MacEwen 1970) have shown that the prevalence of scoliosis among the cerebral palsied is higher than in the general population. The prevalence in the general population has been estimated at 1.9 per 100, of whom only 0.2 per cent have curves of over 35 degrees. Reports vary as to the prevalence among the cerebral palsied. MacEwen (1968*a*) reports that 6 per cent of his patients with cerebral palsy had curves of over 30 degrees, and 21 per cent had curves over 10 degrees. Samilson's study of 906 patients who had cerebral palsy and were in a custodial institution demonstrated that 25.6 per cent had scoliosis. Our own observations of 315 cerebral palsied children (aged 18 months to 21 years) confirms a higher incidence (6.5 per cent) of scoliosis than in the general population. The discrepancies between our data and those of Samilson are probably a reflection of the type of cerebral palsied patient studied. Of Samilson's patients 65 per cent were non-ambulatory; in our patient group only 19 per cent were non-ambulatory.

Location of the Curve

Samilson's data are the most complete, and almost every type of spinal curve is represented. The distribution of the different types of scoliosis in his study is as follows:

Thoracic curve (T5 to L1 with apex at T9 or T10)—16 per cent
Lumbar curve (T12 to L5)—25 per cent
Thoraco-lumbar curve (T8 to L4)—45 per cent
Double main (or primary) curve (T5 to T11 and T12 to L5)—14 per cent

Etiology

Because of the marked differences observed between non-ambulatory and ambulatory cerebral palsied patients with scoliosis, the etiology will be discussed separately for each group.

Scoliosis in the non-ambulatory cerebral palsied. The spinal curvature in non-ambulatory patients appears to be of a similar type to that found in patients with other paralytic diseases such as poliomyelitis and muscular dystrophy (Figs. 1 and 2). Muscle biopsies of the sacrospinalis muscle in two of our cerebral palsied patients with scoliosis have shown evidence of neurogenic atrophy. At surgery not only were these muscles contracted, but the muscle fibers were pale pink, and fatty infiltration was apparent.

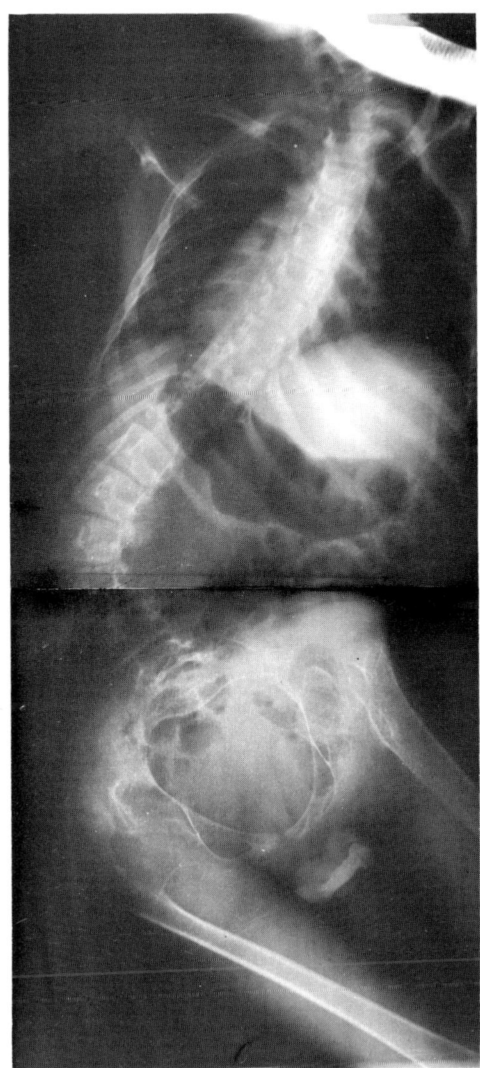

Fig. 1 (*left*). Paralytic scoliosis due to cerebral palsy; quadriplegia, spastic and athetoid type.

Fig. 2 (*right*). Radiograph of patient in Figure 1.

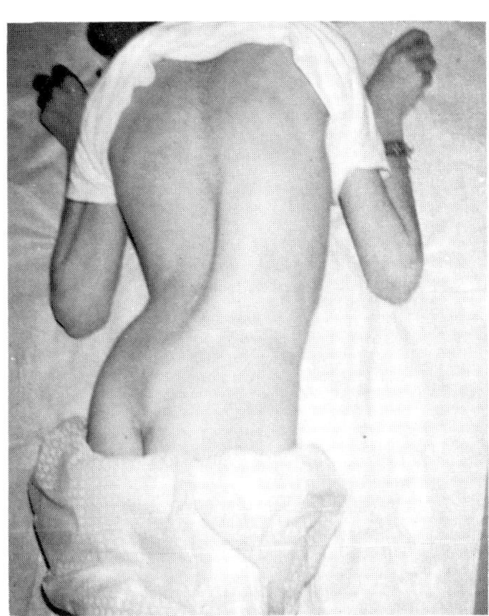

125

Thirty-nine per cent of Samilson's scoliotic patients were confined to bed; 92 per cent had severe spastic quadriplegia and/or tension athetosis. Most of the patients confined to bed had pelvic and hip deformities: 90 per cent had 'windblown' hips, with the femora directed towards the concavity of the curve; 75 per cent had contractures of the iliopsoas and adductors and 59 per cent had subluxated or dislocated hips. In view of these associated pelvic and hip deformities, it might be thought that muscle contractures below the iliac crest are the primary cause of the spinal curvature (Figs. 3 and 4). However, muscle release operations below the iliac crest have not altered the majority of spinal curves. Similar observations were made by James (1956) in his discussion of paralytic scoliosis.

Another possible cause of scoliosis in the non-ambulatory cerebral palsied is the asymmetrical persistence of the infantile incurvatum reflex (Galant's reflex) (see Chapter 4A, figure 14). This reflex is elicited by stroking the dorsal skin alongside the vertebral column, so that the trunk curves with the concavity on the stimulated side. It is present in all newborn infants, and disappears by the ninth day (Beintema 1968). Whether or not the incurvatum reflex persists in severely involved cerebral palsied

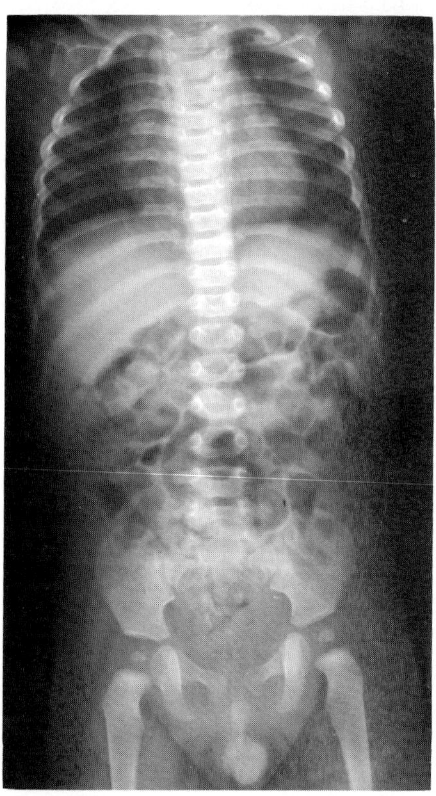

Fig. 3. Case J. F., aged 1 year, with spastic quadriplegia. Radiograph showing normal hips and spine.

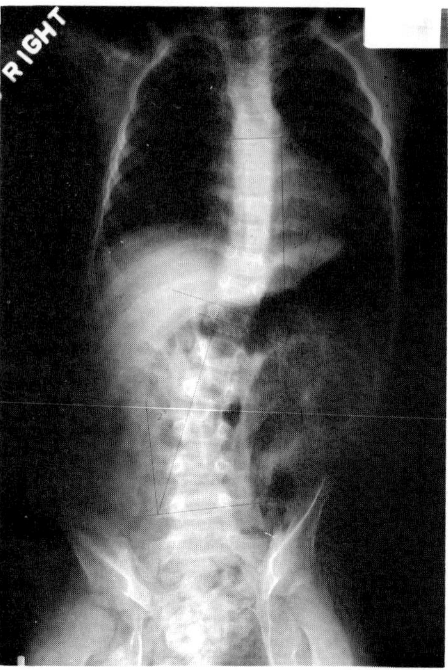

Fig. 4. Case J. F., aged 6 years. Non-ambulatory. Radiograph taken three years after bilateral adductor myotomy and anterior branch obturator neurectomy. Despite the release of hip muscles, he has developed scoliosis.

patients cannot be ascertained without further testing and long term follow-up studies. We tested this reflex in 16 of our patients who had scoliosis, and in 15 it could not be found; however, it was present in one 16-month-old patient with long C-curve of the thoraco-lumbar spine.

Scoliosis in the ambulatory cerebral palsied. Spinal curvatures in the ambulatory patient, though not nearly so frequent as those in the non-ambulatory, afford some interesting thoughts on etiology. The following observations may be pertinent.

(1) The prevalence of scoliosis in the ambulatory cerebral palsied is higher than reported in the general population.

(2) My own observations are that among ambulatory patients with cerebral palsy, those with ataxia most frequently develop scoliosis.

(3) The spinal curvature associated with ataxic cerebral palsy is similar to the idiopathic type (Figs. 5 and 6).

(4) Scoliosis is present in 80 per cent of cases of Friedriech's Ataxia (Farmer 1964).

(5) Animal experiments suggest that a sensory defect exists in cases of scoliosis. Liszka (1961) sectioned five spinal sensory roots on only one side in young rabbits and sheep; no motor paralysis occurred but scoliosis developed. MacEwen (1968b) also produced scoliosis in experimental animals by dorsal root resection.

(6) Brain changes, as demonstrated by EEG abnormalities and enlargement of the third ventricle, were reported in patients with scoliosis by Suzuki *et al.* (1964).

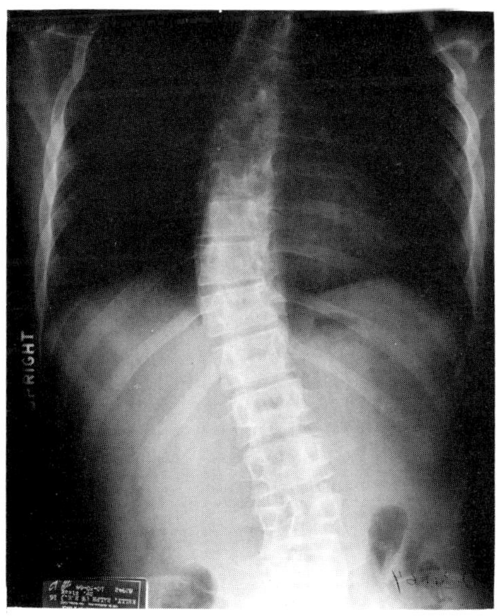
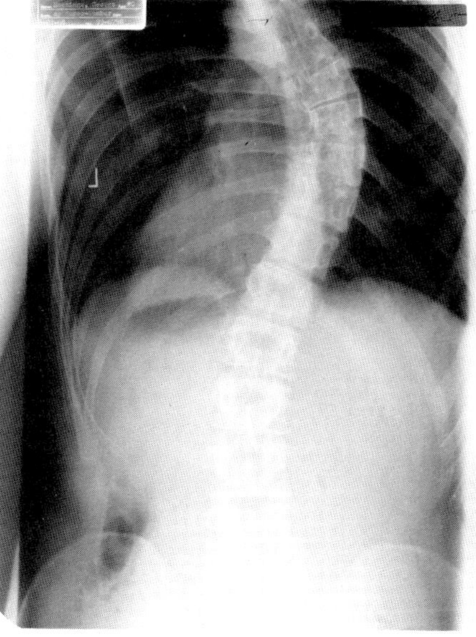

Fig. 5 (*left*). Radiograph, scoliosis, idiopathic type.
Fig. 6 (*right*). Right thoracic scoliosis in an ambulatory patient with the ataxic type of cerebral palsy. The curve location and pattern are indistinguishable from that of the idiopathic type of scoliosis.

(7) Dogs with experimental lesions of the caudate nucleus have developed scoliosis convex to the side of the lesion; destruction of the opposite caudate nucleus resulted in straightening of the spine (Martin 1965).

(8) An electromyographic study of 50 patients with progressive idiopathic scoliosis by Redford *et al.* (1969) demonstrated electrical activity in the sacrospinalis muscle on the convex side of the curve at the apex, but none on the concave side. These patients were tested lying prone. In non-progressive curves or those stabilized by spine fusion, no electrical activity was found with the patients either recumbent or upright.

(9) Enneking and Harrington (1969) reported that the articular cartilage of the inferior articular processes of the spine in cases of idiopathic scoliosis showed more cartilage derangement and retarded enchondral growth on the convex side of the curve. No increased osteoblastic or osteoplastic activity was found. Their study suggested that idiopathic scoliosis was due to extraosseous causes.

All available clinical and experimental data seem to confirm Martin's (1965) hypothesis that idiopathic scoliosis is a positive neuromuscular activity, and that the abnormal posture is due to a particular dysfunction of the central nervous system. The similarity between idiopathic scoliosis and the scoliosis found in ambulatory patients with ataxic cerebral palsy and in patients with Friedreich's ataxia lends further credence to the concept that all these forms of scoliosis are due to abnormalities in postural tone, possibly originating from a cerebral lesion. Some have denied the existence of postural tone, and have claimed that the muscles at rest show no electrical activity. However, the electromyographic study of de Vries (1964), who used highly sensitive electromyographic equipment, indicated that postural tone may be a reality.

That the non-ambulatory cerebral palsied patient has a lack of normal postural control is clear. Our continuing studies on locomotor prognosis in cerebral palsy (Bleck 1965) indicate that an important differentiating feature between those who walk and those who do not walk is the presence or absence of equilibrium reactions. Equilibrium reactions begin to appear normally in the six-month-old infant. Unless equilibrium reactions become sufficiently developed in patients with cerebral palsy, they never walk, despite minimal deformities (Bobath 1966). We have observed that even the most deformed patients will walk if they have normal equilibrium reactions. Those who have border-line equilibrium reactions usually require crutches. Consequently, the two types of cerebral palsied scoliotic patient, the ambulatory and the non-ambulatory, do blend with one common characteristic— namely, a varying deficiency of equilibrium reactions.

Treatment

As in all deformities, preventative measures should come first. No suggestions for prevention can be made, other than that one should attempt to find spinal curvatures early by clinical and radiographic examinations. One can anticipate that the non-ambulatory cerebral palsied child is a likely candidate for scoliosis, and in such cases routine radiographs of the spine would be in order.

The Milwaukee brace has not been used very much in severely spastic and athetoid patients with scoliosis. The brace is not easily tolerated (MacEwen 1968*a*). It

has been used in three of our young cerebral palsied patients, and none have
shown any decrease in the degree of spinal curvature. We have noted that the
Milwaukee brace does provide excellent head and trunk support for children who
cannot sit alone. However, because such children consistently lean to one side, their
necks tend to press uncomfortably against the side bars. We have modified the upper
chin and occipital support connecting bars of the brace, by using a large ring to
connect these two pieces. This ring has helped to relieve the discomfort.

At the age of ten years and over, provided that the spine is flexible, Harrington
instrumentation (1962) and spinal fusion can be performed with fairly good results.
When the curve is severe and rigid, halo-femoral traction prior to Harrington instrumentation has been recommended (MacEwen 1968a, Schmidt 1969). As might be
anticipated, the severely spastic patient is not easy to manage post-operatively. Plaster
casts are not well tolerated. Some athetoid patients have been treated without casts.
In all patients, bed rest of at least six months has been recommended (Figs. 7 and 8).

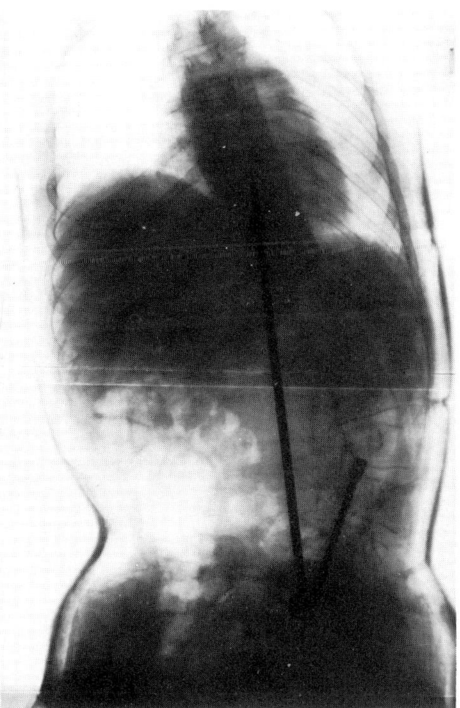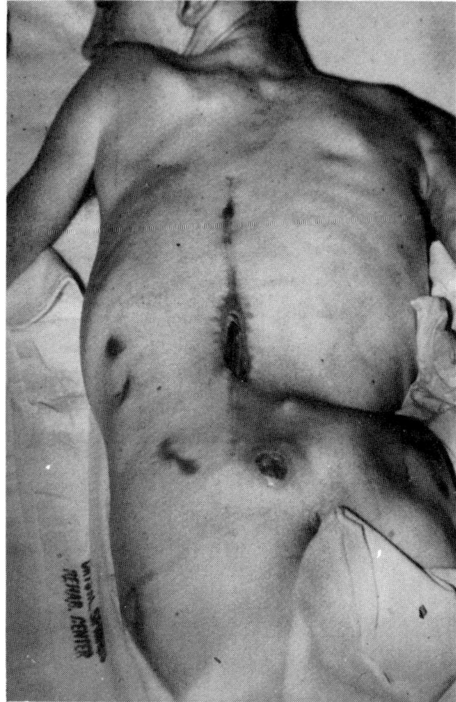

Fig. 7 (*left*). Radiograph of a 17-year-old spastic and athetoid quadriplegic patient after Harrington instrumentation and spinal fusion. The degree of fixed skeletal change precluded significant correction. A better
approach would have been anterior spinal fusion and Dwyer instrumentation followed by a second stage
posterior fusion and Harrington instrumentation. (For contrast in management of a similar case see Figs.
14a, 14b and 15)

Fig. 8 (*right*). Post-operative photograph of patient in Fig. 7. The longer Harrington rod eroded through the
skin, and was removed four months post-operatively.

Diazepam (Valium) does assist in relaxing the patient during this difficult time. Harrington instrumentation and spinal fusion while the curve is still slight seems a logical way of avoiding the difficult and protracted course when surgery is deferred until the curve becomes severe and grotesque (Gaines and Moe 1969). (Figs. 9 and 10). Radiographic analysis of the flexibility of the curve, by taking pictures during side bending and lateral compression, will decide its correctability (Figs. 11 and 12).

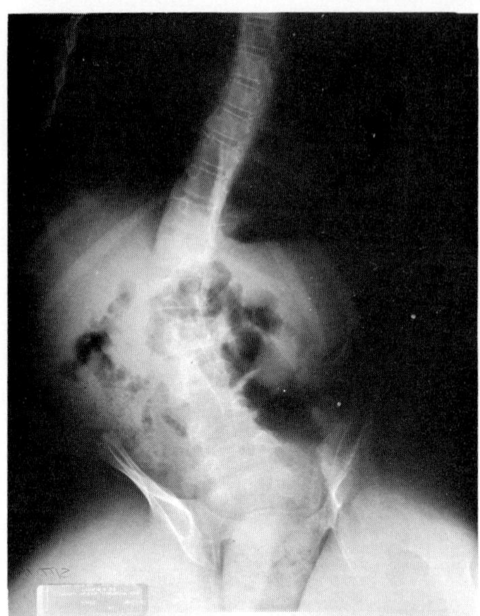

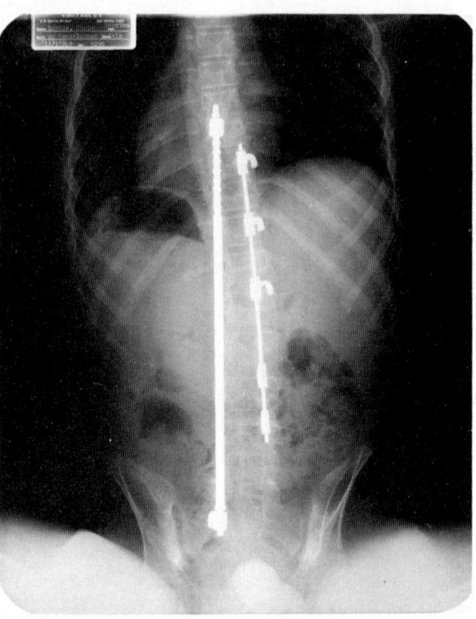

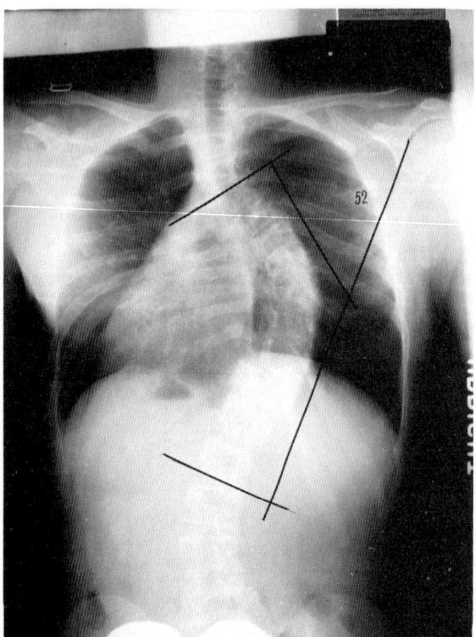

Fig. 9 (*above left*). Radiograph. Case C.L. aged 12 years. Early progressive paralytic scoliosis; the curve was flexible.

Fig. 10 (*above right*). Case C.L. Radiograph taken six years after Harrington instrumentation and spinal fusion into the sacrum. The value of early surgery in progressive paralytic scoliosis seems apparent in this result.

Fig. 11 (*left*). Radiograph showing scoliosis in patient with ataxic type of cerebral palsy.

The ataxic patient presents no special problems as far as Harrington instrumentation and spine fusion are concerned. He can be allowed to move about in a plaster jacket after three months of bed rest (Fig. 13). Because the extra weight of the plaster cast tends to make the ataxic patient top heavy, he may need a cane or walker during the three-month period of post-operative ambulation in the plaster jacket.

Dwyer's technique and instrumentation are a recent innovation in the operative correction of severe curves in children who have cerebral palsy. This technique of anterior interbody arthrodesis and correction using Dwyer's staples and cable system can be used for lumbar curves extending up to the lower thoracic vertebrae. The lower age limit for surgery appears to be between eight and nine years.

The advantages of Dwyer instrumentation in scoliosis in the cerebral palsied seem to be:

(1) better correction of severe lumbar curves;

(2) elimination of the need for a post-operative plaster body cast, and consequent avoidance of the pressure sores so frequently found in cerebral palsy patients (only a light-weight plastic axillary high body jacket is necessary);

(3) a high rate of successful spinal arthrodesis (Bonnett 1972) (Figs. 14*a*, 14*b* and 15).

In Bonnett's (1972) report of 13 cases of lumbar scoliosis corrected and stabilized with the Dwyer technique, there were four who required additional posterior fusion and Harrington instrumentation because of extensive deformity beyond the eight vertebrae corrected anteriorly. Harrington instrumentation and posterior

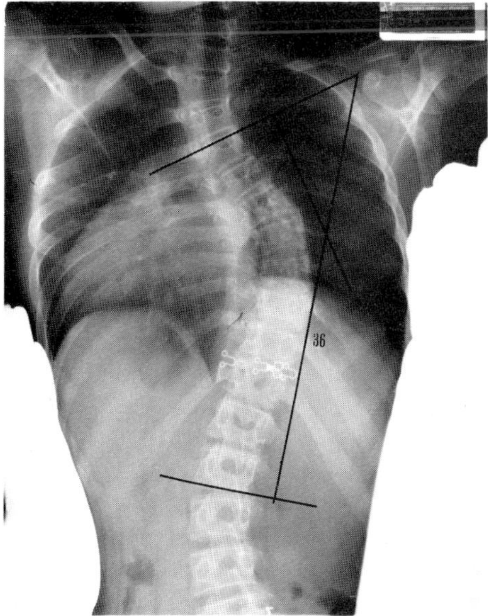

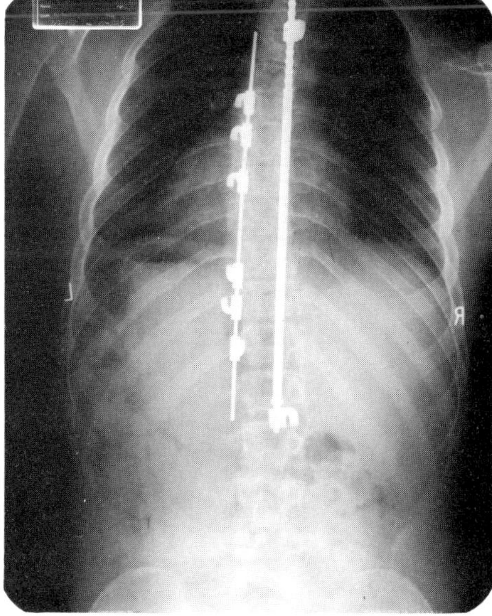

Fig. 13. Radiograph of patient with ataxic type of cerebral palsy, taken after Harrington instrumentation and spinal fusion for scoliosis. Good correction has been obtained, despite late loosening of the distal distraction hook.

Fig. 12. Radiograph. Lateral compression of the spine with gloved hands demonstrates the correctability of the curves shown in Figure 11.

131

spinal fusion may be required to correct co-existent thoracic kyphosis. Because it is impossible to apply the instrumentation lower than the fifth lumbar vertebra, posterior spinal fusion and Harrington instrumentation would be required at a second stage to correct those cases in which the pelvis is part of the curve.

Contractures below the iliac crest should be released. Radiographs of the pelvis, hips and spine of spastic patients from infancy onward will pick up early signs of subluxation of the hip. In a young patient, iliopsoas tenotomy and adductor

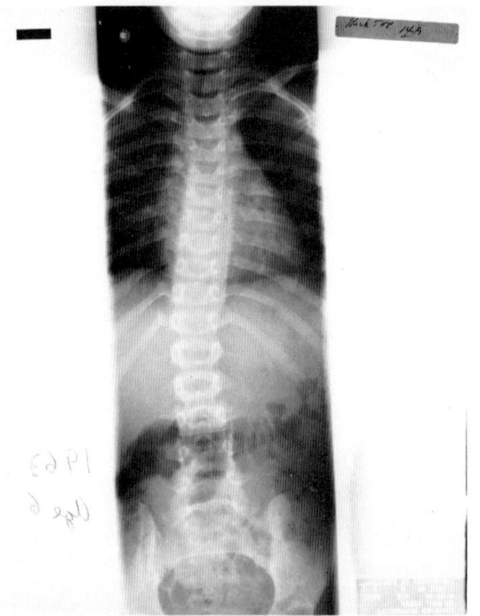

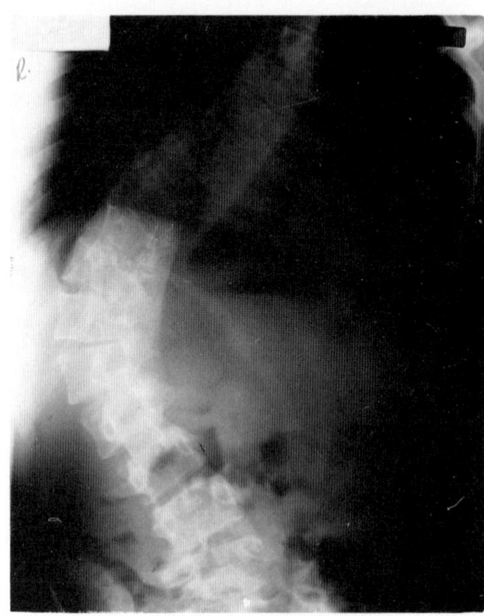

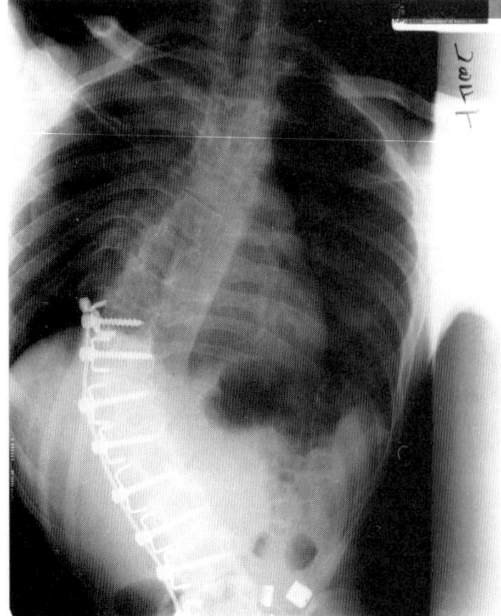

Fig. 14*a* (*above left*). Patient P.D.M. age six years. Cerebral palsy, spastic and athetoid quadriplegia. Radiograph shows a very slight spinal curvature.

Fig. 14*b* (*above right*). Patient P.D.M. age 15 years. Radiograph shows a severe thoraco-lumbar scoliosis. A Milwaukee brace had been worn for three years.

Fig. 15 (*left*). Patient P.D.M. Radiograph one year after anterior spinal fusion and Dwyer instrumentation.

myotomy with anterior branch obturator neurectomy can usually be relied upon to prevent dislocation of the hip and aggravation of the pelvic obliquity (Figs. 16 and 17). After such surgery, continued observation of the spine is essential; we have no proof that hip contractures alone are the initiating factor in scoliosis.

Thoracic Kyphosis

Many cerebral palsied children when first sitting up have a thoracic kyphosis without structural change. Bobath (1966) explained the kyphosis as a compensatory mechanism, to bring the trunk over the pelvis when the child has insufficient flexion of the hips due to extensor hypertonus.

Fixed thoracic kyphosis has been observed in spastic patients with ectodermal dysplasia (Fig. 18). These patients had contracted hamstring muscles, but lengthening of the hamstring tendons did not affect the kyphosis and only caused more lumbar lordosis (Fig. 19). Such patients would be better managed in the Milwaukee brace with a posterior pressure pad over the thoracic spine.

Thoracic kyphosis has developed occasionally in ambulatory patients who have excessive lumbar lordosis. Early correction of the lumbar lordosis by iliopsoas recession may obviate this compensatory kyphosis (Bleck 1971).

Forward cupping of the shoulders and a concomitant high thoracic kyphosis has been frequently observed in spastic patients, particularly in those who use crutches. Attempts to stretch the shoulder girdle into extension have not been successful. However, release of the pectoralis minor muscle in a young patient before fixed changes occur does seem to be a promising method of correcting the forward cupping of the shoulder.

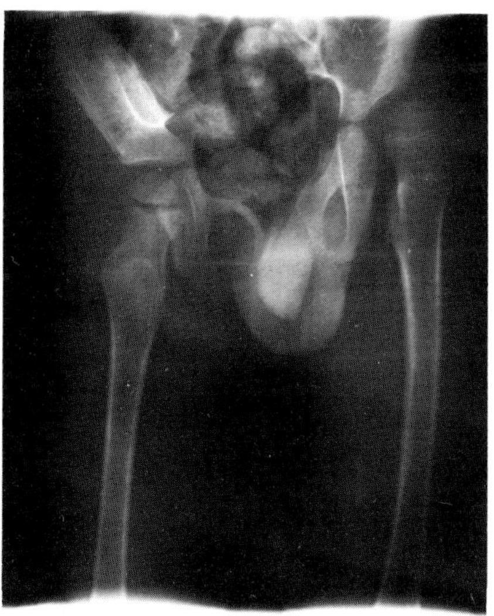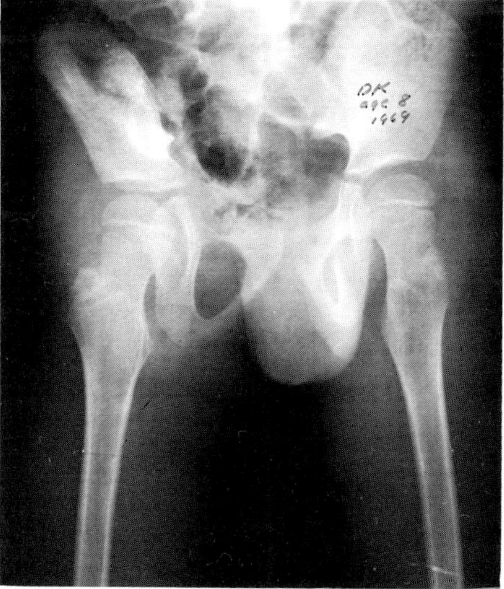

Fig. 16 (*left*). Case J.K., aged 4 years, spastic quadriplegia. Radiograph shows impending dislocation of the hip and pelvic obliquity.

Fig. 17 (*right*). Case J.K., aged 12 years. Radiograph taken after bilateral adductor myotomy, anterior branch obturator neurectomy and iliopsoas tenotomy. The hip has remained stable and normal.

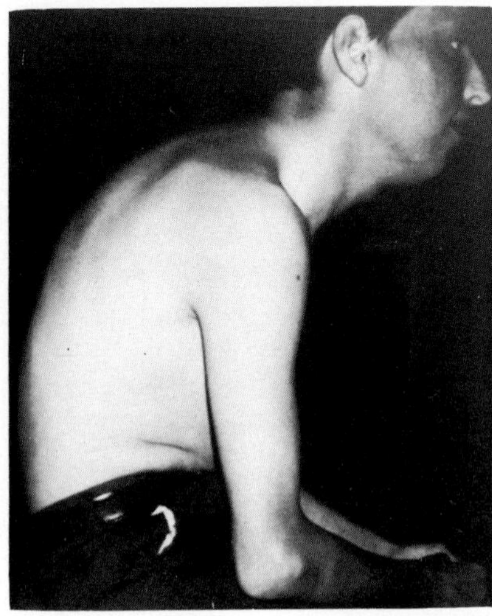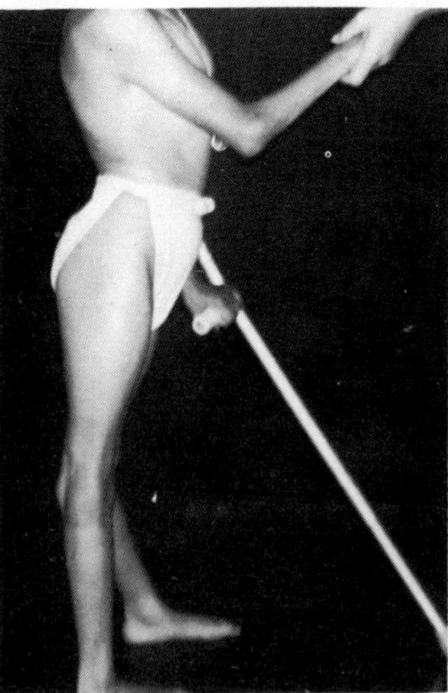

Fig. 18. Case J.R., aged 10 years. Spastic diplegia, ectodermal dysplasia, fixed thoracic kyphosis.
Fig. 19 (*right*). Case J.R., aged 14 years, four years after bilateral hamstring lengthening; spastic quadriceps caused severe back-knee; the thoracic kyphosis was unaltered.

Lumbar Lordosis and Pelvic Inclination

Lumbar lordosis and pelvic inclination are intimately linked in the patient with cerebral palsy, and consequently are discussed together.

Radiographic Measurement

Standing lateral radiographs of the lumbar spine, pelvis and proximal femora may be useful in spastic patients with lumbar lordosis and pelvic inclination for assessing the degree of deformity. The patients should be positioned so as to minimize pelvic and femoral rotation. In our experience, satisfactory radiographs can be made in about 95 per cent of patients (Bleck 1966, 1971). Since the degree of pelvic inclination is a measure of the degree of hip flexion deformity, we attempted in our studies to measure pelvic inclination by the Fick method; however, the pelvic landmarks were difficult to locate on the radiographs, and the method was abandoned. Instead it was decided to measure the sacro-femoral angle. Because the sacrum is part of the pelvis and rotates with it, this method was considered reasonably accurate. (The degree of independent sacral rotation through the sacroiliac joints is no more than four degrees.) With a hip flexion deformity, the relationship of the pelvis to the femoral shaft should be an indication of the severity of the deformity. The measurement was made by drawing one line across the top of the sacrum and a second line through the femoral shaft (Fig. 20). The intersection of these lines was the sacro-femoral angle. In normal children this angle varied from 45 to 65 degrees. In those with hip flexion deformities, standing with flexed knees causes the femoral shaft to become horizontally parallel with the top of the sacrum (Fig. 21), and standing with extended knees caused the top of the sacrum to become vertically parallel with the top of the sacrum (Fig. 22).

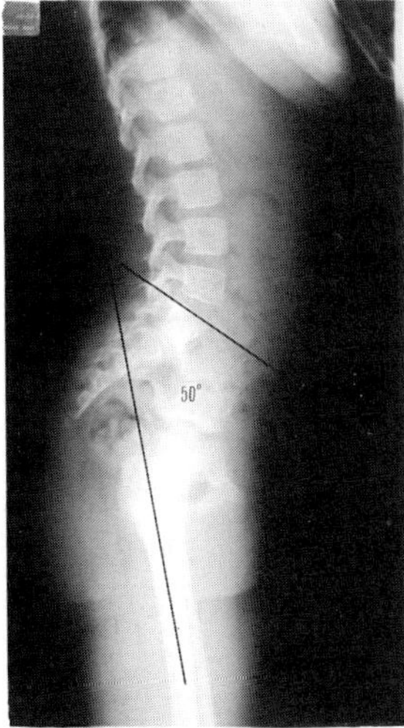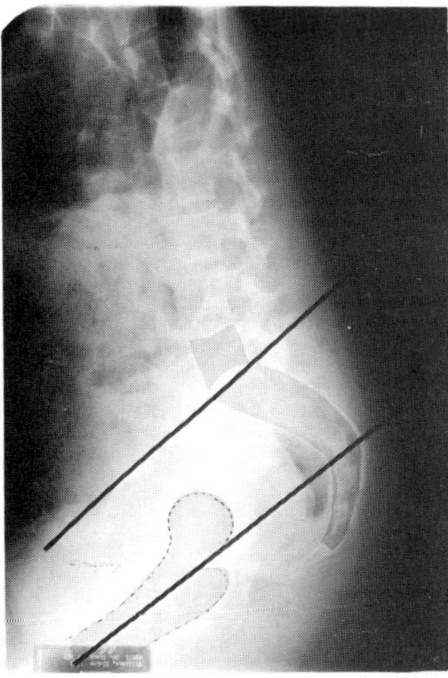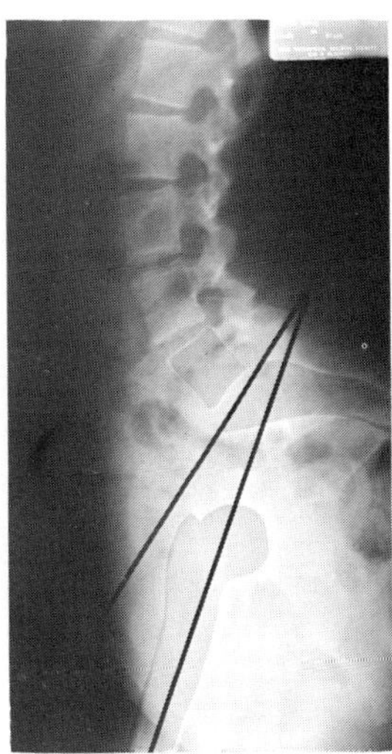

Fig. 20 (*left*). Standing lateral radiograph. The sacro-femoral angle is measured by drawing a line across the top of the sacrum and a second line along the shaft of the femur. The normal angle in children ranges from 45 to 65 degrees.

Fig. 21 (*centre*). Standing lateral radiograph of 12-year-old patient with spastic paraplegia. The hip flexion deformity was 45 degrees, and the knees were flexed 30 degrees. The sacro-femoral angle decreased, and the femoral shaft became horizontally parallel with the top of the sacrum.

Fig. 22 (*right*). Standing lateral radiograph of a 12-year-old patient with spastic paraplegia. The hip flexion deformity was 40 degrees; the knees were hyper-extended due to quadriceps spasticity. The sacro-femoral angle decreased, and the femoral shaft became vertically parallel with the top of the sacrum.

Biomechanical Analysis

The degree of lumbar lordosis in cerebral palsy is dependent upon the degree and direction of pelvic inclination. Pelvic inclination is dependent upon the degree of hip flexion deformity. With a hip flexion deformity, weight-bearing makes the lumbar spine and pelvis conform to the hip flexion deformity. The position of the knee decides the ultimate posture.

In spastic patients, two different compensatory mechanisms to the hip flexion deformity, with two different spastic patterns, can be observed (Bleck 1966, 1970, 1971). One pattern is a spastic quadriceps with a hip flexion deformity. In this pattern the pelvis is inclined anteriorly, the lumbar spine becomes lordotic, and the knees are extended (Fig. 23).

In the second pattern the patient has spastic hamstrings and a hip flexion deformity. The pelvis is inclined posteriorly to the point where it is finally checked by the anterior ligaments of the hip. The lumbar spine becomes flat and the knees flexed. These patients are sitting down while standing up (Fig. 24). In patients who have hip flexion/knee flexion patterns, forced extension of the knees, by bracing or by sectioning, lengthening and transferring the hamstring tendons, tends to increase the disability, by forcing the pelvis to rotate into excessive anterior inclination and so producing lumbar lordosis. The range of extension of the lumbar

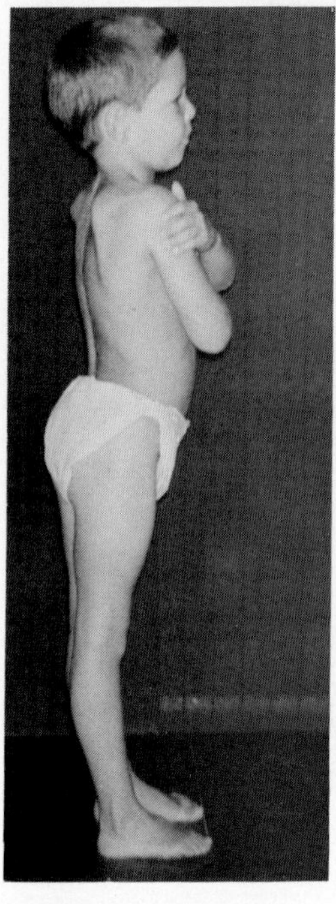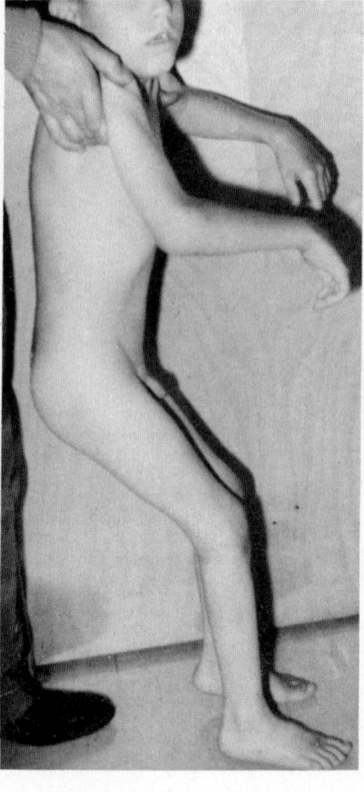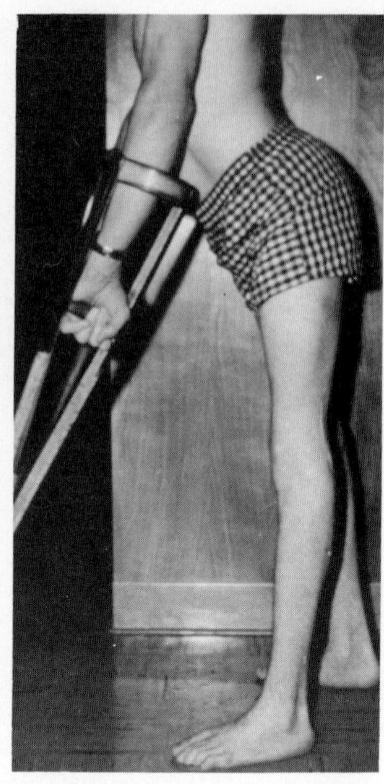

Fig. 23 (*left*). Posture of a spastic diplegic child, aged 7 years. One of two patterns of postural adaptation to the hip flexion deformity. In this child, the hip flexion deformity of 30 degrees was compensated by a severe lumbar lordosis, due to anterior pelvic inclination necessitated by bilateral quadriceps spasticity that kept his knees extended.

Fig. 24 (*centre*). The second type of postural adaptation to the hip flexion deformity. In this 13-year-old spastic diplegic child, the hip flexion deformity of 45 degrees was compensated by flexed knees, due to bilateral hamstring spasm and contracture that pulled the pelvis posteriorly and thus flattened the lumbar spine.

Fig. 25 (*right*). Posture of a 19-year-old patient with spastic diplegia. Picture taken ten years after bilateral hamstring transfer and eight years after Soutter hip muscle slide operation; the 45 degree hip flexion deformity present pre-operatively persisted. To compensate, the pelvis inclined far anteriorly, the lumbar spine became lordotic, and the patient was forced to lean forward on his crutches.

spine in such patients is limited, so that many also lean forward to maintain the center of gravity over their feet (Fig. 25).

Table I shows the sacro-femoral angles and the estimated hip flexion deformity of 45 spastic patients; those patients who had undergone hamstring lengthening, tenotomy or transfer, have had very low sacro-femoral angles. These low angles indicated excessive anterior pelvic inclination and lumbar lordosis. In most cases the lumbar lordosis appeared to take place at the lumbo-sacral articulation. In Figure 26 the angles between the bodies of the second lumbar vertebra and the fifth lumbar vertebra as measured from the standing lateral radiograph are plotted against the sacro-femoral angles of the 45 patients. No correlation between these two angles could be found. In the majority of the patients the lumbar angle was between 45 and 65 degrees.

TABLE I

Sacrofemoral angle of forty-five spastic children
(normals 45 to 65 degrees)

Patient	Age (years)	Surgery	Sacro-femoral angle (degrees)	Estimated hip flexion deformity (degrees)
L.S.	13	Bilateral intrapelvic obturator neurectomy (age 5); bilateral Yount fasciotomy (age 11); bilateral iliopsoas recession and hamstring transfer (age 12)	1	30
F.C.	18	Bilateral hamstring transfer (Eggers) (age 12)	3	20
B.T.	14	Bilateral semitendinosus transfer and semimembranosus lengthening (age 13)	8	10
J.B.	13	Bilateral hamstring lengthening and patellar advancements and rectus femoris release (age 11)	10	0
N.C.	15	Bilateral subtrochanteric derotation osteotomy (age 14); bilateral Yount-Ober fasciotomy (age 9)	11	40
J.B.	8	Bilateral semitendinosus transfer and semimembranosus lengthening (age 6)	16	60
S.H.	11	Bilateral tensor fascia femoris resection; bilateral hamstring lengthening (age 5)	18	30
D.D.	13	Bilateral iliopsoas recession (age 12)	20	60
S.B.	9	Bilateral iliopsoas tenotomy semitendinosus transfer and semimembranosus lengthening (age 8)	22	50
G.V.	7	None	25	15
J.M.	17	None	27	30
K.M.	11	Bilateral iliopsoas recession and rectus femoris release (age 9)	27	20
E.S.	8	Bilateral gastrocnemius lengthening (age 6)	27	30
B.V.	7	Bilateral gastrocnemius lengthening; left obturator neurectomy (age 3)	28	25
S.K.	8	Bilateral hamstring tenotomy (genu recurvatum)	30	25
R.B.	7	Bilateral iliopsoas recession (age 7)	30	40
R.B.	6	None	30	
C.H.	15	Bilateral semitendinosus transfer (age 12)	30	30
E.S.	6	Bilateral iliopsoas recession and rectus femoris release (age 6)	32	10
C.R.	5	None		
R.F.	7	None		
V.R.	7	Bilateral subtalar extra-articular arthrodesis (Grice) (age 6)	34	30
D.M.	9	None	35	40
B.B.	8	Bilateral iliopsoas recession and rectus femoris release (age 7)	35	15
S.A.	8	Bilateral iliopsoas recession and derotation subtrochanteric osteotomy, right (age 7)	38	30
C.C.	9	None	39	5
L.C.	8	None	40	20 (left hip only)

137

Patient	Age (years)	Surgery	Sacro-femoral angle (degrees)	Estimated hip flexion deformity (degrees)
G.R.	13	None	40	10
J.O.	6	None	40	20
W.R.	6	Bilateral subtalar extra-articular arthrodesis (Grice) (age 5)	40	15
J.H.	6	None	40	15
S.V.	4	None	40	5
C.A.	10	None	42	45
L.P.	9	Bilateral iliopsoas recession, semitendinosus transfer and semimembranosus lengthening (age 8)	42	15
J.R.	14	Bilateral hamstring tenotomy (age 7) (severe genu recurvatum)	43	60
R.H.	6	None	45	20
C.D.	6	Right iliopsoas tenotomy and subtrochanteric derotation osteotomy (age 4)	45	20
T.S.	6	None	47	20
P.C.	14	Bilateral iliopsoas tenotomy, hamstring lengthening, patellar advancements, varus subtrochanteric osteotomy (age 9)	47	15
C.R.	18	Bilateral iliopsoas tenotomy, adductor myotomy, anterior branch obturator neurectomy, hamstring lengthening and patellar advancements (age 11)	50	0
G.D.	15	Bilateral iliopsoas tenotomy, adductor myotomy, anterior branch obturator neurectomy, hamstring lengthening and varus subtrochanteric osteotomy (age 10)	50	20
J.H.	9	None	50	20
D.M.	5	Bilateral subtalar extra-articular arthodesis (age 4)	51	5
R.D.	7	Bilateral iliopsoas recession, adductor myotomy, anterior branch obturator neurectomy, rectus femoris release (age 6)	55	15
R.B.	11	None	65	5

Symptoms

Some of our older cerebral palsied patients complained of a low back pain associated with severe lumbar lordosis, and spondylolisthesis was discovered in three of the 100 spastic patients who had lateral radiographs of the lumbar spine. Two of these had undergone hamstring tendon transfer.

Treatment

In our experience, lumbar lordosis in spastic patients responds neither to exercises nor to corsets or braces. Recession or lengthening of the iliopsoas will decrease the lordosis in most cases (Bleck 1971). The sacro-femoral angle increased by a mean of 15 degrees (*i.e.* less lordosis) after iliopsoas recession, in 21 of 25 patients followed two to five years. The mean age of these patients at the time of surgery was seven years. Patients over the age of 12 years had fixed deformities, and reversing the lumbar lordosis by iliopsoas recession was unpredictable.

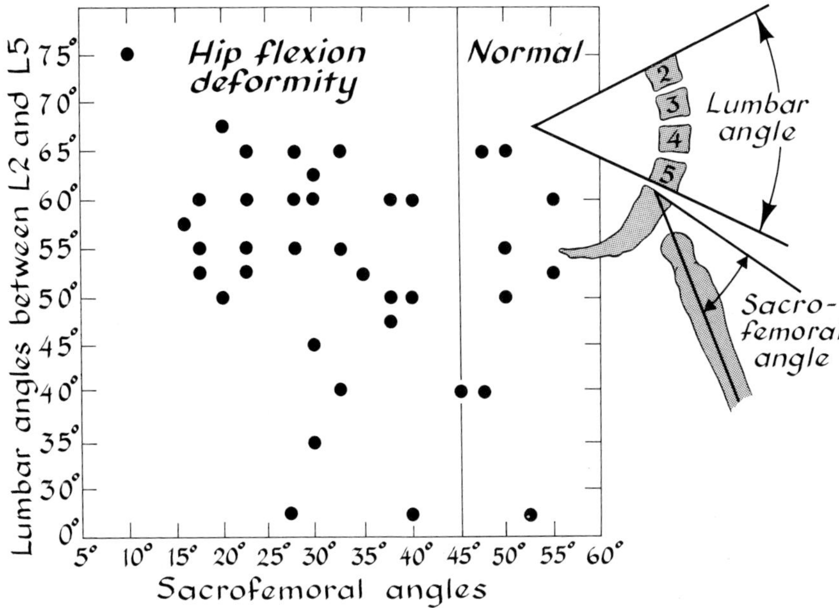

Fig. 26. Graphic representation of the angle between the bodies of the second lumbar and the fifth lumbar vertebrae, plotted against the sacro-femoral angle as measured on a standing lateral radiograph in normal children and those with hip flexion deformities. No correlation between these angles could be found.

Keats (1967) proposed iliopsoas tenotomy as a means of correcting lumbar lordosis. Bleck and Holstein (1963) reported on their experience with iliopsoas tenotomy in 17 spastic patients. A permanent severe loss of hip flexion power was found on 13-year follow-up. This severe weakness of hip flexion is an additional handicap, especially to a patient who never walked with crutches. Fortunately, our patients used crutches pre-operatively, and thus they compensated to some degree for the post-operative weakness of the hip flexion. Because of the observed weakness of hip flexion, I would recommend iliopsoas lengthening or recession rather than tenotomy. With iliopsoas recession the post-operative hip flexion ranged from fair to good.

Severe lordosis after hamstring lengthening or transfer can be prevented by examining the patient for a hip flexion deformity, confirming it with a standing lateral radiograph of the lumbar spine, pelvis and proximal femora, and then treating the hip flexion deformity.

Excessive lumbar lordosis in the spastic patient is a postural adaptation to the hip flexion deformity. The surgeon and the patient must decide if it is objectionable enough to merit surgical treatment. It may be that the existing muscle balance is the best possible, and that since correction of the lordosis will result in some weakness of hip flexion it is not worth doing (Fig. 27).

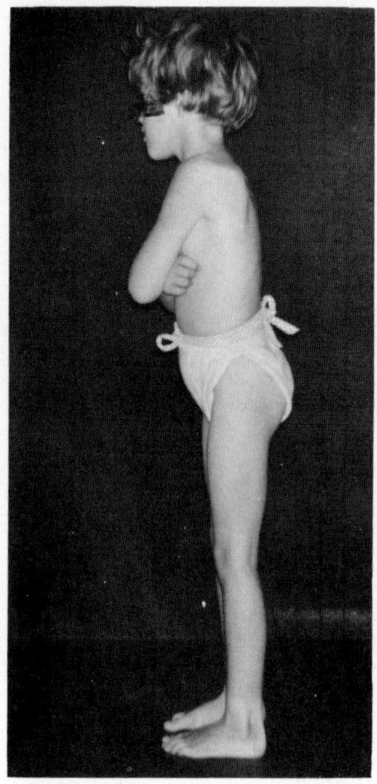

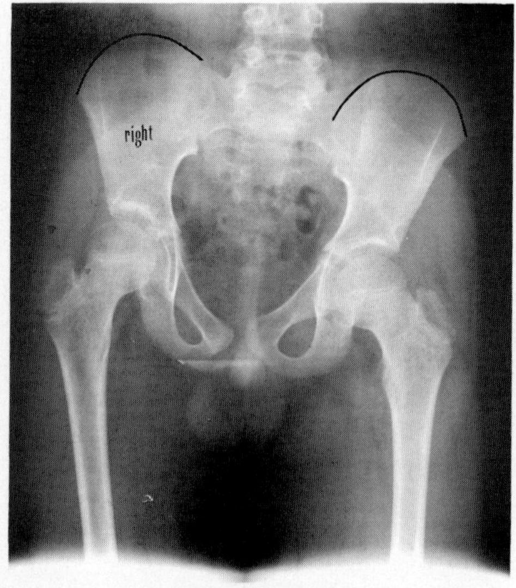

Fig. 27 (*left*). Eight-year-old patient with spastic para-plegia. This girl shows acceptable compensation for hip flexion deformities, spastic hamstrings and spastic quadriceps.

Fig. 28 (*above*). Case D.B. 10-year-old boy with spastic hemiplegia. Pelvic obliquity due to adduction con-tracture of the right hip.

Pelvic Obliquity

Etiology

Obliquity of the pelvis may be due to muscle contractures above and/or below the iliac crest. The most common cause is an adduction contracture of one hip. The mechanics of the adduction contracture, with apparent shortening of the involved extremity, are shown in Figure 28. Most of the severe pelvic obliquities are seen in non-ambulatory spastic or tension athetoid quadriplegic patients. In these patients muscle spasm and contracture occur above the iliac crest, and the pelvic obliquity is part of the scoliosis.

Treatment

In the ambulatory patient who has a pelvic obliquity and no scoliosis, other than a reversible compensatory lateral curve of the lumbar spine, the adduction con-tracture of the hip can be relieved with adductor myotomy and anterior branch obturator neurectomy. In the non-ambulatory patient in whom the pelvis is involved in the scoliosis, skeletal femoral traction, in addition to release of hip contractures, may be necessary to level the pelvis. The fusion of the spine should extend into the sacrum to keep the pelvis level. Surgical release of the quadratus lumborum and the sacrospinalis muscles on the high side of the pelvis has not been rewarding as a pro-cedure for correcting flexed pelvic obliquity.

Pelvic Rotation

Clinical Observation

Lateral (external) rotation of the pelvis has been noted in patients with spastic paralytic dislocations of the hip, the pelvis being rotated laterally on the side of the dislocation (Fig. 29).

Some spastic ambulatory patients who have asymmetrical involvement or hemiplegia have a persistent medial (internal) rotation of the pelvis. In these patients, the entire trunk and the shoulder girdle rotate forward, or they have a hip flexion deformity and limited external rotation of the hip.

Symmetrically involved ambulatory spastic diplegic or paraplegic patients exhibit a gait similar to that of patients who have had an arthrodesis of the hip. These patients can be shown to have pelvic-femoral fixation due to a flexion deformity of the hip. The best way to show this mechanism is to have the patient hold on to a table, stand on one leg, and let the other swing back and forth; as the femur flexes and extends, pelvic roll can be seen. When these patients with partly fixed hips walk, the pelvis rotates medially and then laterally in order to swing the limb through.

Biomechanical Analysis

When the foot is fixed, as in standing or in the stance phase of gait, the pelvis rotates about the head of the femur. Internal rotation of the pelvis in this situation is equivalent to external rotation of the hip. If the hip is limited in external rotation, the pelvis cannot rotate internally and stays behind, so that the opposite side of the pelvis is persistently rotated forward. Persistent unilateral internal pelvic rotation can also occur after too much correction of medial femoral torsion by derotation femoral osteotomy. It is better to leave about 20 degrees of internal hip rotation when performing a derotation femoral osteotomy.

In an attempt to correct persistent medial rotation of the pelvis, we did iliopsoas recessions in four patients. Post-operatively no significant change in the position of the pelvis occurred. In these patients, spastic rotation of the entire trunk precluded further corrective surgery.

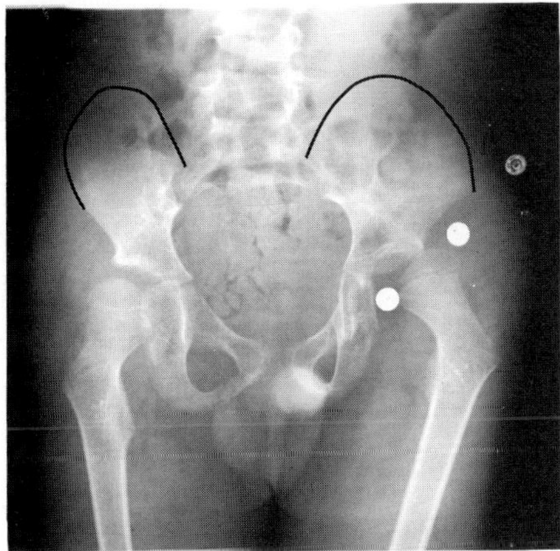

Fig. 29. Radiograph of patient with spastic quadriplegia. The pelvis is rotated laterally on the dislocated side.

Iliopsoas recession in hip flexion deformities has been found to decrease the degree of pelvic-femoral fixation and of pelvic rotation observed during gait.

Degenerative Arthritis of the Spine

Garrett and Stauffer (personal communication) told me in 1969 about several adult athetoid patients whose constant head and neck motion over the years caused neck pain. Narrow intervertebral disc spaces and hypertrophic spurring at the edges of contiguous vertebrae were evident on the radiographs. Immobilization with cervical collars and diazepam in divided doses was the initial treatment. Two of the four athetoid patients observed by Garrett and Stauffer had signs of spinal cord compression due to cervical spondylosis. Four cerebral palsied patients had anterior cervical spinal fusion.

I have had similar experiences with patients who have severe athetosis particularly involving the neck musculature. In one of these patients, constant rotation of the head and neck resulted in intractable unilateral cervical nerve root pain radiating into the hand. Conservative care using a collar, diazepam and cervical traction failed. Myelograms were negative. Tomograms showed a definite assymetry and widening of the intro-articular facets between the fifth and sixth cervical vertebrae. Anterior intervertebral disc excision and spinal fusion promptly relieved the symptoms (Figs. 30 and 31). Prolonged conservative treatment in athetoid patients who have cervical pain should probably be limited, and early surgery might be considered instead.

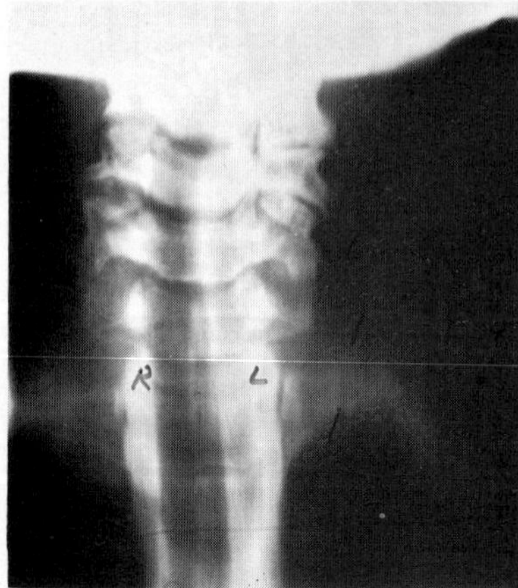

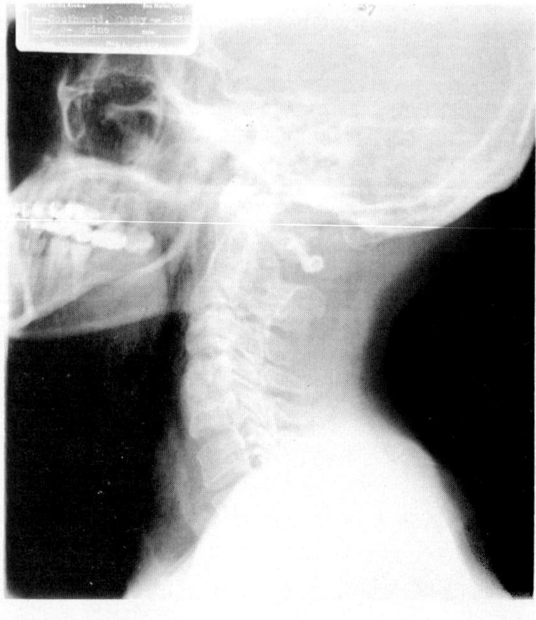

Fig. 30 (*above*). Case C.S., aged 23 years. Tension athetosis and intractable right side of neck and upper limb radiating pain. Tomogram shows asymmetrical intervertebral facets at C5-C6, with widening of the joint on the right.

Fig. 31 (*right*). Case C.S., Radiograph taken after anterior disc excision and spinal fusion at C5-C6 level. Patient asymptomatic.

Summary

Scoliosis in the cerebral palsied is more frequent than in the general population. Scoliosis in the non-ambulatory spastic quadriplegic is similar to scoliosis in other paralytic diseases, so management, while vastly more difficult, is no different. Early recognition, consistent observation, and early surgical treatment should be the program in managing this type of curve.

Scoliosis in the ambulatory cerebral palsied appears similar to idiopathic scoliosis, and the treatment program should be the same: early recognition, consistent observation, the Milwaukee brace, and Harrington instrumentation and posterior spinal fusion, or, if the curve progresses and decompensates. Dwyer instrumentation and anterior spinal fusion.

Thoracic kyphosis in cerebral palsy does occur, and can be treated during growth of the child with the Milwaukee brace.

Pelvic inclination and lordosis are linked together with a single etiology—a hip flexion deformity. Treatment of the lumbar lordosis entails correction of the hip flexion deformity. Lordosis may be prevented if the hip flexion deformity is recognised and treated in time; hamstring lengthenings or transfers are particularly ineffective in this respect unless the hip flexion deformity is corrected at the same time.

Increased internal and external pelvic rotation in spastic patients may be due to:
(1) limited internal hip rotation on one side;
(2) limited external hip rotation on one side;
(3) total trunk rotation as part of the spastic pattern;
(4) pelvic-femoral fixation mocking the gait of a patient who has fused hips.

Degenerative arthritis of the cervical spine has been reported in adult athetoid patients. Unrelieved symptoms have required anterior cervical spine fusion.

REFERENCES

Balmer, G. A., MacEwen, G. D. (1970) 'The incidence and treatment of scoliosis in cerebral palsy.' *Journal of Bone and Joint Surgery*, **52B**, 134.
Beintema, D. J. (1968) *A Neurological Study of Newborn Infants. Clinics in Developmental Medicine, No. 28.* London: Spastics Society with Heinemann.
Bleck, E. E. (1965) 'Locomotor prognosis in cerebral palsy.' *Paper presented at the Annual Meeting of the American Academy for Cerebral Palsy, Cleveland.*
—— (1966) 'Management of hip deformities in cerebral palsy.' *Current Practice in Orthopedic Surgery,* **3,** 75.
—— (1971) 'Postural and gait abnormalities caused by hip flexion deformity in spastic cerebral palsy. Treatment by iliopsoas recession.' *Journal of Bone and Joint Surgery,* **53A,** 1468.
—— Holstein, A. (1963) 'Iliopsoas tenotomy for spastic hip flexion deformities in cerebral palsy.' *Paper presented at the Annual Meeting of the American Academy of Orthopaedic Surgeons, Chicago.*
Bobath, K. (1966) *The Motor Deficit in Patients with Cerebral Palsy. Clinics in Developmental Medicine, No. 23.* London: Spastics Society with Heinemann.
Bonnett, C. (1972) 'Anterior spinal fusion with Dwyer instrumentation for lumbar scoliosis in cerebral palsy.' *Paper presented at the Annual Meeting of the Western Orthopedic Association, Houston, Texas.*
DeVries, H. A. (1964) 'Muscle tonus in postural muscles.' *American Journal of Physical Medicine,* **44,** 275.

Eberhart, H. D., Inman, C. T., Saunders, J. B.de C. M., Levnes, A. S., Bresler, B., McCowan, T. D. (1947) 'Fundamental studies of human locomotion and other information relating to the design of artificial limbs.' *A Report to the National Research Council, Committee on Artificial Limbs, Berkeley, Calif.*

Enneking, W. F., Harrington, P. (1969) 'Pathological changes in scoliosis.' *Journal of Bone and Joint Surgery,* **51A,** 165.

Farmer, T. W. (Ed.) (1964) *Pediatric Neurology.* New York: Hoeber.

Gaines, D. L., Moe, J. H. (1969) 'Scoliosis in cerebral palsy.' *Paper presented at the Annual Meeting of the American Academy for Cerebral Palsy, Las Vegas, Nev.*

Garrett, A. L., Perry, J., Nickel, V. L. (1961) 'Stabilization of the collapsing spine.' *Journal of Bone and Joint Surgery,* **43A,** 474.

Garrett, A. L. (1969) *Personal communication.*

Goldstein, L. A. (1966) 'Surgical management of scoliosis.' *Journal of Bone and Joint Surgery,* **48A,** 167.

Harrington, P. R. (1962) 'Treatment of scoliosis. Correction and internal fixation by spine instrumentation.' *Journal of Bone and Joint Surgery,* **44A,** 591.

James, J. I. P. (1956) 'Paralytic scoliosis.' *Journal of Bone and Joint Surgery,* **38B,** 660.

Keats, S. (1967) 'A simple antero-medial approach to the lesser trochanter of the femur for release of the iliopsoas tendon.' *Journal of Bone and Joint Surgery,* **49A,** 632.

Liszka O. (1961) 'Spinal cord mechanisms leading to scoliosis in animal experiments.' *Acta Medica Polonica,* **2,** (1), 45.

MacEwen, G. D. (1968*a*) 'The incidence and treatment of scoliosis in cerebral palsy.' *Paper presented at the Annual Meeting of the American Academy for Cerebral Palsy, Miami Beach, Fla.*

—— (1968*b*) 'Experimental scoliosis.' *in* Zorab, P. A. (Ed.) *Proceedings of a Second Symposium on Scoliosis; Causation.* Edinburgh: Livingstone. p. 18.

Martin, J. P. (1965) 'Curvature of the spine in post-encephalitic Parkinsonism.' *Journal of Neurology, Neurosurgery, and Psychiatry,* **28,** 395.

Murray, M. P., Drought, A. B. in Kory, R. C. (1964). 'Walking patterns of normal man.' *Journal of Bone and Joint Surgery,* **46A,** 335.

Oi, T. (1966) 'Electromyographic studies on scoliosis.' *Journal of the Japanese Orthopedic Association,* **40,** 71.

Redford, J. B., Butterworth, T. R., Clements, E. L. (1969) 'Use of electromyography as a prognostic aid in the management of cerebral palsy.' *Archives of Physical Medicine and Rehabilitation,* **50,** 443.

Robson, P. (1968) 'The prevalence of scoliosis in adolescents and young adults with cerebral palsy.' *Developmental Medicine and Child Neurology,* **10,** 447.

Samilson, R. L., Bechard, R. (1973) 'Scoliosis in cerebral palsy.' *Current Practice in Orthopedic Surgery,* St. Louis, Mo.: C. V. Mosby Co. p. 183.

Schmidt, A. C. (1969) 'Osteotomy of the fused scoliotic spine and the use of the halo traction apparatus.' *in American Academy of Orthopaedic Surgeons Symposium on the Spine.* St. Louis: C. V. Mosby.

Suzuki, J., Inoue, S., Tsuji, K., Mitsuhasi, M. (1964) 'Studies on the brain changes in scoliosis.' *Journal of the Chiba Medical Society,* **40,** (3), 165.

CHAPTER 8

The Hip in Cerebral Palsy

W. J. W. SHARRARD

Introduction

Deformity at the hip is the second most common orthopaedic problem in cerebral palsy (Pollock and Sharrard 1956). If patients with spastic hemiplegia or with varieties of cerebral palsy other than spasticity are excluded, some measure of hip deformity develops in 95 per cent of patients, notably those with spastic quadriplegia, triplegia or diplegia. In some, the deformity, usually adduction deformity, does not become sufficiently severe to disturb function or to require orthopaedic surgical treatment, but in our experience 72 per cent of patients with spastic or combined spastic and athetoid quadriplegia, triplegia or diplegia have required at least one operative procedure in relation to one or both hips during childhood.

The most serious deformity that can develop in the lower limb in cerebral palsy is dislocation of the hip. Before dislocation develops, progressive limitation of abduction and extension of the hip can be recognized, if the lower limbs of a child known to have cerebral palsy are assessed at regular intervals from as early a date as possible. Dislocation usually takes many months or even years to develop, so it should be possible in most instances to anticipate, and to take measures to prevent, the occurrence of this serious complication. There are, nevertheless, a few children who because dislocation has developed so rapidly or because orthopaedic advice has not been sought sufficiently early, present with established dislocation for orthopaedic management. Persistent neonatal reflexes, such as the Galant response, may increase the likelihood of dislocation.

The Assessment of the Hip in Cerebral Palsy

The function of the hip in cerebral palsy needs to be assessed in respect of gait, stance, posture, passive movements, muscle power and radiological appearances. Cerebral palsied children are easily disturbed by unfamiliar circumstances and surroundings, and they may require to be examined on two or three occasions in order to establish reliable and consistent findings. For formal examination of the hip joint, it is often better that a young child should be examined sitting or lying on his mother's lap rather than in isolation on an examination couch.

Gait

In a child who is able to walk, a study of the gait needs to take note of any dipping when weight is borne on the hip or of a tendency to lurch to one side. A

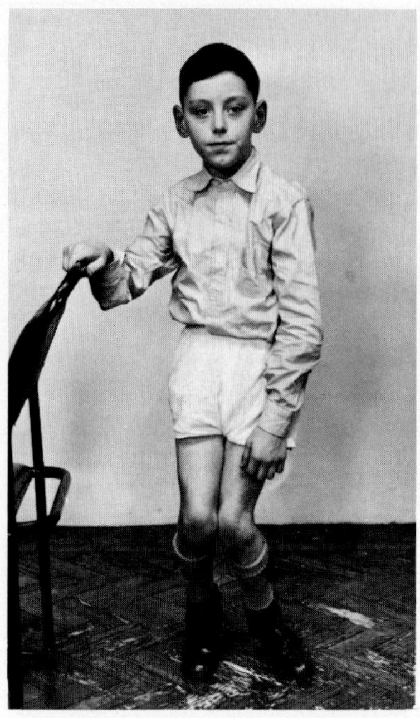

Fig. 1. Stance in a child with bilateral gluteal weakness and flexor and adductor spasticity.

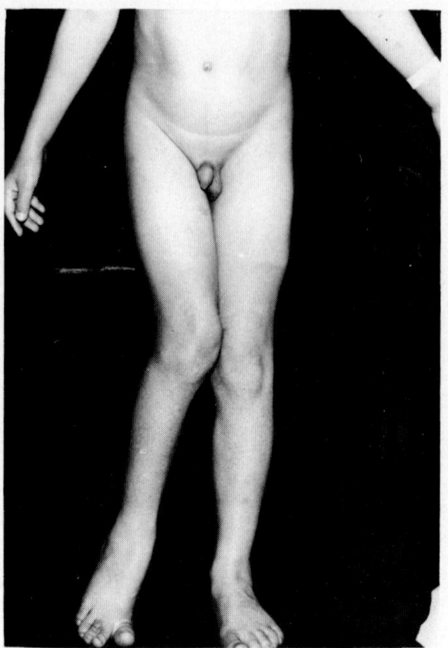

Fig. 2. Stance in a child with asymmetrical spasticity of the right hip flexors and adductors.

dipping gait may be due to weakness of the hip abductors, and this may be confirmed by the presence of a positive Trendelenburg's test. Spasm in, or shortness of, hip extensor muscles may be revealed by a short forward stride and a tendency to rotate the pelvis to increase the length of the stride. (Short stride may also be due to tight hamstrings or activity of stretch reflex in the hip flexors during the swing phase of the gait.) Weakness of hip extension or a fixed flexion deformity of the hip is revealed by a gait with the hips and knees flexed and with an exaggerated lumbar lordosis.

Stance

In a child who is able to stand but cannot walk, or in one who has not yet learnt how to stand but who can be placed on to his feet in a vertical position, observation can be made of the posture of the limbs in the vertical position. In some children the vertical position tends to produce an exaggerated extensor response with the hips in the extended and adducted position, whilst in others, there is a tendency for the hips to go into flexion and adduction. Some children are able to stand erect for a short time and then gradually sink down into flexion and adduction of the hips (Fig. 1). Where the involvement is asymmetrical, the child may be able to stand on one leg whilst the other leg passes over it into flexion and adduction (Fig. 2).

Posture

In any child, whether able to stand or not, the general posture of the limb at rest is significant. The hips should normally lie in 20 degrees of abduction and neutral rotation. Any excessive spasm or shortness of the adductors alters this posture, so that the knees are brought towards each other. The hips too may lie in a position of medial (internal) rotation, while in a few cases they may be externally rotated. The posture of the trunk should be observed at the same time, and particular attention should be paid to any obliquity of the pelvis as shown by the relative levels of the iliac crests. Shortening, true or apparent, of the lower limbs should be measured if there is any clinical suggestion of limb inequality.

The posture of the hips should always be considered in association with the posture of the pelvis and lumbar spine, particularly if there is any lumbar lordosis or scoliosis. If pelvic obliquity or lumbar lordosis is present, the examination of the hips should include an examination of the trunk musculature and trunk reflexes.

Passive Movements and Spasticity

An examination of the range of passive movements at the hip is most important in the determination of the need for surgery in cerebral palsy. The object is not just to discover any limitation of movement at the joint, but to estimate the degree of spasticity and the amount of true shortening of muscle groups or individual muscles controlling the hip.

The movements to be assessed are abduction, adduction, flexion, extension and medial and lateral rotation.

The range of abduction of the hips should be tested with the hips and knees extended. This is because testing with the hips and knees in the extended position is more relevant to future walking, and because it will reveal any limitation of abduction due to shortness of the gracilis or medial hamstring muscles that is masked when the knees are flexed. A comparison between the range of abduction with the hips and knees flexed and that with the hips and knees extended may be valuable in indicating shortness of either of these two muscles. Passive abduction needs to be made slowly and steadily, the aim being to avoid induction of reflex spasm in the adductors until the limits of the range of abduction are reached. In a younger child, attempts to abduct beyond the range allowed by short adductors, will cause pain, and forcing beyond this point should be avoided or the child's confidence will be lost. The position of the two superior iliac spines should be noted whilst abduction is being tested, or gross limitation of abduction in one hip combined with a good range of abduction in the other hip may be taken for a fair range of abduction in both hips.

In most normal children below the age of three years, the range of passive abduction with the hips extended should be at least 80 degrees. Between the ages of three and ten years, the range of abduction should be between 60 and 70 degrees, and at the end of growth it should be 50 to 60 degrees. The degree of spasticity of the adductors can be assessed by bringing the knees together, then abducting the hips as rapidly as possible to determine the point at which adductor spasm blocks abductor movement. If abduction is blocked at 20 degrees, spasticity is severe; if blocked at 35 to 40 degrees, it is moderate, and beyond this range it is mild. Spasticity and shortness are likely to be most evident in the adductor longus and gracilis, whose tendons can be palpated easily in the groin.

The range of passive extension in the normal hip is not great, even in childhood, and the development of limitation of extension or fixed flexion often goes unrecognised in its early stages, especially in the presence of compensatory lumbar lordosis.

The presence of fixed flexion of a hip can be demonstrated by Thomas' test, the opposite hip being flexed fully to eliminate any compensatory lumbar lordosis.* The hip may flex to 45 degrees or more, and some of this flexion may be due to spasm of the flexor muscles, especially the iliopsoas muscle. The true degree of shortening of the flexor musculature must be determined by downward pressure on the front of the opposite thigh by a second individual. In an older child, it may only be possible to discover the precise amount of fixed flexion deformity when the child is anaesthetised. If there is no fixed flexion deformity, limitation of extension may be present; this is best determined with the child lying prone, care once again being taken to ensure that apparent extension of the hip is not arising from extension of the pelvis on the lumbar spine.

Limitation of extension or fixed flexion may be due primarily to shortness of the iliopsoas, the tensor fasciae latae, the rectus femoris or a combination of any of these. The part played by individual muscles can be assessed by discovering the limitation of extension that is present with the hip internally and externally rotated (which affects the length of the iliopsoas), with the hip adducted and abducted (which affects the tensor fasciae latae), and with the knee flexed or extended (which affects the length of the rectus femoris). Spasm in the hip flexor muscles can be demonstrated by eliciting the stretch reflex in the hip flexors during the course of the performance of Thomas' test.

The most common form of limitation of flexion of the hip, that due to shortness of the hamstring muscles, is tested for with the knees extended, and is indicated by a limited range of straight leg raising. Limitation of flexion due to shortness of the gluteus maximus is much less common, and is shown by limitation of hip flexion with the knee flexed.

Limitation of rotation movements of the hip, particularly of external rotation, is commonly associated with combined flexion and adduction deformity. The mechanisms involved in its production are complex. Shortness of the iliopsoas tends to produce limitation of internal (medial) rotation. On the other hand, tightness of the tensor fascia lata produces limitation of external (lateral) rotation, and when the hip is flexed, shortness of the adductors tends to do the same. The range of rotation is best determined with the hips extended as much as possible, and with the hips in neutral abduction, unless there is gross fixed adduction deformity. After testing for limitation of rotation, it is often useful to make a clinical assessment of anteversion, by noting the direction in which the lateral surface of the greater trochanter points relative to the plane of the hip joint, when the knee is facing forwards. Spasm in

the internal (medial) or external (lateral) rotators of the hip may be present, sometimes both the internal and the external rotators may be affected, in which case the
range of movement in both directions is limited.

Muscle Power

In a child who is sufficiently old and sufficiently mentally developed to be able
to perform isolated movements, the power of movements of flexion, extension,
adduction, abduction and rotation in the region of the hip can be determined and
recorded using the accepted system of grading from 0 to 5; however, in a cerebral
palsied child with a hip deformity this can be a difficult procedure.

It is seldom possible to define activity in individual muscles in cerebral palsy, but
the activity in muscle groups and the ability to perform movements can be more
reliably assessed. When there is considerable spasticity of antagonist muscles, for
instance the adductor muscles, the power of active abduction is best shown by preliminary passive stretching of the adductors by the examiner. The child is then asked
to maintain abduction, either against gravity whilst lying on the opposite side, or with
gravity eliminated whilst lying on his back.

In a younger child, or in one who is unable to communicate or to respond to
requests to perform movements, assessment is even more difficult, but it should still
be possible to attempt a provisional assessment of muscle activity in the region of the
hip. Activity in the hip abductor muscles, for example, can be assessed by lying the
child on his side, abducting the hip as far as possible, and then allowing it to fall. A
child who has good power in the hip abductors will bring them into action to prevent
the abducted limb from falling down to strike the opposite limb. If the limb does fall
easily, and particularly if it strikes the other limb, or strikes the ground, this is an
indication of abductor power of less than grade three.

The power of hip extension is more difficult to determine, but an attempt should
be made to do this by placing the child prone on the table with the hips flexed over the
side of the table. The limbs are then lifted up into the extended position and the child is
asked to maintain the hip in extension either with the knee flexed or extended. In a
young child, the thigh is allowed to drop, to assess whether there appears to be any
activity in the gluteus maximus or hamstring musculature. The power of rotation movements is extremely difficult to assess and is seldom of specific value in cerebral palsy.

Radiological Appearances

Radiographs should always be taken of the hips on the first attendance for
orthopaedic examination. Particularly where there is coxa valga or increased femoral
anteversion, radiographs should be repeated at six-month intervals. Ordinarily, an
antero-posterior view with the child lying in his natural posture in the supine position is
sufficient, but, in the presence of apparent valgus of the femoral neck, it may be useful
to take a second radiograph with the hips internally rotated as much as possible. In
certain circumstances, for instance when it is intended to consider the need for rotation
osteotomy, special views to demonstrate anteversion of the femoral neck may be
attempted (Lewis *et al.* 1964). However, as Samilson *et al.* (1972) point out, measurement by the method described by Ryder and Crane (1953) or Magilligan (1956) some-

times cannot be employed because of difficulty in positioning the patient. If there is a suspicion of subluxation of the hip, arthrography may be useful, especially in young children.

The features that need to be assessed are: the position of the femoral head in the acetabulum; the continuity of Shenton's line; the presence of valgus or ante-version of the femoral neck; the slope of the acetabulum; the state of development of the upper femoral epiphyses; the position of the shaft of the femur in relation to the pelvis; the position of rotation of the hip as shown by the visibility of the lesser trochanter; and the obliquity of the pelvis. It is useful also to include the lumbar spine, if the patient shows clinical evidence of obliquity of the pelvis, which may be due to lumbar scoliosis. The features that may be encountered in subluxation or dis-location of the hip will be discussed later.

The Mechanism of Deformity at the Hip

In cerebral palsy, the commonest hip deformity is an adduction and flexion de-formity. Spasticity is commonly present in the hip adductor, hip flexor and ham-string muscles, and these muscles are usually strong as well as over-active. It is tempting to assume that flexion or adduction deformity arises simply because of spasticity in these muscle groups, but this theory fails to explain why, in 20 per cent of spastic quadriplegic patients, no deformity ever develops; it also fails to explain why deformity may develop rapidly in one patient and more slowly in another, though both appear to show the same degree of adductor spasticity and are having the same regime of management.

The key to the development of deformity lies not so much in the spastic muscles but in their opponents. In spastic quadriplegia or diplegia, not only are the adductor muscles spastic, but the gluteal abductors and extensors are often weak, as noted by Mathews *et al.* (1953). If an assessment is made of the power of hip abduction before any deformity has developed, some children show normal or almost normal hip abductor power, many show diminished abductor power at about grade 3 (anti-gravity), and some show considerable weakness, which occasionally amounts to almost complete functional paralysis of abduction. This weakness is primarily weakness of cerebral origin, and does not necessarily imply changes in the abductor muscles such as might be associated with lower motor neurone denervation, though there may be wasting when the abductors are demonstrably weak. A strong correla-tion exists between the degree and rapidity of development of a deformity and the imbalance of activity of agonist and antagonist muscles. Whatever conservative treatment is given, short of permanent application of splintage in the abducted position, adduction deformity will develop whenever there is significant weakness of gluteal abduction relative to the power of strong spastic adductor muscles.

The first element of deformity is usually in the muscles and tendons, particu-larly in the muscles in which there is a large tendinous element, notably the adductor longus, gracilis, iliopsoas, semitendinosus and semimembranosus. Liga-mentous and bony changes follow later, and muscle imbalance in itself may lead to alteration in bony development causing anteversion and valgus of the femoral neck (Morgan and Somerville 1960, Brookes and Wardle 1962). The deformity initially manifests as limitation of movement due to muscle shortening. Muscle shortening arises partly as a result of a predominant posture imposed by the spastic muscle, to which is added the diminished growth of the stronger muscle due to absence of stimulation by its weak opponents.

Once a strong muscle becomes relatively short, and its weaker opponent relatively long, the effective muscle balance is exaggerated. The strong short muscle acts at increasingly efficient mechanical advantage, whilst the weaker paretic muscle becomes increasingly ineffective, especially if it has to work at the outer limits of its range of activity.

A further factor in the development of paralytic deformity in spastic cerebral palsy may be increased sensory input from muscle spindles in the short muscle, which becomes more and more likely to be put under stretch in the course of normal activities. The increased sensory impulses exaggerate the reflex activity of the spastic muscles, and may even produce secondary effects by increasing spasticity in other parts of the lower limb and even in the upper limb. That this is a factor is often demonstrated by improved upper limb function after tight adductor or hamstring muscles have been released.

Conservative Management

It is not appropriate in this section to discuss the merits of various methods of management of cerebral palsy by physiotherapeutic means. However, the specific measures that are required to diminish the risk of hip deformity do merit consideration.

Every effort should be made to maintain the length of muscles that are liable to become short, particularly the hip flexor and adductor muscles. Flexion and adduction deformity could theoretically be prevented by maintaining the hips in full abduction and extension indefinitely, by means of external splintage. To do so would deny the child the possibility of learning the ability to crawl, stand and walk. A further disadvantage of continuous splintage is that it causes even greater weakness of muscles such as the hip abductors by superimposing 'disuse' atrophy. Attempts to maintain spastic muscles in a fully stretched position exaggerate sensory input into the spinal cord, and may even be painful. Except, therefore, for use at night, and then mainly only in early childhood, abduction splintage has limited application.

Measures to maintain the range of abduction and extension of the hip by daily passive movements can be performed by parents under the instruction of a physiotherapist or physical medicine specialist, and, in the author's experience, such measures are just as effective as continuous splintage in maintaining the range of passive movements. Other measures that can minimise the risk of development of deformity are the encouragement of activity in weaker abductor and extensor muscles and the inhibition of activity in strong and spastic muscles. The means to do this are within the province of physiotherapy technique; posture can be employed to diminish reflex activity, and there are a number of activities designed to encourage abductor and extensor activity at the hip.

When the child is able to start bearing weight on the limbs, a special watch needs to be kept for the development of increasing hip deformity, because the upright position may enhance adductor action at the expense of abductor action.

Surgical Treatment of Hip Deformity

This section is concerned with the management of hip deformity short of complete hip dislocation. The indications for surgical treatment are the development of deformity, as shown by limitation of hip movement, sufficient to affect lower limb function or to threaten subluxation of the hip. For most activities, it is not necessary for there to be a full range of hip abduction. Sitting, crawling and walking are quite consistent with a range of abduction that is 40 degrees or more. Once the range of hip abduction becomes less than 20 to 30 degrees, particularly if there is also fixed flexion, early subluxation of the hip is likely to develop and may progress to dislocation, sometimes within a matter of months (Sharrard 1967).

Loss of passive extension of the hip is compatible with most activities, but fixed flexion deformity of more than 15 to 20 degrees produces increasing difficulty in balancing, and the child has to walk with a lumbar lordosis or with flexion of the knees or both. Fixed flexion deformity of more than 40 degrees is quite unacceptable, not only because of the abnormality of gait that it imposes, but also because it is liable to lead to secondary flexion deformity of the knee and, if it is associated with adduction deformity, dislocation of the hip.

Adduction Deformity

Adduction deformity is the commonest deformity that arises at the hip (Lamb and Pollock 1962). Where the neurological pattern is symmetrical, deformity may arise on both sides, at the same time, and to the same degree. In asymmetrical paralysis, one hip may remain with an adequate range of abduction for many years, whilst the opposite hip shows progressive limitation of abduction.

In any child, whatever his age, a diminution of the range of abduction to 40 degrees or less is an indication of surgical treatment to restore length to the adductors and to correct any imbalance of action between the adductor and abductor muscles. Lamb and Pollock (1962), Craig (1967) and Sharrard (1969) all emphasise the importance of good assessment of abductor and adductor activity before operation, and the value of early surgery in the correction of adduction deformity before it has become severe. Assessment of power in the hip abductors sometimes requires preliminary infiltration of the adductor muscles and the obturator nerves with local anaesthetic if spasm is severe.

Adductor division should aim to restore the range of abduction to normal. Subcutaneous adductor tenotomy is seldom adequate for achieving this, and it is doubtful whether it is safe to attempt to divide other than the adductor longus or, occasionally, the gracilis by subcutaneous means. Open division under vision is the safest way of dividing tight adductors accurately and without damage to structures, such as the posterior branch of the obturator nerve, which it is intended to maintain intact. If the gluteal abductor muscles are known to be moderately strong, that is of grade three or four, division of tight adductor muscles alone is indicated. If hip

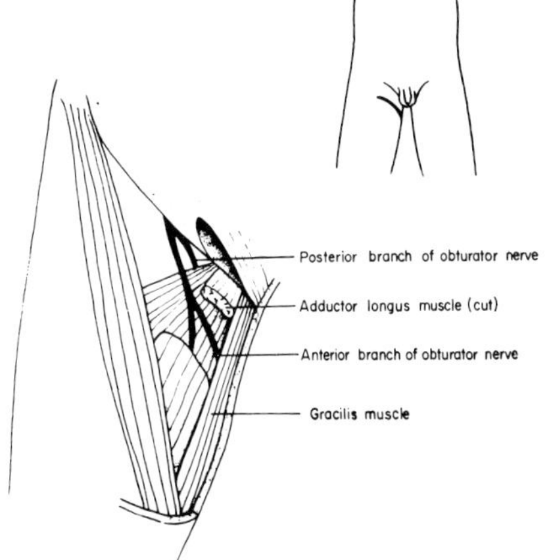

Fig. 3. The anatomy of adductor release and anterior branch obturator neurectomy.

abductor power is weak (equivalent to less than grade three), any short adductor muscles should be released, and the anterior branch of the obturator nerve should be divided. A combination of anterior branch obturator neurectomy and adductor division will reduce the power of the adductors to approximately grade three, and will achieve balanced action against comparably weakened abduction.

Even if it is thought that hip abduction is extremely weak, it is seldom ever wise to divide both branches of the obturator nerve in childhood. There is a considerable danger that marked weakness of hip adduction will lead to fixed abduction deformity, which can often only be corrected by transplantation of the origin of the hamstring muscles to the adductors (Pollock 1958). Intrapelvic obturator neurectomy is, in the author's opinion, rarely suitable for use in childhood, partly because it is impossible to divide other than the whole obturator nerve, and also because it is not possible to perform any release of tight adductors at the same operation. It is indicated occasionally when there is severe adductor spasm without significant adductor contracture, and Samilson *et al.* (1967) did not find that it led to over-correction.

Adductor release (Fig. 3) is performed through a groin incision, made parallel to the groin crease and 2.5 centimetres below it, and centred over the adductor longus tendon. The skin and subcutaneous tissues are divided and mobilised proximally and distally. The fascia overlying the adductor longus is incised longitudinally, and is dissected bluntly to expose the tendons of the adductor longus and gracilis. These two muscles are always short in cerebral palsy. Their tendons are defined close to their attachment to the pelvis, and divided. If the division is made one centimetre from their origin, the obturator vessels and nerves will not be damaged. The origin of the adductor longus is mainly by tendon, but there is some muscle attachment that needs to be divided as well. The gracilis origin is from a thin vertical tendon that is quite extensive, and there is a risk that one will fail to divide the posterior part of the tendon completely. When division is complete, it will almost always be found that a small vessel needs to be coagulated.

The adductor brevis muscle is the visible, and the anterior branches of the obturator nerve and vessels can be identified running downwards and medially across its anterior aspect. The posterior branches of the obturator nerve can be identified similarly on the posterior aspect of the muscle. If the adductor brevis muscle is also tight, it can be divided carefully, but it is quite often possible to stretch the adductor muscle by careful passive abduction. Release of the adductor magnus muscle is seldom needed in cerebral palsy, except when adduction deformity has been allowed to become severe, but, if a range of 80 degrees of abduction cannot be obtained following release of the adductor longus, gracilis and adductor brevis, the adductor magnus should also be divided or stretched. Attention should then be paid to the possibility of tightness of the medial hamstring muscles. This can best be determined by extending the knee fully, and palpating in the depths of the incision to determine whether the tendon of origin of the medial hamstring muscles from the ischial tuberosity is taut. If so, it should be elongated, though with care to avoid the sciatic nerve which lies parallel and close to the tendon.

If pre-operative assessment indicates that the anterior branch of the obturator nerve should also be divided, it can be defined on the anterior aspect of the adductor brevis muscle where it usually divides its two branches. To avoid the occasional hazard of an abnormal anterior course of the whole obturator nerve, the existence of the posterior branch of the obturator nerve should be confirmed before any of the anterior branches are divided. The nerve should be divided with removal of one centimetre or more of nerve, to diminish the risk of re-innervation.

At the end of the operation, the incision is closed in three layers, the vertical layer of fascia defined at the commencement of the operation, the subcutaneous layer and the skin. This measure substantially limits complications such as haematoma or wound infection, which occur commonly if transverse incisions are made through all layers in the exposure (Samilson *et al.* 1967). In older children, suction drainage may need to be used to minimise haematoma formation, but in younger children below the age of seven or eight years, it is unnecessary. Abduction is maintained by plaster casts applied from the groin to the toes and separated by two abduction bars. The hips should be kept in abduction, extension and internal rotation, and not in flexion, abduction and external rotation which is likely to give rise to a persistent 'frog' position (Banks and Green 1960, Samilson *et al.* 1967). The plaster splintage can be removed after three weeks in children below the age of five, and after four weeks in children older than this. As soon as plaster fixation has been removed, physiotherapy treatment to maintain passive abduction and to encourage activity and function in the lower limbs should be instituted; this should be continued daily for four or five weeks.

If adduction deformity recurs after a previous adductor release, it is almost always because there is still a significant muscle imbalance between adductor and abductor power. If several years have elapsed since the previous adductor release, it is reasonable to perform a further adductor release together with a neurectomy of the anterior branch of the obturator nerve (if this has not already been done previously). If recurrent adduction deformity follows an adequate adductor release and anterior branch obturator neurectomy, it is likely that the gluteal abductors are extremely weak, and the possibility may then arise that antero-lateral or postero-lateral iliopsoas transplantation may be needed to supplement abductor power.

The results of adductor tenotomy and myotomy, especially when combined with obturator neurectomy, are good in the experience of most authors (Keats 1957, Green and Banks 1960, Lamb and Pollock 1962, Samilson *et al.* 1967, Sharrard 1969). Unsatisfactory results are likely to be due to inaccurate pre-operative assessment of imbalance between adductors and abductors, so that either too little or too much division is done. Banks and Green (1960) suggest that the hip should be immobilised in abduction splints for a long period, even as long as several years, but the author's experience and that of other authors suggests that, if abductor power is regained by adequate post-operative physiotherapy treatment, prolonged splintage is unnecessary and limits excessively the natural activity of the child. Only where abductor power proves to be very limited or is regained very slowly, may abduction splintage need to be continued for more than six weeks.

Adductor tenotomy may conveniently be combined with posterior transplantation of the divided adductors to the region of the ischial tuberosity (Stephenson and Donovan 1971). This refinement of adductor releases may be of distinct value when there is combined adduction and flexion deformity, and, when flexion deformity is severe, it may be combined with release of the iliopsoas tendon. If this procedure is undertaken, care must be taken to ensure that the suture of the adductors is made with the hip in the desired abducted position.

Flexion Deformity

Flexion deformity often accompanies adduction deformity, though it may present independently or may develop after the adduction deformity has been corrected by an earlier adductor release.

Strong and spastic hip flexor muscles in the presence of weak hip extensors are the usual cause of flexion deformity (Mathews *et al.* 1953). Until recently, most authors have described extensive release procedures for flexion deformity, involving division of tensor fasciae latae, rectus femoris, sartorius, pectineus, iliopsoas tendon and anterior hip capsule (Pollock and Sharrard 1956, Pollock 1962, Hill *et al.* 1966). It is only when fixed flexion has become more than 30 or 40 degrees that there is significant shortening of all the hip flexors. At the earliest stage of flexion deformity, the iliopsoas muscle, which is the most important flexor of the hip, is often the only short structure. In more recent papers, the value of iliopsoas tenotomy or elongation, either alone or in combination with adductor release, has been recognized (Bleck and Holstein 1964, Keats and Morgese 1967, Sharrard 1969).

Surgical correction is indicated when fixed flexion exceeds 20 degrees, and up to 40 degrees of fixed flexion can often be corrected by release of the iliopsoas tendon alone.

The tendon can be approached through the adductor region (Ludloff 1908, Keats and Morgese 1967) or, if the adductors have previously been released or if there is a pure flexion deformity and the possibility of shortness of other hip flexors, it can be approached through an antero-lateral incision made parallel to the sartorius muscle.

When the tendon is approached through a groin incision, it can be found by palpating the lesser trochanter in the depths of the wound, in the interval between the pectineus and adductor brevis muscles. If adductor longus and adductor brevis have been divided in the course of adductor release, exposure is made even more easily. A thin layer of fascia separates the iliopsoas tendon from the plane of the adductor muscles. After this layer has been divided, the *combined* iliopsoas tendon and some fibres of the iliacus that insert into the shaft of the femur separately can be defined. If the approach is made lateral to the sartorius, the dissection proceeds in front of the rectus femoris and behind the femoral nerve and femoral vessels, until the lesser trochanter is reached. The exposure is aided by flexion, external rotation and abduction of the hip, whichever method of exposure is used.

The medial femoral circumflex vessels may pass across the psoas tendon, and, if they obstruct exposure of it, they should be ligated and divided. By appropriate positioning of the femoral shaft, it is often possible to expose three or four centimetres of the tendon. The iliopsoas tendon may insert by two almost distinct tendons, one passing to the lesser trochanter and the other through the femoral shaft posterior to the trochanter. Care must be taken to ensure that both are divided. The iliopsoas tendon can be divided leaving the fibres of the iliacus intact, so that the tendon does not retract too far, or the combined iliopsoas tendon can be elongated by a Z-elongation, with application of sutures to maintain the fragments in apposition. Some authors advocate that the iliopsoas tendon should be divided, and, then either attached to the front of the capsule of the hip or allowed to retract and re-attach to this level. If this is done, the range of function of the iliopsoas will be very considerably diminished, and there may subsequently be a complaint that the patient is unable to flex the hip sufficiently strongly to climb upstairs.

The wound is sutured in layers, and a hip spica applied to maintain the hips in an abducted and extended position. Fixation should be retained for approximately four weeks, after which time active physiotherapy can be instituted (Fig. 4).

Flexion deformity of 45 degrees or more requires the release of other flexor muscles in addition to the iliopsoas tendon, and among the structures that may need to be divided are the tensor fasciae latae and its sheath, the sartorius, the pectineus, and sometimes the anterior capsule of the hip and the ilio-femoral ligament. All these structures can be exposed through the oblique antero-lateral incision described.

The extent to which flexion deformity can be corrected by flexor release depends on the tightness of the femoral nerve or femoral vessels or both. It may be possible to correct up to 60 degrees of flexion deformity by release of soft tissues alone. However, a more severe flexion deformity is almost always impossible to correct adequately by soft tissue release alone, because of tightness of the femoral nerve and vessels. After division of the soft tissues and healing of them, the residual flexion deformity may need to be corrected by extension osteotomy of the femur at the inter-trochanteric level with internal fixation using a nail-plate. If the deformity is severe, it may be necessary to remove one or two centimetres of the femoral shaft. Fixation in a plaster spica with the hip extended needs to be maintained for about six weeks. Iliopsoas tenotomy or flexor release diminishes the power

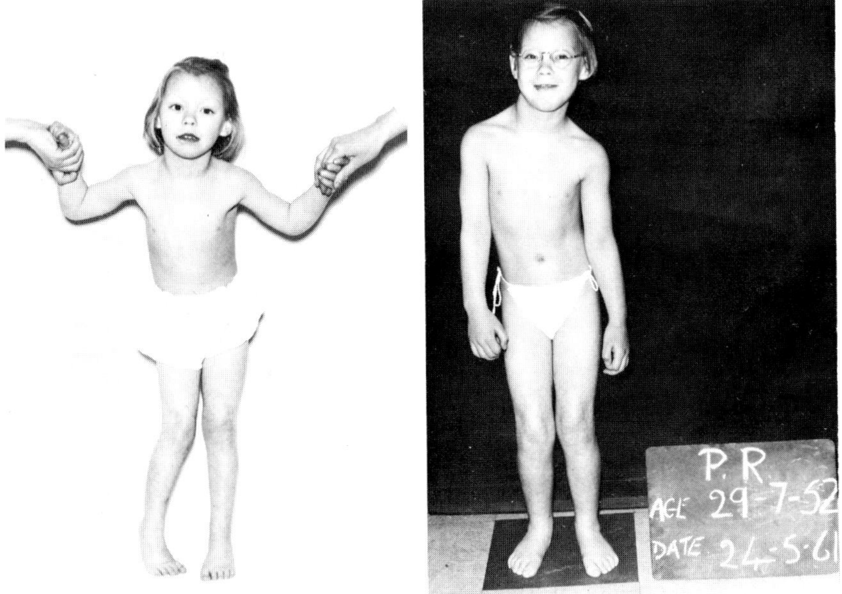

Figs. 4 *a* **and** *b*. Improvement in gait and stance after bilateral adductor release and iliopsoas tendon lengthening.

of hip flexion, and this alone may be sufficient to balance the power of flexion and that of extension. If recurrent flexion deformity develops, it may be appropriate to consider transplantation of the iliopsoas tendon posteriorly or postero-laterally (see page 167). Alternatively, posterior transplantation of the origins of adductor muscles to the ischium, or of the hamstring muscles to the posterior aspect of the lower end of the femur (Eggers 1952), may be sufficient to supplement extensor power, provided that hip flexion contracture of 15 to 20 degrees does not exist. Flexion deformity of the hip that has been allowed to progress to more than 45 degrees is often associated with flexion deformity of the knee. Once this has occurred, it may be difficult to determine whether the primary deformity was at the knee or at the hip. The author's experience has been that, ever since early flexion deformity of the hip has been treated by performing iliopsoas tenotomy before the deformity becomes excessive, flexion deformity of the knee has become a relatively uncommon problem.

Internal Rotation Deformity

Internal rotation deformity often accompanies flexion and adduction deformity at the hip in cerebral palsy. The development of this deformity is unlikely to be a result of the action of the iliopsoas muscle, which, by itself, is more usually an external rotator. The most obvious internal rotator muscles of the hip are the anterior fibres of the gluteus medius and the tensor fasciae latae, but neither of these is particularly liable to be spastic or strong in cerebral palsy. Studies of the action of the adductors and medial hamstring muscles, however, indicate that they can be quite powerful internal rotators of the hip when the latter is flexed. It seems likely, therefore, that the adductors and medial hamstring muscles are responsible in the majority of instances for internal rotation deformity of the hips when there is fixed flexion and adduction deformity. If this is so, the implication is that correction of flexion and adduction deformity is likely to correct any internal rotation deformity; in fact, this is what happens in many patients in whom the three elements of deformity are combined together.

In other instances, internal rotation deformity may exist by itself, or persist after flexion and adduction deformity have been corrected. In most such patients, clinical and radiological examination will usually show that the deformity arises in association with anteversion of the femoral neck. If this is the case and the patient's gait is embarrassed by internal rotation with in-toeing, the deformity can be corrected by external rotation osteotomy of the femur; this will be performed either in the sub-trochanteric region or in the lower third of the shaft of the femur, depending on whether valgus of the femoral neck is also present and requires correction at sub-trochanteric level. Hill *et al.* (1966) advise that one or more of the medial hamstrings at the knee should be transplanted postero-laterally to the anterior aspect of the lateral femoral condyle, where they may become capable of acting as external rotators. Their power as external rotators is not unduly great, and it seems likely that the effectiveness of this transplant is as much derived from release of the internal rotating action on the hamstring muscles as from the action that these muscles develop in their new insertion. Furthermore, in the presence of increased femoral anteversion, transfer of medial hamstrings to the lateral femoral condyle cannot be expected to correct the bone deformity.

External rotation osteotomy of the femur is performed through a lateral incision made either over the upper third of the femoral shaft or over the lower third, the shaft being exposed after incision of the fascia lata and mobilisation of the quadriceps muscle forwards. Guide marks should be made or guide-pins inserted above and below the proposed level of osteotomy, so that after the femoral shaft has been divided the degree or rotation that is being imposed can be determined accurately. The shaft is divided transversely with an oscillating saw or osteotome, and the position after correction of the rotation deformity is held by a six-hole plate in the lower third of the femoral shaft or by a nail-plate if the osteotomy is done at sub-trochanteric level. The incision is closed in two layers. Internal fixation alone should never be relied upon in spasticity, because of the tendency for strong and spastic muscles to break or bend the plate or to pull out screws. Fixation should be supplemented by a hip spica plaster from the chest to the toes, with the knee in 20 degrees of flexion and the rotated position maintained.

Extension Deformity

Fixed extension deformity in cerebral palsy is very rare, but limitation of flexion of the hip occasionally arises in the presence of short hamstring muscles. Some shortness of the hamstring muscles is very common in quadriplegic and diplegic cerebral palsy, and its usual effect is to cause flexion deformity of the knee. If, however, the quadriceps is strong, the main effect of the short hamstrings is to limit the range of flexion of the hip, as shown by limited straight leg raising. If the range of straight leg raising becomes less than 30 degrees, disability results. The patient cannot sit with the legs straight out in front of him, he is unable to take a full forward stride, and he has to walk with a characteristic rotation of the pelvis.

This situation is substantially relieved by proximal elongation of the tendon of origin of the hamstrings (Seymour and Sharrard 1968). The condition often occurs bilaterally. The operation is performed with the patient prone. An incision is made lateral to the ischial tuberosity over a distance of about five centimetres. The lower border of the gluteus maximus is defined and retracted upwards, to expose the tendon of origin of the hamstring muscles from the ischial tuberosity. The sciatic nerve is identified and retracted. The tendon of origin of the hamstring muscles is divided obliquely and the distal end allowed to retract. The ends of the tendon are sutured with two or three sutures to prevent excessive retraction that can lead to unbalanced weakness of hip extension. The incision is closed in two layers.

The patient is nursed in the half-sitting position with the knees extended, and is gradually encouraged to sit up during the course of the next two or three weeks. The patient can be allowed to recommence walking after three weeks.

Dislocation of the Hip

Dislocation of the hip in cerebral palsy is practically always a paralytic dislocation. When it is found in early life, for instance at the age of six or nine months, it may be thought to be a congenital dislocation, since the radiological features of a sloping acetabulum and a small upper femoral epiphysial nucleus simulate completely the appearances of congenital dislocation. In other respects, the dislocation is completely different. The hip is adducted and flexed with short adductor and flexor muscles.

Incidence

Very varied figures have been given for the incidence of dislocation of the hip in cerebral palsy. Gherlinzoni and Pais (1950) reported an incidence of 4.6 per cent, Mathews *et al.* (1953) reported an incidence of 2.6 per cent, Tachdjian and Minear (1956) reported an incidence of 4.2 per cent and Phelps (1959) reported an incidence of 17 per cent. These variations are probably due to differences in the age at which the assessment was made, in the type of populations studied, in the type of cerebral palsy, and in management and treatment. If attention is specially directed towards spastic quadriplegic or diplegic cerebral palsy, the proportion of dislocations is much higher. Pollock and Sharrard (1958) found an incidence of 23 per cent of subluxation or dislocation in such patients, and Samilson *et al.* (1971) recorded an incidence of 28 per cent of subluxation or dislocation of the hip in a selected population of severely involved cerebral-palsied patients.

Aetiology and Pathology

Watson-Jones (1926) was the first to point out that paralytic dislocation of the hip arises when the hip flexor and adductor muscles are strong and short and the gluteal muscles are weak or paralysed. All authors are agreed that in cerebral palsy muscle imbalance, particularly that due to relatively strong hip adductors in the presence of weak abductors, is a constant factor in the production of subluxation and dislocation (Tachdjian and Minear 1956, Pollock and Sharrard 1958, Phelps 1959, Samilson *et al.* 1972); but there is some disagreement as to the mechanism by which the dislocation develops.

Valgus and anteversion of the femoral neck are present in almost all hips that develop subluxation or dislocation (Phelps 1959, Baker *et al.* 1962, Samilson *et al.* 1972). The two almost always occur together, with anteversion as the most important feature. Anteversion and valgus deformity, either separately or in combination, occur very commonly in all paralytic conditions associated with weakness of the hip, and even in children without paralysis but with brain damage of such severity that they do not walk. The degree of anteversion of subluxated hips in cerebral palsy was found by Samilson *et al.* (1971) to average 69 degrees, while the valgus deformity, as shown by the neck shaft angle, averaged 154 degrees in subluxations and 160 degrees in dislocations. Similar findings have been described by all authors in subluxated and dislocated hips in cerebral palsy (Phelps 1959, Tachdjian and Minear 1956).

Somerville (1959) and Samilson *et al.* (1971) consider anteversion and valgus of the femoral neck to be a more important factor in the production of dislocation than the presence of muscle imbalance. Femoral neck deformity undoubtedly aggravates the liability to dislocate, because the hip is not centred in the acetabulum when the limb is in neutral adduction, and because the greater trochanter comes to lie almost directly below, instead of lateral to, the origin of the gluteus medius and this diminishes the effective force of the gluteus medius as an abductor. That valgus and anteversion of the femoral neck are not by themselves responsible for dislocation is shown by the many instances in which weakness of the hip musculature results in the development of valgus and anteversion of the femoral neck, yet the hip does not dislocate because there is no unbalanced activity of the hip flexors and adductor muscles against the gluteal muscles (Fig. 5). Jones (1962) states that correction of valgus and anteversion by osteotomy alone, without correction of muscle imbalance, often fails to prevent recurrent dislocation, even when adequate correction of the bony deformity has been made. On the other hand, correction of imbalance between adductor and abductor action, even without osteotomy, can correct and prevent subluxation successfully (in the absence of excessive femoral anteversion or coxa valga) (Sharrard 1971); however, in a neglected and severely affected hip with established dislocation, soft-tissue operations alone will not be sufficient to maintain correction of the dislocation, unless valgus and anteversion of the femoral neck are also corrected.

The mean age at which dislocation occurs in cerebral palsy is seven years (Samilson *et al.* 1971), but it can be seen as early as the sixth month of life, or as late as the twelfth year. Except in patients in whom the dislocation occurs during the first year of life, shallowness of the acetabulum is not a constant feature of dislocation of the hip in cerebral palsy; nor is there so great a liability to the development of limbus formation or infolding of the hip capsule into the acetabulum as in congenital dislocation.

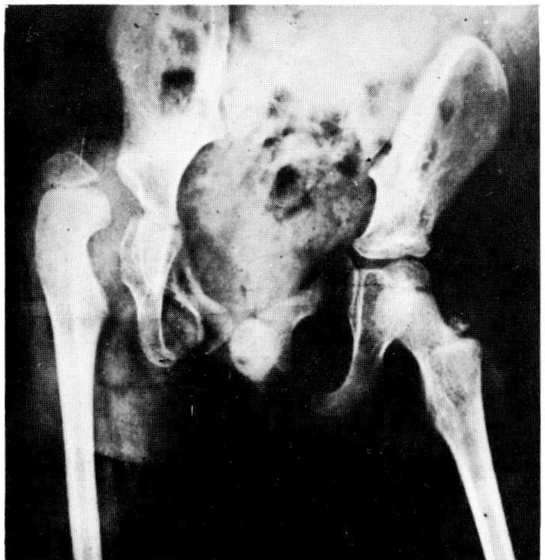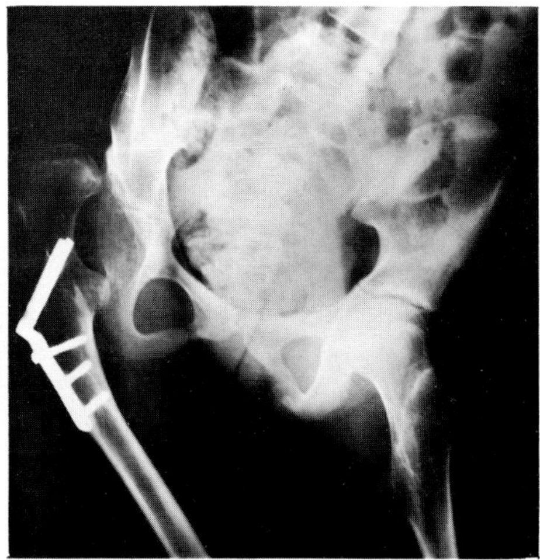

Fig. 5a. Severe valgus and anteversion deformity of the femoral neck of both hips; the right hip has dislocated, but the left has remained in joint. On the left side, gluteal power was adequate; on the right side, it was severely paretic.

Fig. 5b. Two years after varus osteotomy and reduction of the dislocation on the right side. An adequate adductor release and muscle balance procedures had not been perfomed. The dislocation has recurred rapidly.

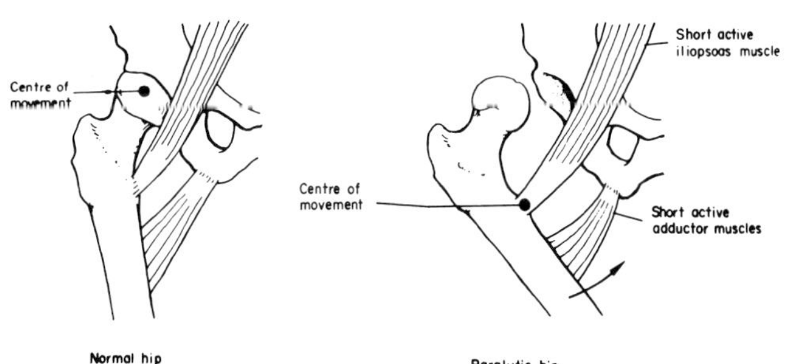

Fig. 6. The mechanism of spastic dislocation of the hip. Shortness and over-activity of the iliopsoas and hip adductors in the presence of weak hip abductors and extensors transfers the center of movement of the hip from the head of the femur to the level of the lesser trechanter. Antero-lateral forces apply to the capsule of the hip which stretches and the hip dislocates.

The mechanism of dislocation is discussed by Sharrard (1971). In the course of development of paralytic dislocation, there is a stage at which the hip, when extended, dislocates in and out of joint on adduction and abduction. When the hip is flexed, adduction and abduction does not result in dislocation. Radiological analysis using image intensification and cine-radiography shows that during the development of paralytic dislocation the axis of movement at the hip moves distally from the centre of the head of the femur to a point in the region of the lesser trochanter (Fig. 6). Adduction and abduction leads to lateral and upward displacement of the femoral head; this stretches the capsule of the hip and eventually results in dislocation. Once adduction becomes fixed and severe, the dislocation remains permanently.

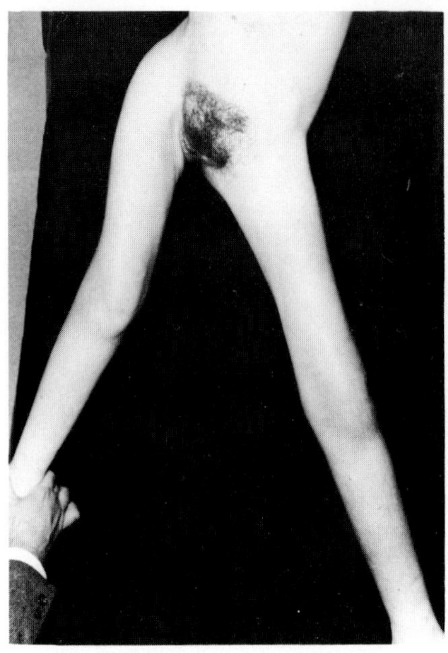

Fig. 7. Flexion and adduction deformity with shortening of the right lower limb in a dislocated hip. Perineal care becomes extremely difficult, sitting balance is markedly impaired, and hip movement is painful.

If, during the course of development of dislocation, the iliopsoas tendon is divided, a more normal axis of movement is restored, and, if the adductors are also released from their origin, the axis of movement returns to the centre of the head of the femur. Thus it is believed that the primary mechanism in the development of paralytic dislocation is a relative shortening of the hip flexor and adductor muscles, occurring as a paralytic phenomenon in a patient with strong hip flexor and adductor muscles and a weak gluteal musculature. The presence of valgus and anteversion of the femoral neck aggravates the tendency and the longitudinal shortening of all pelvi-femoral muscles contributes to the proximal displacement of the femur.

Once the hip has dislocated, the nursing of a cerebral-palsied patient becomes increasing difficult (Fig. 7). Perineal care becomes a severe problem, especially if both hips are involved. Sitting balance is impaired, and the patient may develop pressure ulceration over the trochanters. A child who, with slowly developing nervous maturity, might have become able to walk, is totally unable to do so because of the dislocation. In adolescence and early adult life, the subluxated or dislocated hip becomes painful, and initiates strong reflex spasms in the flexor and adductor muscles, grinding the head of the femur against the side of the pelvis. The ligamentum teres or the hip capsule may cause notching of the femoral head. Eventually, the articular cartilage becomes eroded and pitted, and the femoral head becomes grossly mis-shapen.

Dislocation of the hip in cerebral palsy develops more rapidly and becomes more severe in neurologically immature patients, the most severe varieties presenting in patients showing combined athetosis and spasticity. Scoliosis considerably aggravates the liability to dislocation. Fixed pelvic obliquity, especially when

162

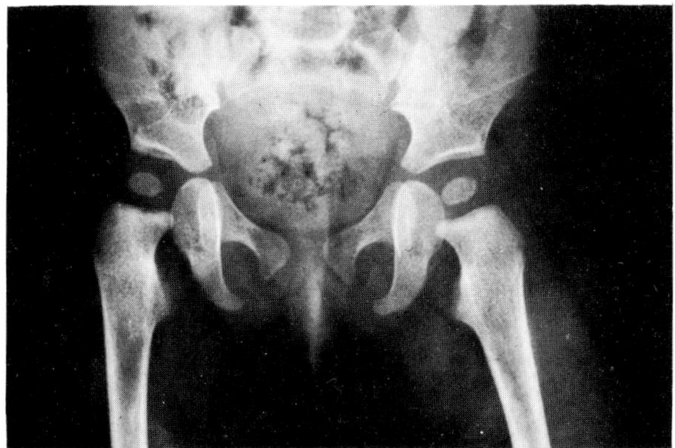

(a)

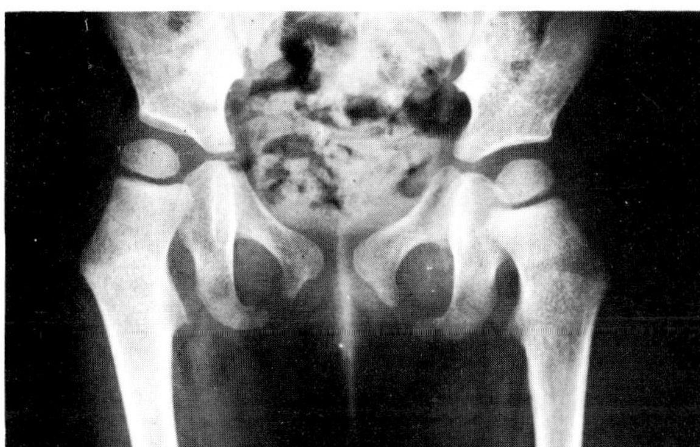

(b)

Figs. 8a and 8b. Radiographs of the hips in cerebral palsy. There was limitation of abduction to 30 degrees on the right and to 70 degrees on the left.

(a) *Upper radiograph.* The first sign of hip subluxation is present with a break in Shenton's line and slight upward and lateral displacement of the femoral epiphysis. The left hip is in joint. There is anteversion and valgus of the femoral neck on both sides.

(b) *Lower radiograph.* Nine months later, the right hip has subluxated further; adductor release is indicated on the right side.

associated with a thoraco-lumbar C-curve due to asymmetrical over-activity of the lateral trunk muscles and the preservation of the incurvatum reflex, causes one hip to lie in adduction and the other to lie in abduction. In this situation, even a moderate imbalance between adductors and abductors combined with valgus of the femoral neck can result in dislocation, and the retention of primitive adductor reflexes at the hip also aggravate the liability to dislocation in the neurologically immature (Samilson *et al.* 1971).

Radiological Features of Subluxation and Dislocation in Cerebral Palsy

A high proportion of patients with cerebral palsy affecting the hip joints show anteversion of the femoral neck, and in certain instances some degree of true valgus of the femoral neck. This sign alone is not indicative of subluxation. The first radiological sign of subluxation is a break in Shenton's line (Fig. 8). If this is present, the hips should be examined radiologically in adduction and abduction to demonstrate any abnormal pattern of movement. With progressive subluxation, the femoral head displaces proximally and laterally relative to the acetabulum, and this appearance is aggravated when the hip comes to lie in fixed adduction. The hip eventually dislocates, with the shaft of the femur in gross adduction and flexion. In a very young child, the acetabular roof may appear to be sloping and the nucleus of the upper femoral epiphysis is small, the picture simulating congenital dislocation of the hip. Arthrograms demonstrate that, even in young children, there is a relatively minor degree of deficiency in the acetabular roof during the early stages of dislocation, and reduction of the dislocation will usually result in spontaneous reformation of the bony acetabular roof. When dislocation occurs after the age of three years, the acetabulum has already been fully formed, and any defect of the acetabular roof is usually relatively mild.

Prevention of Dislocation

Once subluxation of the hip has commenced (as evidenced radiographically by a break in Shenton's line), it is doubtful whether any conservative method of treatment can prevent the slow insidious progress of subluxation and dislocation, though this may take two or more years to become complete. Maintenance of passive abduction, by stretching or by splinting in abduction, can diminish the rate at which subluxation progresses, but this management, by itself, is inadequate, and always needs to be supplemented by surgical treatment at some time.

Clinical and radiological evidence of subluxation of the hip is always accompanied by a moderate or severe degree of limitation of abduction and, often, of extension and also by clinical evidence of significant weakness of the gluteal abductors. Traction in the management of subluxation is not effective, is poorly tolerated by the patient, and frequently aggravates the stretch reflex in the psoas and adductor muscles.

In the early stages of development of subluxation, adductor release, elongation of the iliopsoas tendon and anterior branch obturator neurectomy are sufficient to prevent the progress of subluxation towards dislocation in a high proportion of patients (Fig. 9). In 101 of 134 hips with early clinical and radiological evidence of the development of subluxation, this procedure alone was sufficient to prevent any further deterioration of the hip (mean length of follow-up 5 years) (Sharrard *et al.* 1969). In 28 of the hips, a further adductor release was needed five or six years later, but the hips reached maturity without further deterioration. In two patients, adduction and flexion deformity recurred rapidly, in association with very severe weakness in the gluteal abductors. At a second operation, the iliopsoas muscle was transplanted postero-laterally in these patients, and this additional measure was sufficient to maintain the hip joint until maturity. The technical features of iliopsoas transplantation will be described in the section devoted to the management of complete hip dislocation (page 167).

The management of the hip after flexor and adductor release is the same as that described earlier in this chapter; however it may sometimes be valuable to maintain abduction splintage at night for three to six months following release from plaster fixation, to encourage the correction of looseness of the antero-lateral hip capsule.

In an older child, *i.e.* over the age of seven or eight years, who has had flexion and adduction deformity with slowly progressing subluxation for two or three years, flexor and adductor release should be supplemented by distal transplantation of the gluteal insertion. Through an incision on the outer side of the greater trochanter,

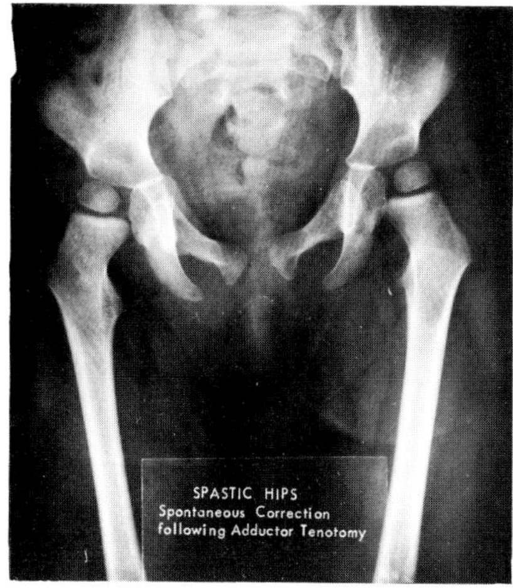

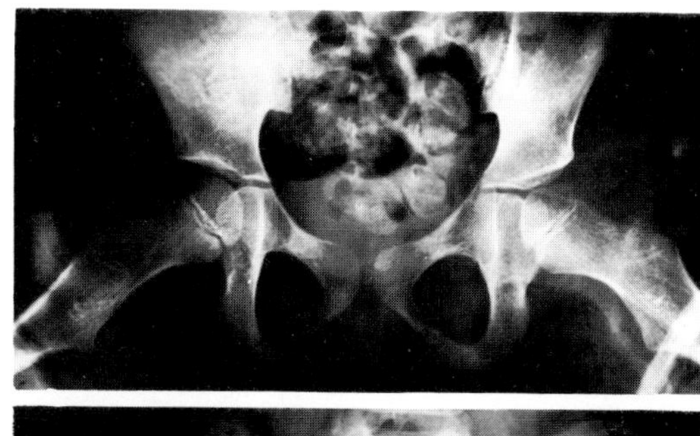

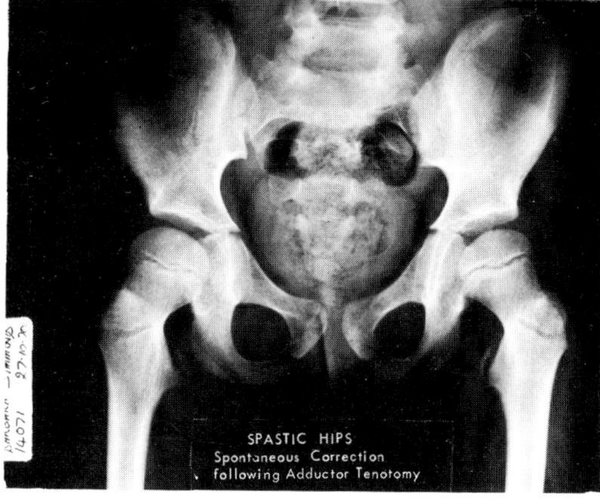

Fig. 9. Radiograph of spontaneous correction of subluxation and anteversion of the femoral neck by adductor tenotomy alone. (a) (*above left*) Before operation. (b) (*above right*) Immediately following bilateral adductor release and anterior branch obturator neurectomy. Plaster fixation was maintained for four weeks only. (c) (*right*) Two years later there is no trace of subluxation and much of the valgus and anteversion has corrected spontaneously.

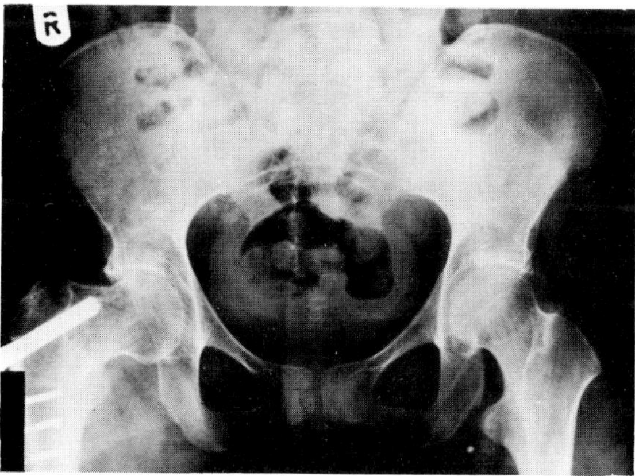

Fig. 10. Spastic quadriplegia five years after adductor tenotomy, iliopsoas tendon lengthening and varus osteotomy for marked subluxation of the right hip.

the tendon of insertion of the gluteal muscles is detached from the upper part of the trochanter, displaced downwards as far as possible with the hip in abduction and extension, and sutured two or three centimetres further down the greater trochanter. It may be useful to hold the tendon at its new site with the help of a staple.

If, after adequate soft tissue release, there is doubt about hip stability (except in full abduction) and the acetabulum is still adequate, varus osteotomy combined with some degree of external rotation may be needed (Fig. 10). The position of the

osteotomy should be held by internal fixation using a nail-plate or a bent plate with
screws.

The Management of Severe Subluxation or Dislocation of the Hip

If a patient presents to the orthopaedic surgeon with an established severe
subluxation or dislocation of the hip, the orthopaedic management is much more
difficult. However, an attempt should always be made to reduce the dislocation or at
least to correct the deformity. Provided that complete dislocation has not been
present for more than two or three years, satisfactory reduction can be achieved in a
remarkably high proportion of patients, even those who are aged ten years or more.
This is possible because the acetabulum is relatively slightly affected, particularly
when the dislocation has occurred in later childhood.

Surgery is almost always indicated, and, even when the dislocation cannot be
reduced, improvement in the position of the femur following adductor release helps
perineal care, improves sitting balance, and reduces pain. Ideally, an attempt
should be made to reduce any dislocation in a spastic child, provided that it has not
been present for more than four years.

When the hip is completely dislocated posteriorly, there is often severe
adduction deformity and moderately severe flexion deformity. The gluteal musculature is elongated and ineffective, and the hip capsule is also stretched and
voluminous. There is usually marked anteversion and valgus deformity of the
femoral neck, and there is occasional shallowness and inadequacy of the acetabulum.

The aim of treatment is to correct all the elements of deformity, and to correct
muscle imbalance in order to prevent recurrence of dislocation. As far as the soft
tissues are concerned, the tight structures are the hip adductors and flexors, whilst
the lengthened structures are the glutei and the hip capsule, and the imbalance is due
to considerable weakness of the gluteal abductors and extensors in the presence
of strong flexors and adductors. When the hip has been dislocated for a while, it
may be riding very high, and articulating with the outer surface of the ilium.

In a long-standing case, a preliminary period of traction for two or three weeks
may be helpful, but it is seldom useful to continue for longer than this, and conservative means or manipulation will not achieve reduction. Through an incision in the
groin, a radical adductor release should be performed, dividing, as necessary, the
adductor longus, gracilis, adductor brevis and, sometimes the adductor magnus, the
medial origin of the hamstrings and the pectineus. The anterior branch of the
obturator nerve should be divided, but the posterior branch should be left intact,
since some adductor power will be needed later to act as balancing force against the
transplanted iliopsoas muscle. Once the adductors have been adequately released,
the hip will sometimes reduce in flexion, but the psoas will almost always be
found to be extremely tight. In many patients, the psoas muscle bridges across
the front of the lower part of the acetabulum, infolding the capsule at this point and
preventing any downward displacement of the femoral head to reduce it into the
acetabulum. It is convenient to expose the iliopsoas tendon and the lesser trochanter
through the incision in the groin, and to lengthen the iliopsoas tendon to allow
reduction of the dislocation. A plaster spica is applied and kept on for three or four
weeks.

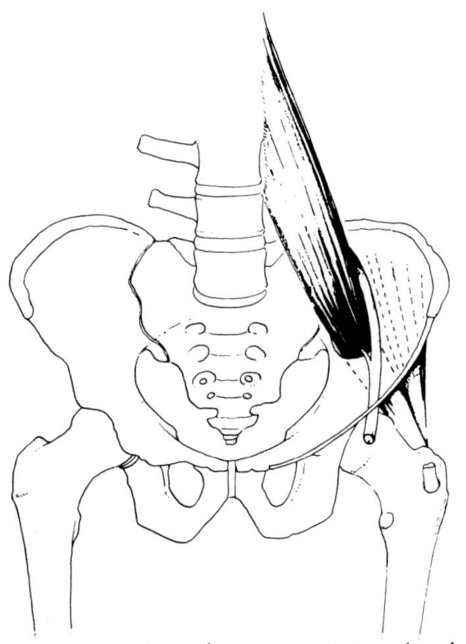

Fig. 11. Postero-lateral iliopsoas transplantation.

Muscle imbalance can be corrected by postero-lateral iliopsoas transplantation (Sharrard 1967, 1971). This operation can be done when the elongated tendon has healed. The site of transfer of the psoas muscle is indicated in Figure 11. Through an incision along the anterior two thirds of the iliac crest, and passing obliquely along the lateral side of the sartorius muscle, the tensor fasciae latae and gluteal muscles are exposed through the gluteal part of the incision. The gluteal muscles and tensor fasciae latae are separated extraperiosteally to expose the ilium, particularly its posterior two thirds, and the capsule of the hip joint. If flexion deformity is severe, the rectus femoris may be divided just distal to its origin by an oblique incision. The reflected head can be used to identify the position of the acetabular roof. The hip capsule is mobilised from the outer surface of the ilium, and the hip joint opened through a T-shaped incision, one limb of which runs parallel to the acetabular margin from the superior part of the acetabulum along its anterior border to its infero-medial aspect, and the second limb of which is placed anteriorly parallel to the femoral neck. The acetabulum can then be identified, and is usually found to be adequate, with a reasonable acetabular roof. The ligamentum teres may be elongated, thickened or completely stretched and ruptured; if present, it may present a bar to reduction so it should be removed. By extension, abduction and internal rotation, it should be possible to reduce the dislocation if this has not been achieved at the first operation. If this does not prove to be possible, it will usually be found that a portion of the iliopsoas or of the inferior capsule requires further release. A triangular portion of redundant capsule can be removed prior to suture of the capsule, which should be done at the end of the operation.

The dissection is continued on the medial side of the sartorius, exposing the femoral nerve as it emerges from beneath the inguinal ligament. The branches of the femoral nerve are dissected carefully, and retracted laterally. A triangle, formed by the femoral vessels medially, the femoral nerve laterally, and the inguinal ligament proximally, is exposed. Crossing this triangle are the lateral femoral circumflex vessels, which are isolated carefully, ligated and divided. Medial retraction of the femoral vessels and lateral retraction of the femoral nerve allow the iliopsoas tendon and lesser trochanter to be exposed and visualised. The iliopsoas tendon, which has previously been detached through a groin incision, can now be mobilised proximally.

The pelvis is opened by incising the cartilage of the anterior two thirds of the iliac crest and allowing the abdominal musculature to be retracted proximally. The pelvis is entered on the medial side of the iliacus muscle, exposing that muscle and the psoas muscle, with the femoral nerve lying between them. The iliopsoas tendon is mobilised into the pelvis, and transposed deep to the femoral nerve to its outer side. The iliacus is detached, by blunt dissection, from the inner surface of the ilium extra-periosteally. A foramen is made in the ilium, just lateral to the sacro-iliac joint. The foramen should be approximately one third of the width of the false pelvis and oval in shape, with a long axis parallel to the sacro-iliac joint. The iliopsoas tendon and the whole of the iliacus are passed through the foramen into the gluteal region.

The anterior aspect of the greater trochanter is exposed by an incision through the fascia lata, and by mobilisation of the quadriceps forwards from the front of the greater trochanter. A hole is made in the greater trochanter passing upwards, posteriorly and a little medially, using a burr or drill. A tendon cannula is passed through this hole to emerge in the gluteal region. A suture is applied to the iliopsoas tendon after it has been trimmed to the size of the hole in the greater trochanter. The suture is passed through the tendon cannula, so as to hold the hip of the lesser trochanter onto the end of the cannula, which can then be withdrawn through the greater trochanter. When this is done, the tip of the greater trochanter will emerge to the front of the greater trochanter. If the hip capsule was opened earler in the operation, it should be sutured at this point. The hip is put into moderate abduction and extension, and the transplant is sutured to the front of the greater trochanter with strong silk sutures. Movements of the hip joint are tested to ensure that the hip does not now dislocate on adduction; the transplant itself should prevent adduction beyond the neutral position. The wound is closed in three layers, and a plaster spica applied with the hip extended and abducted. Spica fixation is maintained for four to six weeks, depending on the age of the patient, and the hip is then allowed to mobilise freely.

In a relatively recent dislocation, even if there is valgus and anteversion of the femoral neck, the stability of the hip may be so adequate that no further procedures are needed (Fig. 12). After two or three years, the valgus and anteversion of the femoral neck will diminish as a result of the action of the transplant on the greater trochanter. In more long-standing dislocations, additional bony correction may be needed, either of the femoral neck to correct valgus and anteversion, or of the acetabulum to improve cover of the femoral head. Valgus and anteversion of the

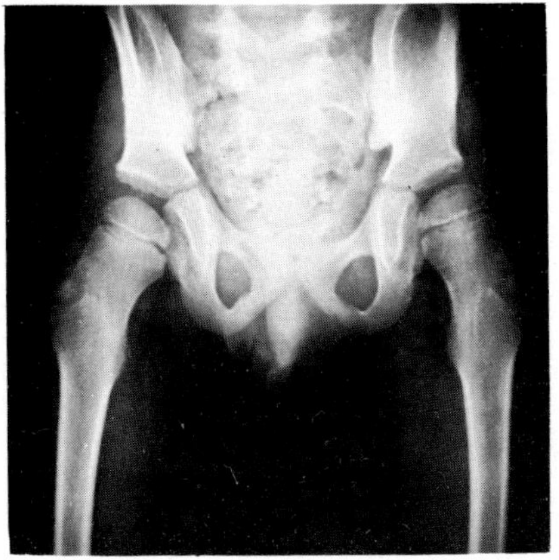

Fig. 12. Stable hips six years after bilateral adductor release and postero-lateral iliopsoas transplantation for complete dislocation of both hips. The acetabular roofs on both sides are slightly deficient, but sufficiently adequate to prevent further subluxation or dislocation.

femoral neck can be corrected by varus and rotation osteotomy through the inter-trochanteric region; there are various techniques for achieving this, the common essential feature being removal of an appropriate wedge of bone based medially, and to some extent posteriorly, followed by internal fixation with a nail-plate or other internal fixation device. The osteotomy can be combined with the soft tissue procedures already described, or can be undertaken three or four weeks after the soft tissue operations have been performed.

In very long-standing dislocation, with a very high displacement of the femoral head, a combination of varus osteotomy with removal of up to two centimetres of femoral shaft may make reduction possible when the pelvi-femoral musculature is short. Smith (1969) is an advocate of combined multiple soft tissue and bony procedures at one operative session.

Inadequacy of the acetabular roof may occasionally benefit from innominate osteotomy somewhat similar to the Salter (1961) type, the main aim being to rotate the acetabulum downwards to provide additional cover for the femoral head. The operation can be combined with iliopsoas transplantation. With a small amount of additional exposure of the anterior part of the ilium and the anterior superior iliac spine, a Gigli saw can, after subperiosteal dissection, be passed through the greater sciatic notch at its most anterior part. The Gigli saw is used to divide the innomin-ate bone antero-posteriorly from the anterior part of the sciatic notch to the anterior inferior iliac spine. The distal part of the innominate bone, including the aceta-bulum, is displaced laterally and downwards to open up a wedge-shaped gap between the upper and lower fragments of the osteotomy. The gap so opened up can be filled with a triangular piece of bone, and it may be useful to use the piece of bone which has been removed from the iliac wing in the course of the iliopsoas transplantation. The fragments are held by two pins or by Kirschner wires trans-fixing all the fragments (Fig. 13).

After osteotomy, either of the femoral neck or of the innominate bone, or of both, fixation in a plaster spica in abduction, extension and some medial rotation needs to be maintained for six weeks.

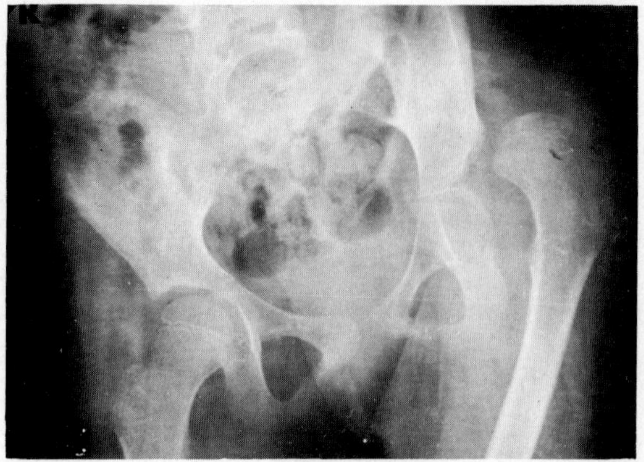

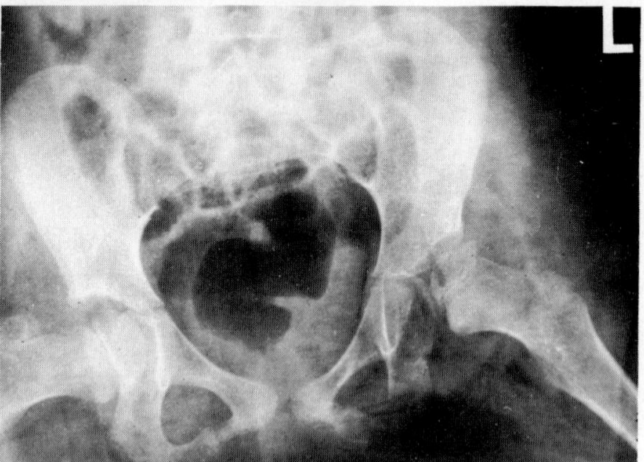

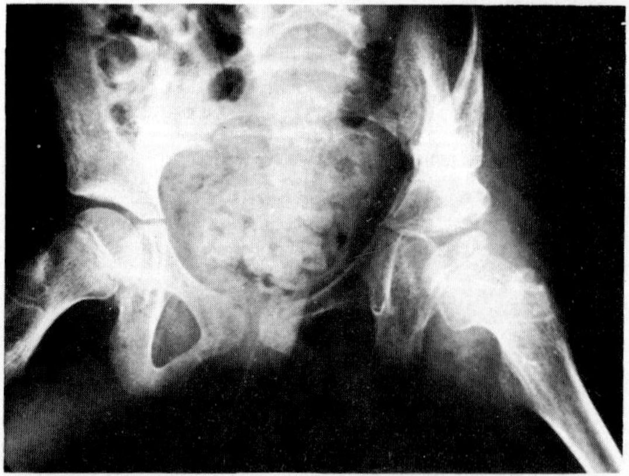

Fig. 13. Dislocation of the hip treated by adductor release, postero-lateral iliopsoas transplantation and Salter innominate osteotomy. (a) Before operation. (b) Three weeks after adductor release and partial reduction. (c) Eight months after postero-lateral iliopsoas transplantation combined with innominate osteotomy. The upper femoral epiphysis is deformed to some degree, but this deformity was present before operation. The hip is clincally stable, and the child is able to walk without any supports.

Intravenous blood transfusion is required during operation to replace blood loss, and intravenous glucose saline infusion should be continued post-operatively for 24 to 48 hours, until the possibility of paralytic ileus has been eliminated and fluid intake and output has been restored to normal. When the plaster is removed, a complication that may occur is fracture of the femur, usually in the supracondylar region, either in the limb that has been operated upon or in the opposite limb. An over-extensive derotation of the femoral neck for correction of valgus and ante-version may lead to recurrent posterior dislocation. In some patients, avascular necrosis of the femoral head may occur, following the need for extensive mobilisation and open reduction of a long-standing dislocation.

Results suggest that correction in dislocation is well worth attempting, even in patients who are fairly severely affected and is certainly worthwhile in patients with a moderate degree of neurological maturity. Samilson *et al.* (1972) were able to reduce 75 per cent of dislocations and 87 per cent of subluxations in a severely affected group of individuals.

The Treatment of Painful Subluxation or Dislocation of the Hip

Pain developing in an unreducable chronically subluxated or dislocated hip in cerebral palsy can sometimes be severe, even in a patient who is confined to sitting, and the pain is often difficult to relieve. Very rarely it may be appropriate to consider the possibility of correcting the deformity and of arthrodesing the hip either in the subluxed position or even in the dislocated position. An alternative is to perform abduction osteotomy of the upper end of the femur to correct the deformity, and this, in itself, will sometimes relieve pain. In patients with long-standing dislocation and gross deformity, who are confined to a wheel-chair, excision of the head of the femur can be performed as a last resort, but the operation is not an entirely satisfactory one and the stump of the femoral neck is still likely to lie beneath the skin and to be a source of irritation or even skin ulceration.

REFERENCES

Baker, L. D., Dodelin, R., Bassett, F. H. (1962) 'Pathological changes in the hip in cerebral palsy: incidence, pathogenesis and treatment.' *Journal of Bone and Joint Surgery,* **44A,** 1331.
Banks, H. H., Green, W. T. (1960) 'Adductor myotomy and obturator neurectomy for the correction of adduction contracture of the hip in cerebral palsy.' *Journal of Bone and Joint Surgery,* **42A,** 111.
Bleck, E. E., Holstein, A. (1964) 'Iliopsoas tenotomy for spastic paralytic deformities of the hip.' *Journal of Bone and Joint Surgery,* **46A,** 1375.
Brookes, M., Wardle, E. N. (1962) 'Muscle action and the shape of the femur.' *Journal of Bone and Joint Surgery,* **44B,** 398.
Craig, J. J. (1967) 'Cerebral palsy.' *in* Graham, W. D. (Ed.) *Modern Trends in Orthopaedics—5.* London: Butterworths, p. 44.
Eggers, G. W. N. (1952) 'Transplantation of the hamstring tendons to femoral condyles in order to improve hip extension and to decrease knee flexion in cerebral spastic paralysis.' *Journal of Bone and Joint Surgery,* **34A,** 827.

Gherlinzoni, G., Pais, C. (1950) 'Trattamento della lussazione patologia dell'anca.' *Chirugia degli organi di Movimento,* **34,** 335.

Hill, L. M., Bassett, F. H., Baker, L. D. (1966) 'Correction of adduction, flexion and internal rotation deformities of the hip in cerebral palsy.' *Developmental Medicine and Child Neurology,* **8,** 406.

Jones, G. B. (1962) 'Paralytic dislocation of the hip.' *Journal of Bone and Joint Surgery,* **44B,** 573.

Keats, S. (1957) 'Combined adductor-gracilis tenotomy and selective obturator-nerve resection for the correction of adduction deformity of the hip in children with cerebral palsy.' *Journal of Bone and Joint Surgery,* **39A,** 1087.

—— Morgese, A. N. (1967) 'A simple anteromedial approach to the lesser trochanter of the femur for release of the iliopsoas tendon.' *Journal of Bone and Joint Surgery,* **49A,** 632.

Lamb, D. W., Pollock, G. A. (1962) 'Hip deformities in cerebral palsy and their treatment.' *Developmental Medicine and Child Neurology,* **4,** 488.

Lewis, M. R., Samilson, R. L., Lucas, D. B. (1964) 'Femoral torsion and coxa valga in cerebral palsy. A preliminary report.' *Developmental Medicine and Child Neurology,* **6,** 591.

Ludloff, K. (1908) 'Zur blutigen Einrenkung der angeborenen Hüftluxation.' *Zeitschrift für orthopädische Chirurgie,* **22,** 272.

Magilligan, D. J. (1956) 'Calculation of the angle of anteversion by means of horizontal lateral roentgenography.' *Journal of Bone and Joint Surgery,* **38A,** 1231.

Mathews, S. S., Jones, M. H., Sperling, S. C. (1953) 'Hip derangements seen in cerebral palsied children.' *American Journal of Physical Medicine,* **32,** 213.

Morgan, J. D., Somerville, E. W. (1960) 'Normal and abnormal growth at the upper end of the femur.' *Journal of Bone and Joint Surgery,* **42B,** 264.

Phelps, W. M. (1959) 'Prevention of acquired dislocation of the hip in cerebral palsy.' *Journal of Bone and Joint Surgery,* **41A,** 440.

Pollock, G. A. (1958) 'Treatment of adductor paralysis by hamstring transposition.' *Journal of Bone and Joint Surgery,* **40B,** 534.

—— (1962) 'Surgical treatment of cerebral palsy.' *Journal of Bone and Joint Surgery,* **44B,** 68.

—— Sharrard, W. J. W. (1958) 'Orthopaedic surgery in the treatment of cerebral palsy.' *in* Illingworth, R. S. (Ed.) *Recent Advances in Cerebral Palsy.* London: Churchill, p. 286.

Ryder, C. T., Crane, L. (1953) 'Measuring femoral anteversion: the problem and a method.' *Journal of Bone and Joint Surgery,* **35A,** 321.

Salter, R. B. (1961) 'Innominate osteotomy in the treatment of congenital dislocation and subluxation of the hip.' *Journal of Bone and Joint Surgery,* **43B,** 518.

Samilson, R. L., Carson, J. J., James, P., Raney, F. L. (1967) 'Results and complications of adductor tenotomy and obturator neurectomy in cerebral palsy.' *Clinical Orthopedics and Related Research,* **54,** 61.

—— Tsou, P., Aamoth, G., Green, W. T. (1972) 'Dislocation and subluxation of the hip in cerebral palsy. Pathogenesis, natural history and management.' *Journal of Bone and Joint Surgery,* **54A,** 863.

Seymour, N., Sharrard, W. J. W. (1968) 'Bilateral proximal release of the hamstrings in cerebral palsy.' *Journal of Bone and Joint Surgery,* **50B,** 274.

Sharrard, W. J. W. (1967) 'Paralytic deformity in the lower limb.' *Journal of Bone and Joint Surgery,* **49B,** 731.

—— (1969) 'The orthopaedic surgery of cerebral palsy and spina bifida.' *in* Apley, A. G. (Ed.) *Recent Advances in Orthopaedics.* London: Churchill, p. 265.

—— (1971) *Paediatric Orthopaedics and Fractures.* Oxford: Blackwell.

Smith, E. T. (1969) 'Hip dislocation in cerebral palsy.' *Developmental Medicine and Child Neurology,* **11,** 291.

Somerville, E. W. (1959) 'Paralytic dislocation of the hip.' *Journal of Bone and Joint Surgery,* **41B,** 279.

Stephenson, T., Donovan, M. M. (1971) 'Transfer of hip adductor origins to the ischium in spastic cerebral palsy.' *Developmental Medicine and Child Neurology,* **13,** 247.

Tachdjian, M. O., Minear, W. L. (1956) 'Hip dislocation in cerebral palsy.' *Journal of Bone and Joint Surgery,* **38A,** 1358.

Watson-Jones, R. (1926) 'Spontaneous dislocation of the hip.' *British Journal of Surgery,* **14,** 36.

CHAPTER 9

The Knee in Cerebral Palsy

E. BURKE EVANS

In cerebral palsy there are two important knee problems: either the knee is not straight enough or it is, in a sense, too straight. Of these two problems—knee flexion and genu recurvatum—the former is the more common. And although loss of extensibility of the knee is found among patients with dyskinesia, particularly those with tension or increased resistance to passive motion, it is observed most often in those with spasticity or with a mixed motor affection of which spasticity is a conspicuous component.

Medial inclination of the knee may occur in patients with cerebral palsy, as may torsional deformity of the tibia or femur, which affects the knee. Genu valgum appears more frequently in combination with flexion deformity than as an isolated phenomenon, but it will be considered briefly as a separate entity.

KNEE FLEXION DEFORMITY

Genesis

It is convenient to assume that all deformity at the knee is by nature secondary—that the knee accommodates to affection at the hip and ankle. For example, the spastic infant who, when held aloft, adducts the hips, extends the knees and points the toes will be obliged when weight-bearing to flex or to hyperextend his knees in order to remain upright. To what degree and with what consistency the knee is affected by deformities of the hip and ankle is best determined by those who have worked with the cerebral palsied patient from infancy. Likewise they know best to what extent the knee deformity is preventable. Other factors are involved in the genesis of knee flexion deformity apart from the strength, length and spasticity of muscles, but these characteristics of muscles are at least reasonably assessable. In the standing or gravity-imposed position, all of the muscles affecting the lower extremity may be implicated, and it is possible for knee flexion deformity to accompany any one, or any combination, of the following states:

(1)   abdominal muscle weakness;
(2)   hip extensor weakness;
(3)   hip flexor contracture or spasticity;
(4)   hip adductor contracture or spasticity;
(5)   tensor fasciae latae contracture or spasticity;
(6)   quadriceps weakness;

173

(7) hamstring contracture or spasticity;
(8) triceps surae contracture or spasticity;
(9) triceps surae weakness.

Physical Examination

The illustrated test methods described and illustrated below have been found useful in determining the character, cause and severity of knee-flexion deformity.

In the testing of all muscle groups the examiner should get some impression of strength and length. A third factor to be considered is the readiness with which the patient initiates action after command. A slow response is a negative prognostic indicator.

Testing as described is essential to total pre-surgical evaluation. However, an experienced examiner will learn as much from observation of the patient walking and in other functional activities as from testing on a table. Predictions based on these observations are usually quite accurate.

Quadriceps (Fig. 1.)

For testing of quadriceps strength it is best to have the patient lying on his back with his legs over the edge of the table. If the examiner desires, the trunk may be supported slightly to relieve lordosis. To have a patient sitting would put the quadriceps at a disadvantage, as a result of hamstring tightness and spasticity and because of relaxation of the rectus femoris. It is easier for a child to extend both extremities simultaneously than to extend one at a time. Individual extremity testing with resistance can be accomplished with both extremities extended. Additional information as to the functional strength of the quadriceps can be gained by observing the patient's ability to ascend stairs or to correct knee flexion while standing.

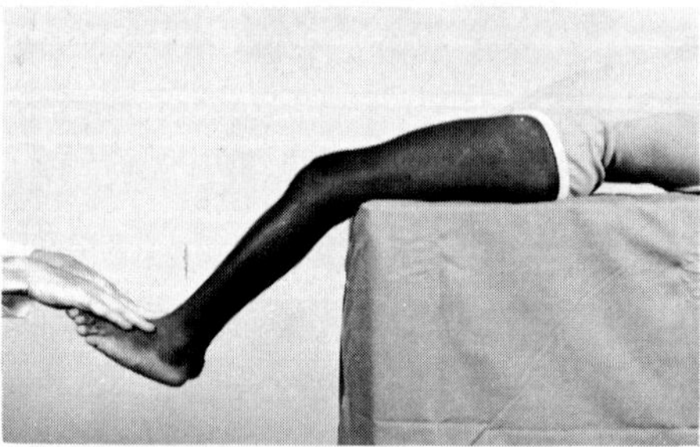

Fig. 1.

Rectus Femoris

Rectus femoris resistance is usually tested with the patient prone and with knees extended (Fig. 2a). The knees are then flexed passively to at least 90 degrees (Fig. 2b). The hips will flex abruptly and the buttocks will rise, because of the triggering of the stretch reflex of the rectus femoris. The hips will then gradually extend (Fig. 2c). The degree of the remaining hip flexion in excess of that present before testing is presumed to be due to rectus tightness. The initial hip flexion,

174

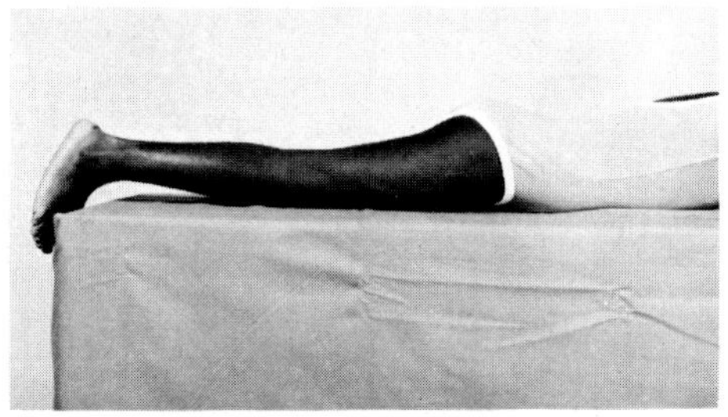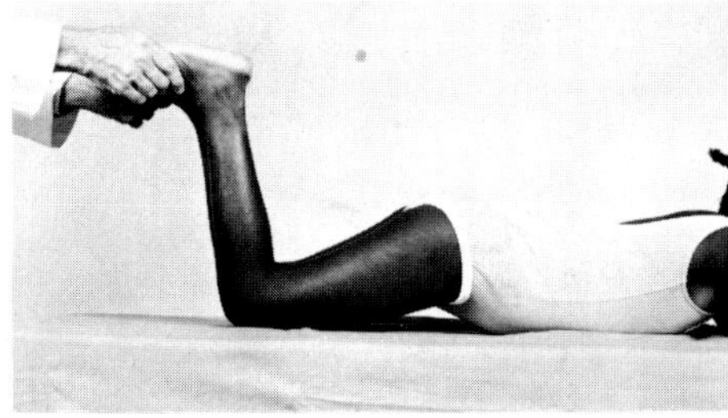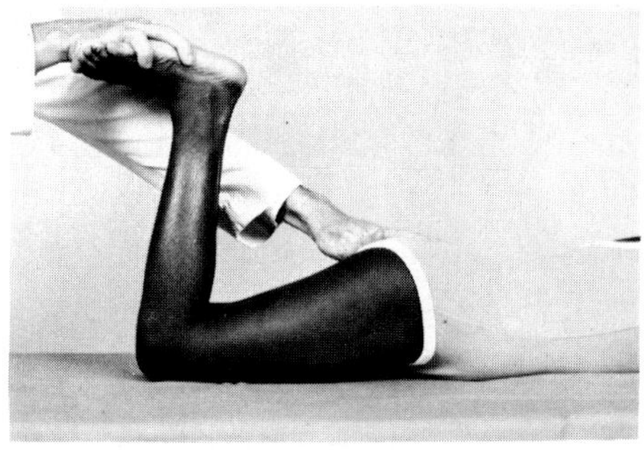

Figs. 2a *(above left)*, 2b *(above right)* **and** 2c *(right)*.

however, may be due to the action of other hip flexors. The tensor fascia femoris in particular is affected by knee action, but it is not put on the stretch by knee flexion. The examiner may get a better idea of rectus resistance and tightness by simply observing how much passive flexion of the knee increases as the hip is flexed.

Hip Flexion

The Thomas test serves well enough for the cerebral palsied. The examiner should be sure, however, that he stabilizes the opposite hip and the pelvis at that point at which the lumbar lordosis is just corrected (Fig. 3a). There is no advantage in rolling the pelvis. In fact the measurement may then be erroneous. There are often two measurements to be made: the first being the natural position of the thigh without pressure (Fig. 3b), and the second being the position gained after pressure has been applied on the dorsum of the thigh to the point of resistance (Fig. 3c). A measurement obtained by forcing the hip into additional extension is of no use. Usually, the thigh will remain adducted because of tight adductors. If it should fall into abduction, however, it must be brought at least to neutral for the maneuver. In those cases in which abduction can be obtained, the tensor fasciae femoris can be partially eliminated as an offender if the hip is extended in abduction. With the hip adducted, both the iliopsoas and the tensor fasciae are tested, and the tensor, alone, can be palpated. The effective hip flexor fixation of the pelvis can be roughly assessed by holding the lower extremities together with knees extended, flexing the hips until the back is flat, and then extending them until the lordosis begins to return (Figs. 3d and 3e). For simultaneous bilateral gross testing in a slender patient, there is nothing easier than placing the patient in the prone lying position on a flat surface.

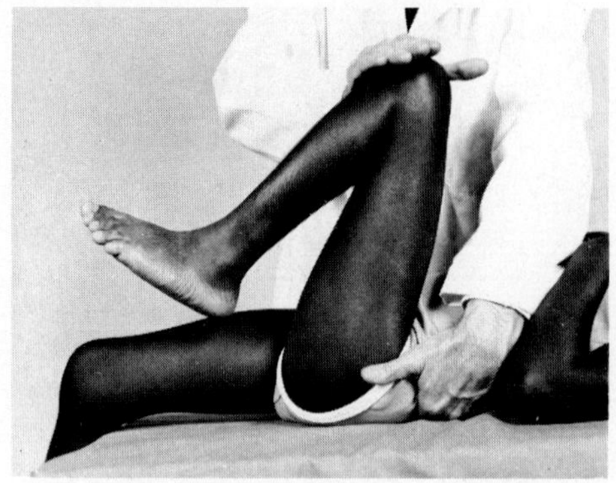

Fig. 3*a*.

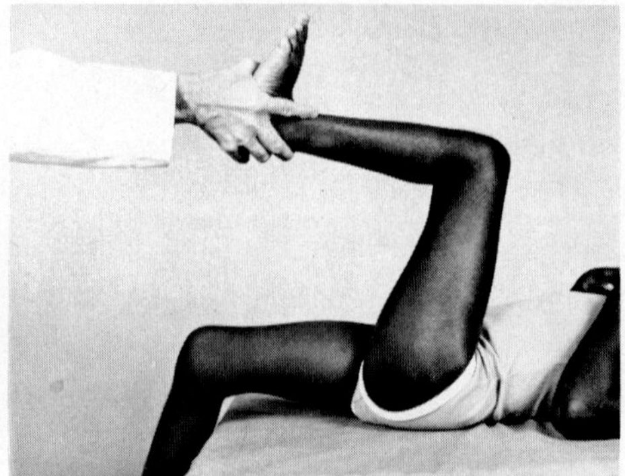

Fig. 3*b*.

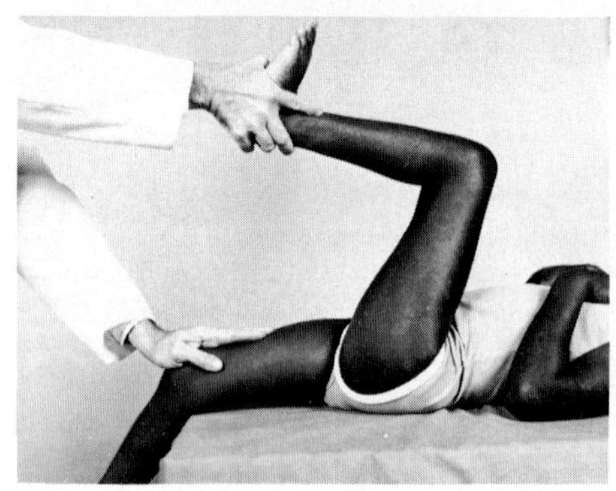

Fig. 3*c*.

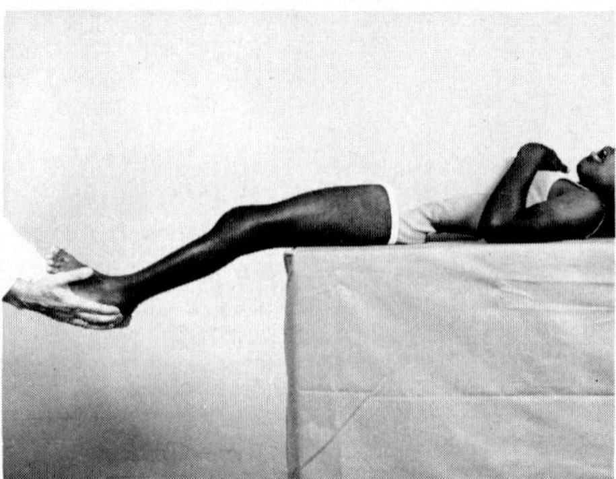

Fig. 3*d*.

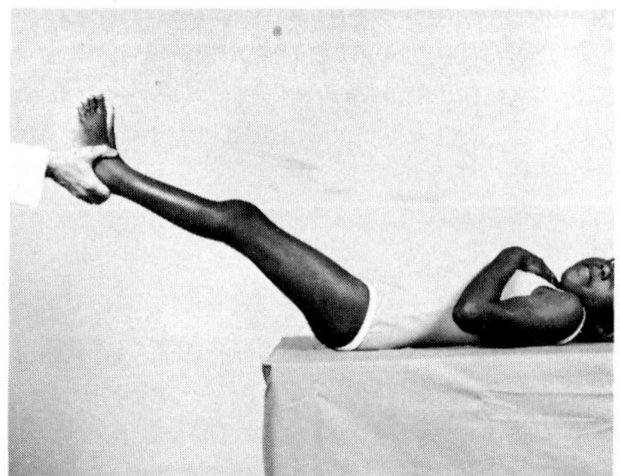

Fig. 3*e*.

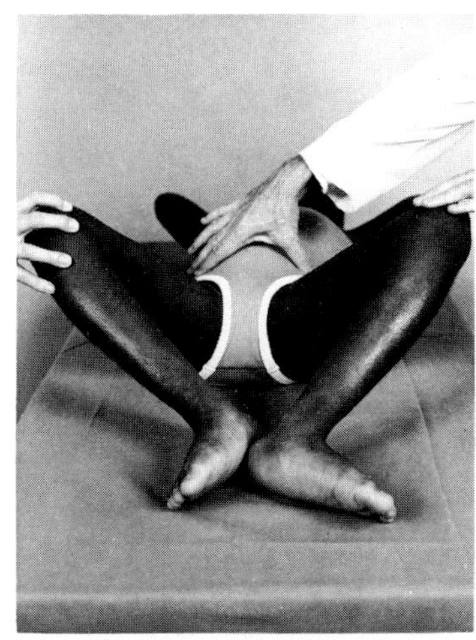

Fig. 4a.

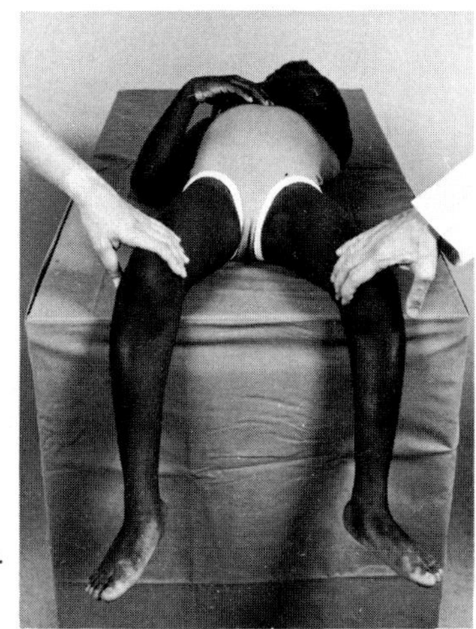

Fig. 4b.

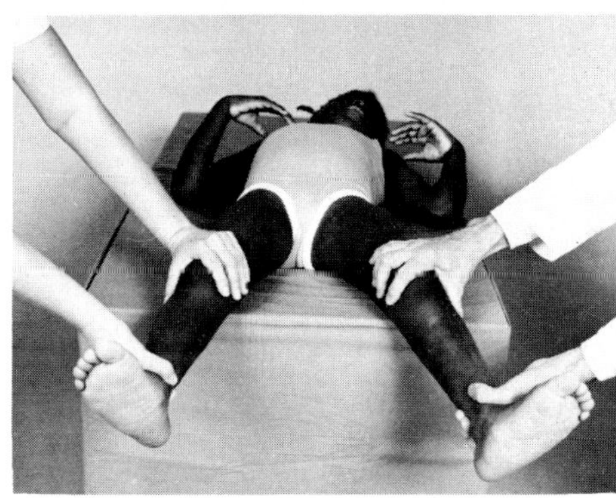

Fig. 4c.

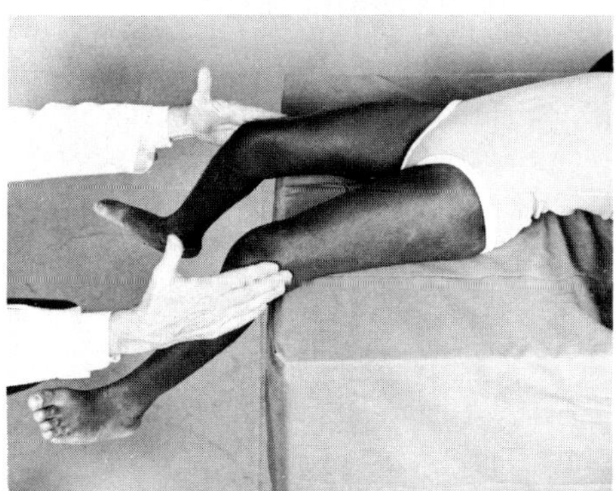

Fig. 5.

Hip Adductors (Figs. 4*a*, *b* and *c*)

Adductor tightness must be checked in three positions: (1) with knees and hips flexed (Fig. 4*a*), (2) with hips extended and knees flexed (Fig. 4*b*), and (3) with knees and hips extended (Fig. 4*c*). Hip flexion relaxes the anteriormost adductors, which are also hip flexors. Knee flexion relaxes the gracilis, which inserts below the knee. There may thus be three measurements as the muscles are successively put on the stretch.

Hip Abductors (Fig. 5)

To best determine hip abductor power, the examiner should position the patient so as to gain as much hip extension as possible. This writer prefers having the patient on his back. If there is a knee flexion contracture, the legs must be free of the table, since the contracture at the knee will impose additional flexion at the hips. The patient is then asked to spread his thighs. At maximum abduction, resistance is applied. An assistant may be used to watch for tilt of the pelvis. The

177

patient may tend to flex the hips slightly in the abduction effort. This is usually tensor action, the flexion component of which can be dissipated by gentle anterior pressure on the thigh by the assistant. The side-lying position for testing abductors is useless if there is any degree of hip flexion contracture or if there are tight adductors. In this position, apparent abduction is likely to be due to the action of trunk muscles and tilt of the pelvis.

Hip Extensors

In the testing of hip extensors it is possibly more important to determine the quality of contraction than to be concerned with excursion. Excursion will, after all, be limited by hip flexion contracture. The patient is positions prone, with the hips flexed at the edge of the table, and the thighs free (Fig. 6*a*). He is asked to raise both extremities at once, and the gluteal contraction is observed and palpated (Fig. 6*b*). If the examiner wishes, he may hold the knees flexed to eliminate the hamstrings, but this simply increases hip flexion by tensing the rectus femoris. Testing hip extension with the patient prone but with the thighs on the table will give an indication of the ability of the patient to hold the amount of extension already passively achieved. Any apparent additional extension will be due to elevation or tilting of the pelvis and to the action of trunk extensors. Hyperextension of the hip is a rare enough feat among normal persons.

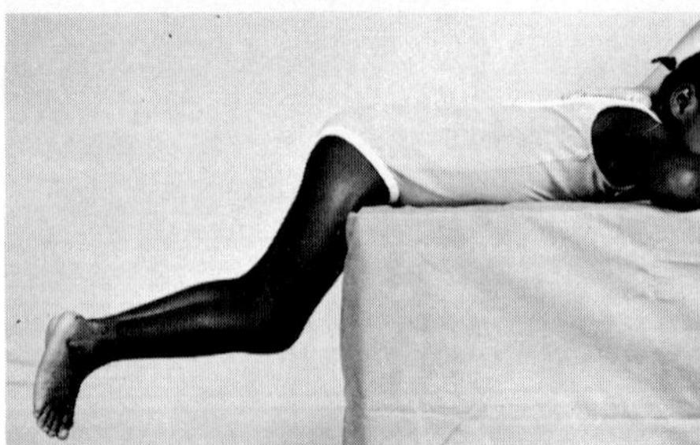 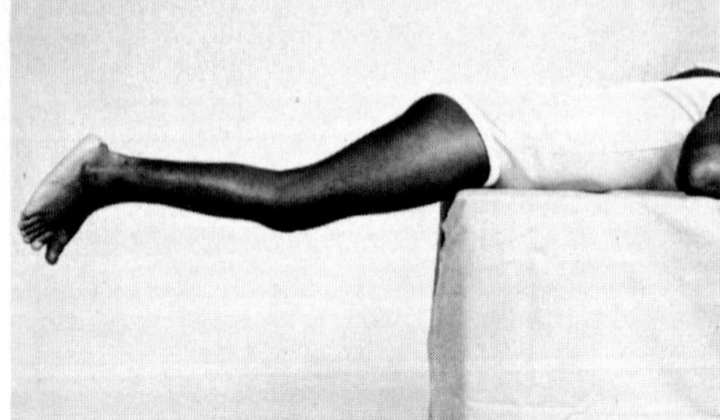

Fig. 6*a*. **Fig. 6*b*.**

Hamstrings

Hamstring extensibility should be assessed in three ways. (1) With patient prone or recumbent and hips fully extended, the knees are passively completely extended. Any remaining flexion is due to what may be called 'absolute' hamstring contracture (Fig. 7*a*). (2) With the patient recumbent, one hip is held firmly in extension. The opposite hip is flexed to 90 degrees and the knee is then extended to the point of resistance. The flexion angle remaining is the apparent contracture (Fig. 7*b*). (3) In the same position, one hip is flexed until the lumbar lordosis is relieved. The opposite hip is flexed to 90 degrees, and the knee is then extended (Fig. 7*c*). In this maneuver the pelvis is tilted to correct for hip flexion contracture, and the angle of knee flexion remaining is thus more nearly accurate than that of the second test.

178

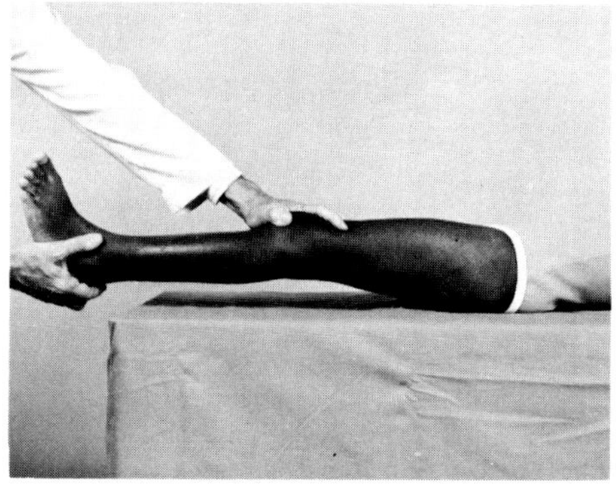 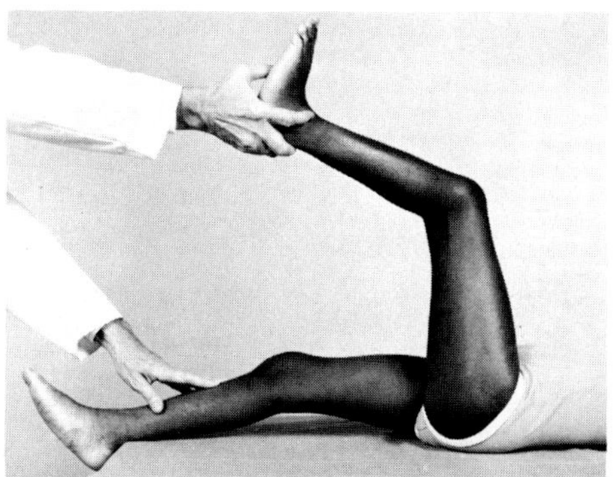

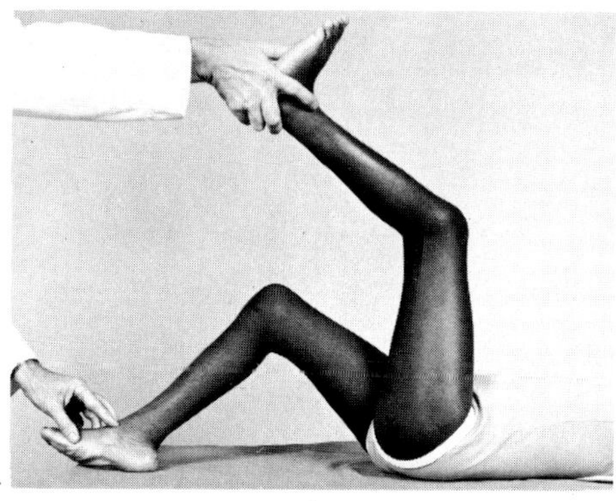

Figs. 7a (*above left*), 7b (*above right*) **and** 7c (*left*).

For testing hamstring strength, the patient sits upright on the edge of the table and is asked to bend both knees. Resistance is applied to each calf separately. Prone testing of hamstring strength is not feasible, because of the natural active incompetence of the muscles and because of quadriceps tightness.

Triceps Surae

If the ankle can be passively dorsiflexed with the knee flexed (Fig. 8b) but not with the knee extended (Fig. 8a), it is understood that of the two major parts of the triceps surae the gastrocnemius is the more offensive. If knee flexion does little to relieve tension, then both the soleus and gastrocnemius are participants in the contracture.

This standard test is for extensibility. It gives no clue as to the strength of the muscles, but the examiner may get some idea of their resiliency. For proper control, the foot should be held as shown. The heel is in the neutral position or slightly inverted, and as the dorsiflexion force is exerted the heel is actually pulled by the grasping fingers. The dorsiflexion force is exerted by the heel of the hand. Only with this kind of stabilization can the examiner be sure that part of the dorsiflexion is not taking place in the mid-foot. Figure 8c shows the resistance encountered to passive knee extension when the ankle is held firmly in dorsiflexion.

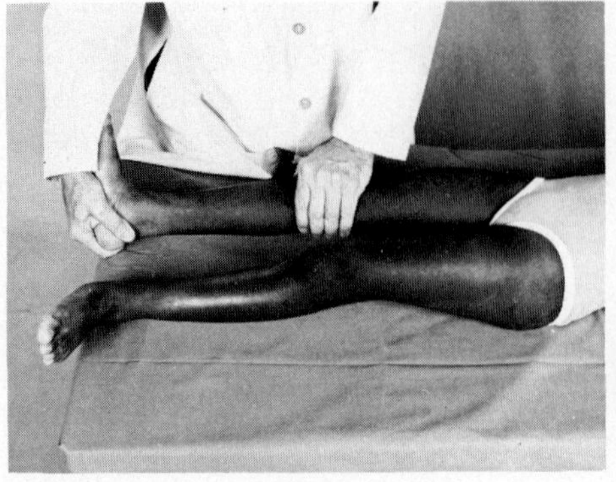

Fig. 8*a*.

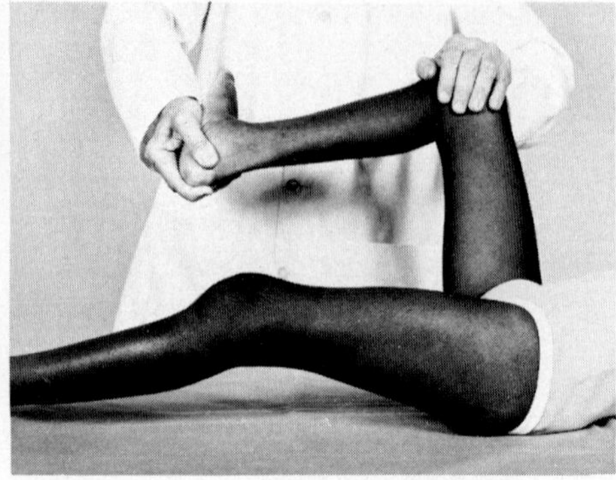

Fig. 8*b*.

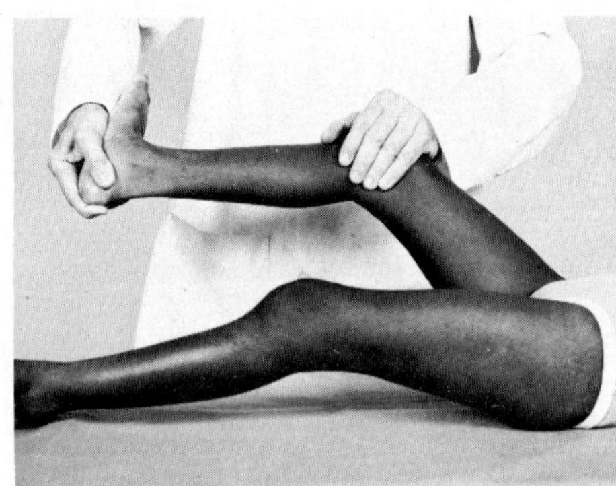

Fig. 8*c*.

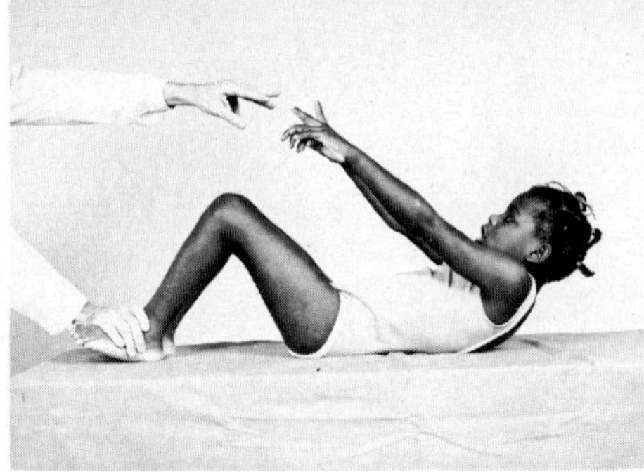

Fig. 9.

Triceps surae strength is often difficult to assess. Many children with tight or spastic muscles will be unable to walk on their toes or to rise on them. Manual testing will give but a gross idea of strength. It must not be assumed that because of contracture the triceps surae are strong—more often the reverse is true. It is helpful to palpate the muscle bellies during testing. If there is little change in the quality of resistance during contraction, the muscles may be assumed to be weak and in-efficient. In such cases, muscle lengthening procedures may lead to calcaneous deformity and thus must be performed with caution.

Abdominals (Fig. 9)

With the patient on his back, knees and hips flexed and feet stabilized, he is asked to reach above his knees, raising first the head and then the shoulders. The quality and symmetry of abdominal contraction is observed and palpated. With certain patients, it is necessary to raise and support the head and shoulders slightly, to favor initiation of the contraction.

Hamstring Anatomy

Because of the consistent implication of the hamstrings in knee flexion deformity, it is appropriate to review the anatomy and function of these muscles.

From the point of view of the anatomist, the hamstrings are those three muscles—the biceps femoris, semitendinosus, and semimembranosus—which arise from the ischial tuberosity and insert into the tibia. By virtue of similar nerve supply and anatomic position, the longest fibers of the adductor magnus belong to the group. The gracilis is popularly included.

The biceps femoris has two distinct muscle bellies. Its ischial portion is a thick, flat muscle, the fibers of which arise from the short tendon which it shares with the semitendinosus. These fibers gain final insertion into the undersurface of its aponeurosis at the level of the lower one-third of the femur, where they are replaced by fibers of the femoral portion. The fibers arising from the femur continue with the aponeurosis to within one or two inches of its insertion into the head of the fibula. The two muscle bellies are approximately the same size, and each is about two-thirds as long as the entire muscle.

The semitendinosus shares its tendon of origin with the biceps. Its round, fleshy portion begins near the ischial tuberosity and continues for two-thirds of the length of the muscle. The semitendinosus lies on the posterior surface of the semimembranosus, except at the distal extreme, where its tendon extends beyond the termination of the semimembranosus to insert deep to the gracilis and sartorius on the upper part of the medial surface of the tibia. A proximal extension of the tendon of insertion gives the muscle belly a fibrous septum for much of its length.

The semimembranosus at its proximal end has a wide, flat aponeurosis, which lies deep to the semitendinosus and which gives origin to broad bipennate diagonal fibers. There are two distinct portions, the fibers of which are roughly parallel. The proximalmost is medial and deep to the semitendinosus. The distalmost is deep and lateral to the semitendinosus. The muscle inserts on the medial side of the back of the tibia, just distal to the knee joint. Strong connective tissue fibers fan out from the muscle on the posterior surface of the knee, giving secondary insertion into the capsule.

Function

The three muscles (the biceps femoris, semitendinosus and semimembranosus) act as a group to flex the knee and to extend and adduct the hip. Under special circumstances (which are discussed on page 187), the hamstrings may aid in extension of the knee.

The biceps femoris, acting through its ischial fibers, may function singly as a weak lateral rotator of the hip. It is encumbered in this action by its femoral fibers. When the knee is flexed and the extremity free, the biceps is a prime lateral rotator of the leg. When the foot and leg are fixed, this same action can medially rotate the femur, and thus the trunk, on the leg. In both of these latter actions, the femoral portion participates.

The semitendinosus is a medial rotator of the hip and a medial rotator of the leg when the knee is flexed. The semimembranosus shares in these two functions.

The adductor magnus and gracilis both take part in hip adduction. The gracilis also acts as a knee flexor. The adductor magnus, through its most distal attachment, extends and medially rotates the hip.

Biarticular Function

The hamstrings, because of their biarticular nature, have a distinct functional relationship with the rectus femoris, the only biarticular muscle of the front of the limb. The example cited by Steindler (1955) is that of shortening the extremity by drawing the heel toward the buttock. In this situation, the hamstrings, acting distally, flex the knee; the rectus femoris, acting proximally, flexes the hip, but cannot extend the knee because of the action of the hamstrings. The two muscles thus shift position—the rectus femoris downwards and the hamstrings upwards—but each retains its original length. There is a similar shift in the crouch position.

The hamstrings are too short to permit simultaneous full flexion of the hip and full extension of the knee. This is known as 'passive insufficiency.' On the other hand, the hamstrings are too long to effect simultaneous full extension of the hip and full flexion of the knee. This is termed 'active insufficiency.'

Thus the shift with the rectus femoris is essential to retain the muscle at its optimum length for maximum tension.

Excursion

The amplitude of a muscle is proportional to the length of its parallel fibers. A straight-fibered muscle can shorten to roughly 50 per cent of its maximum length. It is also true that the tension which a muscle develops is proportional to its average cross-sectional area. The semitendinosus, a straight-fibered muscle, has, therefore, a greater excursion than does the semimembranosus; but the semimembranosus, by virtue of its cross-sectional area, can develop greater tension. The biceps is straight-fibered, but is limited by the femoral attachment. Its combined cross-sectional area is greater, however, than that of either of the other two muscles.

Tendon-tagging Experiment

In order to learn more about the excursion of the hamstrings, and to determine to what extent their tendons retract after surgical division, three cases of spastic cerebral palsy were selected for hamstring tendon division only. The tendons were tagged with stainless steel wire—one loop being placed in the gracilis, two in the semitendinosus, three in the semimembranosus, and four in the biceps femoris. The tendons were divided half an inch distal to the line of tags. Roentgenograms were taken before division, with the knees in flexion and in extension. After division, roentgenograms were taken at regular intervals up to one year.

The pattern of retraction was the same in the three cases. The gracilis and semitendinosus retracted to the level of the middle third of the femur. The biceps femoris and semimembranosus were restricted to the lower third. This pattern thus reflected accurately the anatomic features of each of the muscles.

Relation of Hamstrings to Abnormal Postures: the Crouch Position

In cerebral palsy of the spastic type the most common posture is the crouch. In this position the hips and knees are flexed. The ankle may be plantar flexed, or dorsiflexed. There is usually adduction and internal rotation of the thighs.

Individuals who stand with a crouch posture may in recumbency lie flat, or nearly so. It is with the imposition of gravity, the stimulus of contact with the floor, or the effort to remain upright or balanced, that the crouch is assumed. Apart from gravitational force, factors which may cause the crouch posture to be assumed are a strong plantar thrust at the ankle, a flexion contracture at the knee or hip, or a combination of these. The associated adduction and internal rotation of the thighs may be secondary to strong muscular thrust or contracture, or may be a stabilizing mechanism.

In this complex situation, the separate rôle of the hamstrings can be identified with reasonable clarity. It is apparent from observation of the interaction of the rectus femoris and the hamstrings that flexion at the hip will impose a stretch on the hamstrings, which in turn will flex the knee. In the spastic state, this chain of events is exaggerated by an increased insufficiency of the hamstrings, in the form of contracture or hyperreflexic resistance. Thus the hamstrings are, in effect, too short to allow simultaneous extension at the knee and flexion at the hip. Similarly, the rectus femoris cannot allow flexion of the knee and extension at the hip.

In the crouch position, any adductive force produces internal rotation of the hip: thus all hip adductors become internal rotators. The rotation is facilitated if the floor contact is with the ball of the foot only. The hamstrings, however, in addition to adducting, exercise a positive internal rotating force, which is independent of the patient's position, and which is augmented by the action of the medial-most fibers of the adductor magnus. The rotary action of the hamstrings is brought prominently into play when the crouch posture is adopted. The prime offender in producing this rotation is likely to be the semitendinosus, by virtue of its greater leverage due to its insertion well forward on the tibia. The semimembranosus has less leverage, but is a more powerful muscle. It has been found to be solely responsible for rotary deformity occurring after section or transfer of the semitendinosus.

The biceps, in acting at the flexed knee to rotate the tibia laterally, must, when the foot is fixed, augment internal rotation of the hip by stabilizing the tibia and by internally rotating the femur on the leg.

In most patients with a crouch gait, the rectus femoris and hamstrings are of about equal strength. Occasionally one observes patients in whom the rectus femoris is relatively weak. These individuals will have a deep crouch and, because of the weak rectus, will have a somewhat more erect trunk. This combination of factors— the flexed knee and the extended hip—results in an absolute hamstring contracture, in that even in recumbency the knees cannot be passively extended to 180 degrees.

Acquired Dislocation of the Hip. In the crouch position, the hamstrings, through their adductive and internal rotary action, exert strong lateral and posterior forces on the hip, which, in combination with the vertical force, favor displacement of the head of the femur. The hamstrings must, then, be implicated along with the gracilis and the other adductors in the genesis of hip subluxations and dislocations in cerebral palsy. We are of the opinion that their rôle in the production of these acquired deformities is a major one.

Relation of Hamstrings to Abnormal Postures: the Extension Stance

Another common posture in spastic cerebral palsy is that in which the feet and ankles are in equinus, the knees in extension, and the hips in varying degrees of flexion. In addition, there is often a prominent adductor thrust. When these patients begin to walk, they lean forward on their crutches. Foot contact is toe-heel; the triceps surae, the rectus *and* the hamstrings then combine to extend the knee. The triceps surae or the fixed equinus initiates the thrust. The hamstrings may produce internal rotation at the end of the thrust. Again the lack of heel contact facilitates rotation. Many of these patients have hamstring contractures, and may, following surgery for relief of equinus, assume a crouch posture.

When equinus is the only problem in a relatively mild case, the gait will be toe-heel, and again the hamstrings will help to extend the knee and may cause internal rotation. In this instance and in the one cited in the preceding paragraph, the extensor action of hamstrings is dependent upon toe contact and ankle equinus and upon resistance of a superincumbent pelvic level, which is fixed by the foot-flat length of the opposite extremity.

In the hemiplegic patient with heel-cord contracture, the heel will touch the floor only if the knee is hyperextended. The hamstrings again work as extensors. If there is a severe hamstring contracture in combination with the tight heel cord, the knee does not extend and the heel does not come into contact with the floor.

When there is double hemiparesis, the pattern may be much like that of hemiparesis; however, the less involved of the two sides may assume the position of the more involved. In this situation, what appears to be a symmetrical dynamic response is simply a matter of mimicry or accommodation by the less affected side.

Conservative Treatment of Knee Flexion Deformity

If knee-flexion posture is a secondary phenomenon, it should be preventable and, in its less severe forms, even correctable by conservative means. Prevention involves (1) the maintenance of extensibility by passive and active means, (2) the avoidance of prolonged periods spent in static positions, such as sitting, which would favor contracture, and (3) the achievement of sufficient balance and security in standing as to make knee flexion unnecessary. These goals are difficult to attain.

In an older child with moderately severe contractures, active stretching, combined with balance and gait training, may reduce the contracture sufficiently to make surgical relief unnecessary, or optional. Often, however, the child has contractures at the hip and ankle, and so long as these persist the knees will continue to be a problem.

Surgical Correction of Knee Flexion Deformity

Non-contractural knee flexion, which is proved to be secondary to deformity at the hip or ankle, may be relieved by operation at either or both of the other two levels; that is, by surgical correction of hip flexion contracture and/or equinus.

As straightforward and uncomplicated as this correction formula may seem, there are distinct hazards. If equinus is corrected in a patient who, in spite of passive and active extensibility of the knee, has tight hamstrings, the knee-flexion posture may persist or recur because of triceps surae weakness. If there is relative quadriceps incompetence, there may be a significant knee flexion sag after correction of the equinus, due to the loss of the stabilizing effect of the tight or spastic triceps surae. If the hip flexion contracture is not corrected with the equinus, knee flexion will still be required for upright posture. If the hip flexion contracture is inadequately corrected, as is most often the case, the patient may continue to prefer that degree of knee flexion which accommodates to the hip flexion and relieves the lumbar lordosis.

Correction of Hip Adduction Contracture

Isolated hip adduction contracture may cause knee flexion in two ways. (1) The gracilis attaches below the knee and this may cause knee flexion directly. (2) In the scissoring gait, standing and walking are facilitated by knee flexion. However, once the knees are flexed, the hips are likewise flexed and as previously noted, all adductor forces, when the foot is in contact with the floor, become internal rotation forces as well—just as all internal rotation adducts.

Adductor tenotomy alone may therefore relieve moderate knee flexion deformity and moderate internal rotation deformity of the hip. Another procedure, transposition to the ischial tuberosity of the tendons of origin of the principal adductors, seems a better, more positive means of solving the problem of hip adduction and internal rotation combined with moderate hip and knee flexion (Stephenson and Donovan 1970). The procedure gives excellent correction of adduction and internal rotation; knee and hip flexion, if not immediately relieved, likely to become progressively less troublesome, probably due to the posterior pelvic stabilizing effect of the transposed adductors. The procedure will not correct severe knee-flexion deformities.

Hamstring Weakening

An established knee flexion contracture, whether primary or secondary, is corrected as a rule by surgical weakening of the hamstrings. Hamstrings may be weakened by tenotomy, lengthening, proximal recession or transfer, or by a combination of these methods—there being a sufficient number of muscles to permit variation. It is likely that the means of weakening is less important than the amount.

It should not be the aim in any hamstring surgery to get the knee straight. Rather the aim should be to accomplish just sufficient weakening to balance knee flexion and extension power. Any hamstring weakening procedure will, to some degree, increase lumbar lordosis, because of the decrease in the posterior stabilizing effect of the hamstrings on the pelvis. It will decrease knee flexion power, and it may cause troublesome back-knee.

It is unwise to weaken hamstrings in the presence of a fixed equinus or a strong plantar thrust, as this will most surely lead to genu recurvatum. If the knees are straightened surgically in the presence of hip flexion contracture, the victim will be unable to stand erect without severely accentuating his lordosis, and he will often be forced to lean forward acutely, using crutches to make a three-point base of support.

For good alignment with the knees fully extended in the upright position, the hips must be fully extensible—a feat difficult to accomplish among patients with spastic cerebral palsy. Furthermore, for those with persisting hip flexor tightness of even minor degree, posture is better if the knees remain slightly flexed. There follows a review of hamstring weakening procedures.

Tenotomy. This procedure has the advantage of ease of performance. It is useful for patients who will not walk, and for patients in whom an improvement in knee extension is desirable to facilitate handling or nursing care. Selective tenotomy may still be performed by some surgeons in ambulant patients. The two muscles most often tenotomized are the gracilis and the semitendinosus. These muscles can be shown by palpation and by testing to be the most consistent offenders. The disadvantages of tenotomy are loss of knee flexion power and loss of posterior pelvic stability.

Lengthening. This procedure is a popular one because it allows graded correction without loss of muscle continuity. The gracilis and semitendinosus must be lengthened in a step-cut or sliding fashion. The biceps and semimembranosus may be lengthened either by division of the aponeurosis or by step cutting, but aponeurotic section is often favored, because in both muscles the muscle belly extends to the level of the knee, and free tendons of insertion are short. Division of the aponeurosis of the biceps femoris lengthens mainly the ischial portion of that muscle. It may be assumed that as early as 1942 Green and McDermott had resolved the problem of knee flexion contracture by means of selective step-cut and fractional aponeurotic lengthening. This procedure, selectively executed, may be used safely for all degrees of knee flexion deformity. Knee flexion power is retained.

Transfer (Eggers). In its full form this procedure involves: (1) transfer of all hamstrings from their insertions below the knee to the ipsilateral femoral condyles, and (2) division of the medial and lateral patellar retinacula. It was originally used by Eggers (1952), in patients with moderately severe or severe spastic diparesis who had fixed knee flexion contractures. There was good rationale for the procedure. It corrected the knee flexion deformity, and it converted the hamstrings to one-joint muscles which could extend the hip and augment knee extension when the foot was fixed.

The procedure proved to be most useful for patients with severe knee flexion contractures. It had the advantage of permanency of correction. But it had the previously listed disadvantages of eliminating knee flexion power, of allowing back-knee, and of accentuating lumbar lordosis.

The procedure has since been modified by Dr Eggers (Eggers and Evans 1963, Evans and Julian 1964) to accommodate all grades of involvement, and the full hamstring transfer is now rarely performed. The modification of the procedure and suggested criteria for their use are as follows (see Fig. 10).

(A) The full hamstring transfer may be indicated for absolute knee flexion contractures of 20 degrees or more. It can be determined at the time of surgery whether or not hamstrings participate in the contracture. With long-standing deformity of this severity, knee extension will be facilitated by division of the patellar retinacula.

(B) The semimembranosus is the stoutest proximal defender of the back of the knee. It can be left intact, so long as it can be adequately lengthened by aponeurotic section. The other hamstrings have more distal attachments, and it may be better to transfer these in cases where there is a fixed absolute contracture of 10 to 20 degrees. The patellar retinacula may be divided as well.

(C) The gracilis and semitendinosus are consistently the most offensive of the medial muscles. The gracilis may be sacrificed, as shown in Figures 10*b, c* and *d*, by section of five centimetres or more of its tendon, because it is usually not needed as a hip adductor. The semimembranosus and biceps are lengthened by aponeurotic division in patients with 5 to 10 degrees of absolute contracture when all muscles are to some extent offensive.

(D) More often than not, the medial hamstrings are more offensive than the biceps femoris. If their division or lengthening accomplishes sufficient passive extension, the biceps should be left intact. This is the most commonly performed modification of the hamstring transfer procedure.

(E) Patients with slight knee flexion contracture and a tendency to rotate the lower extremity medially when walking, may be substantially benefited by transfer of the offending semitendinosus to the lateral femoral condyle. This procedure was described by Eggers in 1963 and by Baker in 1964. It is not performed by the writer if hip flexion contracture exceeds 10 degrees, nor is it performed in combination with other surgery at the knee.

Similar modifications of the hamstring transfer procedure have been advocated by other surgeons, who have found that in most cases transfer of all hamstrings is neither necessary nor desirable. The writer presently lengthens hamstrings as often as he transfers them. The results, initially at least, are indistinguishable.

Recession

The only report of experience with release of hamstrings from their ischial origin is that of Seymour and Sharrard (1968), who limited use of the recession procedure to those patients who could extend the knee completely but who had a short stride due to hamstring tightness. They were favourably impressed with the results.

Lachman and Steel (personal communication) state that they favor proximal hamstring myotenotomy in patients who have excessively spastic quadriceps with strong resistance to passive motion. In these patients the knees bend slowly, and the

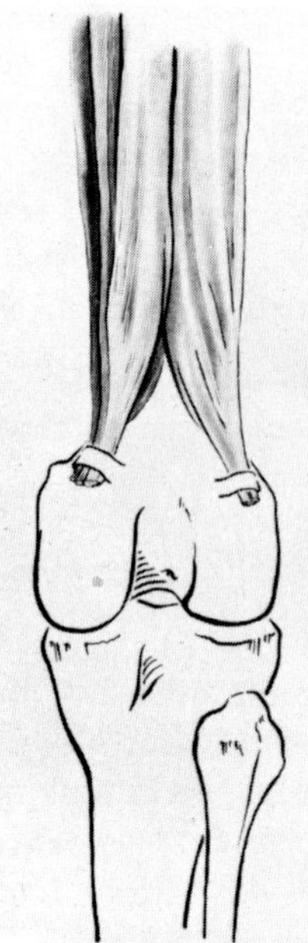

Fig. 10*a*.

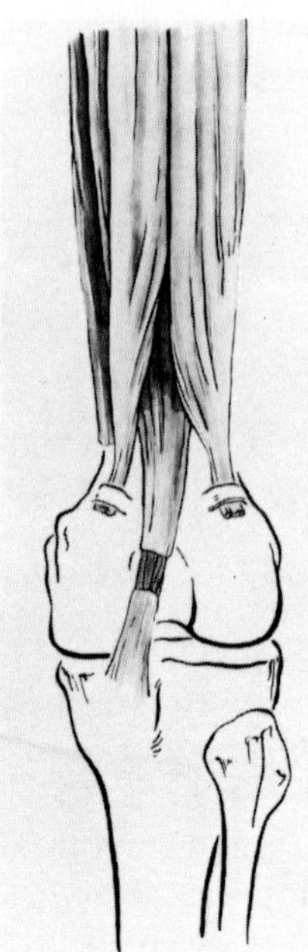

Fig. 10*b*.

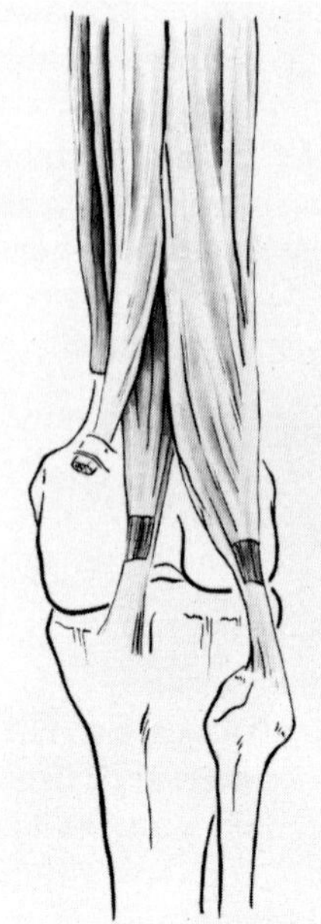

Fig. 10*c*.

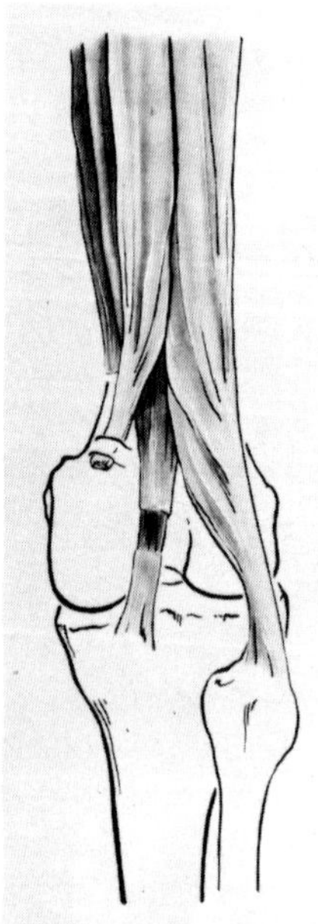

Fig. 10*d*.

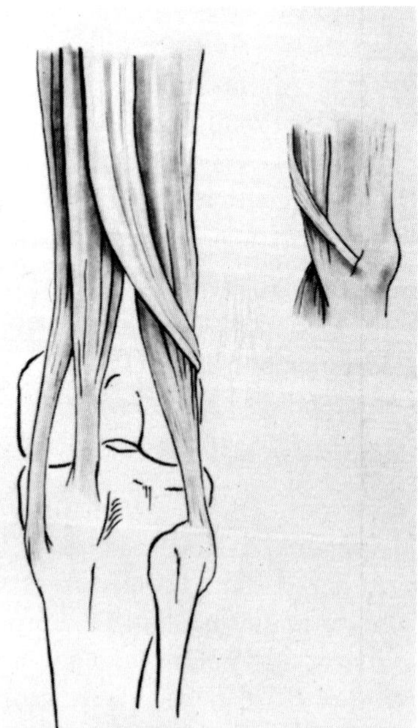

Fig. 10*e*.

patella is often high-riding. They believe that the procedure should be accompanied
by a rectus femoris tenotomy to reduce the hip flexion contracture and the tendency
toward lordosis. They have noted that if hamstrings are lengthened at the knee when
quadriceps are quite spastic, the patient afterwards has extreme difficulty bending
the knees.

Moore (personal communication), who has routinely lengthened hamstrings by
proximal myotenotomy for fifteen years, has not found accentuation of lumbar
lordosis to be a troublesome post-operative problem. He corrects any persisting knee
flexion contracture with wedging plaster casts.

Quadriceps Augmentation

The chronically flexed knee may fail to extend completely because of the
resistance or tightness of the hamstrings, because of incompetence of the quadriceps, or for both of these reasons. Active extension may be limited to one degree
and passive extension to quite another. If there is an active extension lag of 10 or
more degrees and if the quadriceps are found by test to be weak, it may be desirable
to augment extensor power.

The procedure advocated by Dr Eggers (1950) for restoration of the central pull
of the quadriceps was division of the patellar retinacula as an accompaniment to
hamstring transfer. The retinacula, under the circumstances described, may be
sufficiently tight to encumber otherwise functional quadriceps. To what extent
release of the patellar retinacula is now performed it is impossible to say. At the
University of Texas Medical Branch it has been found to be unnecessary in most
cases which require hamstring weakening, but it is still performed if there is
demonstrable extension lag and/or weak quadriceps.

Other procedures for augmenting quadriceps power are transfer of hamstrings
into the patella or quadriceps, and patellar tendon advancement. The latter of these
two procedures has retained popularity among those surgeons who have found it
useful in patients with high-riding patellae or with persisting knee extension lag
after other surgery for correction of knee flexion (Roberts and Adams 1953, Baker
1956, Keats and Kambin 1962).

Patellar tendon advancement was described and modified by Chandler (1933),
and further modified by Baker (1956). It has not been used in the surgical treatment
of cerebral palsy at The University of Texas Medical Branch. Duncan (personal
communication) believes that any distal advancement of the patellar tendon should
be accompanied by rectus femoris release to avoid accentuation of hip flexion and
restriction of knee flexion.

Post-operative Care

Following all surgery in the region of the knee or ankle for correction of knee
flexion deformity, the extremities should be immobilized in circular plasters from
toe to groin, with the ankles at neutral and the knees in the amount of extension
surgically attained. A crossbar may be used for stability and for holding the
extremities in easy hip abduction and external rotation. If the surgery has included
hip flexor release, a spica may be used if desired in place of the long-leg plasters.

The patient may be stood in his plasters on the third post-operative day. Trunk and upper extremity exercises should be started as soon as the patient will co-operate. In most instances, plaster immobilization need not be continued for more than three weeks.

Post-operative bracing may be used for gait training, for support, or for further correction. (Long-leg braces are used for training purposes only. They are discarded as soon as the desired gait pattern has been established.) If the knee requires external support because of quadriceps weakness, the brace is retained until strength is sufficient to allow its removal. If it was impossible or impractical to gain full knee extension surgically, the remaining few degrees may be gained post-operatively through the use of calibrated knee locks.

For the child who had an effective crouch gait prior to surgery, it may be functionally advantageous to brace the knees at 160 degrees or with as much as 20 degrees of flexion, even if the knees can be fully extended. He will have an immediately secure gait with this posture, and be can gradually be trained into a more extended one.

It is improper for walking or standing to force the knees into full extension in braces. Rarely, as previously noted, are the hips so free of flexion as to be able to accommodate to the fully extended knee. More often the accommodation will be in the lumbar spine, while the hips remain flexed. It is the writer's opinion that the real key to good posture post-operatively in spastic cerebral palsy is the fully extensible hip.

It is unwise to require the patient to walk before he has gained good standing tolerance, balance and alignment. An insecure and inefficient gait will become more so as deformities recur.

If minimum surgery for hamstring weakening and correction of knee flexion has been performed, then there is no alternative to a continuing post-operative program of active hamstring and hip flexor stretch and strengthening of all trunk and lower extremity muscles, including hamstrings. Patients who have undergone total hamstring lengthening or transfer are obviously in less danger of early recurrence of knee flexion deformity.

In programming for home care, it is essential that the patient avoid long periods of unrelieved sitting (as in school) and that he continue with prescribed exercises and prescribed periods of standing and walking. Responsibility for exercises should be shifted to the patient when this is possible.

Comments on Surgery for Correction of Knee Flexion Deformity in Cerebral Palsy

There is seldom complete agreement among surgeons as to the most suitable surgical procedure or pre-operative and post-operative program for any one knee flexion problem. The following list of rules may be useful.

(1) Discounting the effect of contractures at the hip and ankle, the key to determining the right amount of compromise of the hamstrings is the evaluation of quadriceps strength and spasticity.
(2) Only that amount of surgery necessary to obtain knee extension should be performed.
(3) It is not essential to gain full knee extension surgically.

(4)   In physical assessment of active motion, the longer the lag between command and execution, the less promising the outcome of surgery.

(5)   If there are offensive contractures at the hip, knee and ankle, simultaneous surgical correction at all three levels is technically feasible and functionally advantageous.

(6)   Persistence of hip flexion or ankle equinus affects the corrected knee adversely.

(7)   Persisting moderate knee flexion can be corrected post-operatively with bracing and exercise.

(8)   Post-operative immobilization must be kept to a minimum as regards both dimension and time.

(9)   Bed confinement and inactivity must be avoided post-operatively.

(10)   Active exercise is distinctly better than passive exercise.

(11)   Post-operatively, the patient should stand before he walks.

Multilevel Surgery

The topic of multilevel surgery merits some elaboration. If contractures at the hip and ankle are mild, it is possible that the change in postural alignment brought about by knee straightening will affect the other levels favorably, and that no surgery at the hip or ankle will be required. Gradual correction of hip flexion has been observed among patients who have had hamstring transfers and have remained ambulatory, with or without lateral support.

Similarly, with correction of adductor thrust, both hip and knee flexion con tractures often become less of a problem. Whether this improvement at other levels is reflex or mechanical in nature (or a bit of both) is difficult to say, but the fact that it does occur speaks for conservatism in surgery.

On the other hand, there are probably more patients who are functionally hampered by strict surgical conservatism than there are patients who benefit. In the interest of expediting the post-operative program, more than one level may be approached in patients who would obviously need corrective surgery at each one of these levels, were that the only level involved.

It was a positive dictum of Dr Eggers that knee surgery should be done as an initial measure, with other surgery, if necessary, being reserved for later. Other surgeons have felt equally strongly that the knee should be reserved for the last.

Knee Extension and Total Function

Although full knee extension may be cosmetically appealing, it is not always functionally desirable in persons with spastic muscles. The surgeon, therefore, must remember that there are patients who will function better with slightly bent knees than with knees which fully extend. A patient who has a stable, balanced independent gait with flexed knees may require crutches after knee-straightening surgery. If he has poor upper extremities, he may require a wheelchair. The moderately involved patient can often achieve, through exercise, the amount of additional knee extension and the balance of flexion and extension power appropriate to his gait. A softly extended knee is generally preferred to one that is hyper-extended.

Back-knee as it occurs in cerebral palsy, may be classified as: (1) apparent, (2) mechanical, (3) hypotonic, and (4) iatrogenic.

Apparent Back-knee

In certain patients, when the knee and hip are extended, the extremity is in internal rotation. In this position the medial femoral condyle is quite prominent, and the knee has the appearance of being hyperextended. If the internal rotation is controlled, it will often be found that the amount of knee extension is normal.

Mechanical Back-knee

This may be a misnomer, for it has to do with seeming muscle imbalance accentuated by mechanical forces. In patients with tight heel cords and strong quadriceps, the knee may be forced into hyperextension with each step and with standing. Hamstrings may even participate in this extension posture.

Because of the fixed equinus, the patient must lean forward for balance, and there is usually hip flexion contracture as well. Cautious surgery at hip and ankle and post-operative brace protection will usually correct the back-knee. These patients may be converted to a crouch posture by injudicious surgery because of tight hamstrings.

Hypotonic Back-knee

Among patients with hypotonic muscles, whether athetotic, ataxic or spastic, a degree of recurvatum of the knee may be essential to stability in standing and walking. Although these patients may be taught to walk in braces which prevent back-knee, they are probably better left alone.

Iatrogenic Back-knee

Back-knee is a frequently encountered problem among patients who have had hamstring weakening procedures. It is particularly troublesome if heel cords remain tight or if there is an uncontrolled plantar thrust. It is likely that hip flexion contracture also accentuates this problem. Relief of the contractures at hip and ankle may solve it.

If there is no remaining knee flexion power—that is, if all hamstrings have been transferred or tenotomized, it may be possible surgically to retrieve hamstring tendons for reattachment to the tibia. This is not, however, a particularly rewarding procedure. Bracing is then necessary, with restrictions of knee extension to 160 or 170 degrees. In severe cases, with or without surgical re-attachment of the hamstrings, bracing may be required indefinitely, and the knees must be splinted in flexion at night. Eventually, most patients retain a relatively soft knee and can then be brace-free.

The sharply hyperextended knee often observed after hamstring surgery should be controlled with braces set at 170 degrees, as previously suggested, until, with the new posture, the knees are under better voluntary control.

Medial Inclination (Genu Valgum)

In cerebral palsy, valgus position of the knees is often observed, varus position seldom. Patients may assume the knee-to-knee position because of tight adductors; in such cases the knees will flex and the hips accordingly flex and internally rotate; eventually there will be not only an apparent valgus deformity, but possibly a bit of lateral tibial torsion in addition. In this circumstance the tensor fasciae latae and the iliotibial band are likely to be to blame.

The knee-to-knee posture is assumed in other patients, especially the weak, for stability. Patients who cannot extend the knees well can often adduct quite strongly and they thus secure themselves.

Surgical correction of the imbalance and brace support will, as a rule, cause the genu valgum to disappear. The torsional defects will however remain, and must be corrected by osteotomy.

The Rectus Femoris and Knee Function

The functional interrelationship of the rectus femoris and the hamstrings has been discussed (see section on Hamstring Anatomy, page 181). Tight hamstrings may limit the stride in walking, and a tight rectus femoris may limit knee flexion or knee swing. Duncan (1955) noted that some patients could not flex the knee without flexing the hip. For this problem he recommended division of the rectus femoris at its origin. If after hamstring surgery a patient cannot walk with a freely swinging knee; he will probably benefit from rectus femoris release. Following the release, there is no functional deficit.

The Problem of Asymmetry

Rarely in spastic cerebral palsy is there truly symmetrical affection of the lower extremities. The most decidedly asymmetrical pattern is called 'hemiparesis', but among many diparetics and paraparetics there is an assessable difference between the two extremities. However slight or extreme the difference, recognition of it is important in planning for surgical treatment, since the lesser involved of the two extremities often mimics the other, and the knee flexion deformities will appear to be the same. The surgical procedure must be appropriate, or the result may be an accentuation of the asymmetry. Whereas decisions are comparatively simple for the hemiparetic, they can be difficult when the asymmetry is more subtle.

REFERENCES

Baker, L. D. (1956) 'A rational approach to the surgical needs of the cerebral palsy patient.' *Journal of Bone and Joint Surgery,* **38A,** 313.

Chandler, F. A. (1933) 'Re-establishment of normal leverage of patella in knee-flexion deformity in spastic paralysis.' *Surgery, Gynecology and Obstetrics,* **57,** 523.

—— (1940) 'Patellar advancement operation: revised techniques.' *Journal of the International College of Surgeons,* **3,** 433.

Duncan, W. R. (1955) 'Release of rectus femoris in spastic paralysis.' *Paper presented at the Annual Meeting of the American Academy for Orthopedic Surgeons, Los Angeles.*

Eggers, G. W. N. (1950) 'Surgical division of the patellar retinacula to improve extension of the knee joint in cerebral spastic paralysis.' *Journal of Bone and Joint Surgery,* **32A,** 80.

—— (1952) 'Transplantation of hamstring tendons to femoral condyles in order to improve hip extension and to decrease knee flexion in cerebral spastic paralysis.' *Journal of Bone and Joint Surgery,* **34A,** 827.

—— Evans, E. (1963) 'Surgery in cerebral palsy.' *Journal of Bone and Joint Surgery,* **45A,** 1275.

Evans, E. B., Julian, J. D. (1964) 'Modifications of the hamstring transfer operation.' *Paper presented at a Meeting of the American Academy for Cerebral Palsy, New York City.*

Green, W. T., McDermott, L. J. (1942) 'Operative treatment of cerebral palsy of spastic type.' *Journal of the American Medical Association,* **118,** 434.

Keats, S., Kambin, P. (1962) 'An evaluation of surgery for the correction of knee-flexion contracture in children with cerebral spastic paralysis.' *Journal of Bone and Joint Surgery,* **44A,** 1146.

Mortens, J. (1965) 'Orthopaedic operations in the treatment of children with cerebral palsy.' *Danish Medical Bulletin,* **12,** 22.

Pollock, G. A. (1962) 'Surgical treatment of cerebral palsy.' *Journal of Bone and Joint Surgery,* **44B,** 68.

—— (1965) 'Transplantation of the hamstring muscles in cerebral palsy. (Revised version.)' *Paper presented at the Study Group on Orthopaedics and Physical Medicine in Cerebral Palsy, Bristol.*

Roberts, W. M., Adams, J. P. (1953) 'The patellar-advancement operation in cerebral palsy.' *Journal of Bone and Joint Surgery,* **35A,** 958.

Seymour, N., Sharrard, W. J. W. (1968) 'Bilateral proximal release of the hamstrings in cerebral palsy.' *Journal of Bone and Joint Surgery,* **50B,** 274.

Steindler, A. (1955) *Kinesiology of the Human Body.* Springfield, Ill.: C. C. Thomas pp. 78, 438.

Stephenson, C. T., Donovan, M. M. (1970) 'Transfer of hip adductor origins to the ischium in spastic cerebral palsy.' *Paper presented at the Annual Meeting of the American Academy for Cerebral Palsy,* Houston, Texas.

CHAPTER 10

The Foot and Ankle in Cerebral Palsy

HENRY H. BANKS

When determining the needs of the foot and ankle in cerebral palsy, it is clearly important not to make an assessment of the lower extremities in isolation, but to consider the patient as a whole (Banks and Panagakos 1966).

Equinus (Fig. 10), equinovalgus (Fig. 12), equinovarus (Fig. 16), calcaneus (Fig. 17), hallux valgus (Fig. 19) and toe deformities are the commonest problems requiring attention in this area. The majority of patients have mild deformities that respond well to non-operative, conservative measures, including active and passive exercises, night support (Fig. 9) and minimal bracing (Banks and Panagakos 1967).

Without preventive measures, mild deformities may, with time and growth, become severe. Where spasticity is severe, conservative measures are unsuccessful. Under these circumstances, the possibility arises of correcting the deformity with surgery. Yet, surgical procedures have had a poor reputation in cerebral palsy. The indications are often vague, the types of procedures are innumerable, and the recurrence rate is often quoted as being too high (Phelps 1957).

Criteria for Selection for Surgery

(1) The patient should be old enough to co-operate with physician and therapist, and to take advantage of the surgical procedure. This is usually four years of age.

(2) Patients with spasticity are more likely to be improved by surgery than those with athetosis.

(3) The patient should show some ability to assume the erect position (so-called 'balance'). He should present some evidence of being able to sit and stand with minimal or no assistance. Deformities usually will not prevent walking, but may interfere with precarious 'balance'.

(4) The patient's intelligence should be such as to make him trainable after his operation. A patient with a low intelligence quotient, however, may have his nursing care greatly simplified by a surgical procedure.

(5) There should be a deformity to correct. This may be fixed or functional. In testing for equinus for example, it is important to note where the exaggerated stretch reflex comes into play. This is where the foot functions in gait, and not where it can be passively forced toward dorsiflexion.

(6) Pre-operatively conservative treatment is important to indoctrinate the patient and family in the use of exercises and night support.

(7) There should be a good home situation, and adequate facilities for careful follow-up after the operation. The patient must receive proper post-operative care, as only in this way can one prevent recurrence.

(8)   The reader is referred to Chapter 4 for principles of assessment of the foot and
ankle.

Equinus

The most common foot deformity in cerebral palsy is equinus (Fig. 10). For well
over a hundred years now, the exaggerated stretch reflex of the triceps surae has been
weakened, and its length re-established, by various procedures performed from
its proximal to its distal limits. Quite clearly, assuming that each of these procedures has been well performed, the result is more related to the choice of patient
and the standard of post-operative care.

Although Delpech (1823) began to perform subcutaneous tenotomy of the tendo
achilles in 1816, the procedure became popular for the correction of equinus from
any cause, due to the efforts of Strohmeyer in 1831 (Strohmeyer 1838). While the
initial results in cerebral palsy were brilliant, the long-term results were poor, because of inadequate post-operative care.

Stoffel reported in 1913 that selective motor neurectomies could correct muscle
imbalance due to spasticity. Neurectomy of one or more branches of the tibial nerve
to the gastrocnemius-soleus was advocated for the correction of equinus. The procedure which was popularized by Phelps (1951) and later by Eggers (1952)—soleus
neurectomy (Fig. 1)—should, in theory, be effective in correcting functional equinus

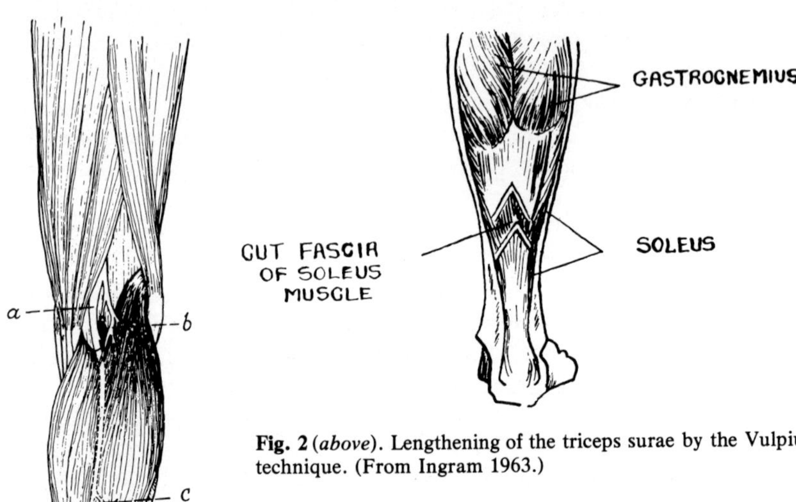

Fig. 2 (*above*). Lengthening of the triceps surae by the Vulpius
technique. (From Ingram 1963.)

Fig. 1. (*left*). Diagram showing the insertion of nerves into the
soleus muscle; (*a*) = the tibial nerve, (*b*) = proximal and major
branches to the soleus (divided in soleus neurectomy) and (*c*) =
small distal branch to the soleus (not divided in soleus
neurectomy). (From Eggers 1952.)

caused by spasticity of one or both muscles, but will be ineffective when there is a fixed contracture of the triceps surae. Banks and Green (1958) noted the difficulty, when doing a neurectomy, of avoiding too much or too little motor paralysis. Neurectomy is not a popular procedure for correction of equinus at this time, but may be indicated in the presence of sustained ankle clonus.

In 1913, Vulpius and Stoffel described the correction of equinus by transverse section of the gastrocnemius tendon just below the middle of the leg posteriorly and by transverse section of the soleus tendon, leaving the underlying muscle fibers intact (Fig. 2). Passive dorsiflexion of the foot then stretches the soleus fibers without affecting their continuity.

Baker modified the Vulpius procedure by a tongue and groove lengthening of the gastrocnemius aponeurosis in the middle third of its fibers (Fig. 3) (Baker 1956, Bassett and Baker 1966). Table I records the recurrence rates following baker's procedure for the correction of equinus. Baker has emphasized the need for adequate post-operative care, including long-term splinting during the growing period, to prevent recurrence.

TABLE I

Results obtained by Baker in correcting equinus. (From Bassett and Baker 1966.)

	Trips to OR	*Extremities operated*	*Recurrences*	*Percentage of recurrences*
Neurectomy	45	85	21	26
Gastrocnemius recession	36	62	10	16
Mid third lengthening of gastrocnemius aponeurosis	283	447	20	4
TOTAL	364	594	51	

Because of his disappointment with the results of the previously described procedures for the correction of equinus, Strayer (1950) described a procedure similar in principle to that of Vulpius (Fig. 4). The aponeurotic tendon of the gastrocnemius was divided transversely near its junction with that of the soleus, the foot was passively dorsiflexed to neutral, and the retracted proximal portion of the tendon was sutured to the underlying soleus (Fig. 4). In 1958, Strayer reviewed his results in 23 patients, and rated them as good or excellent in 16.

Silfverskiöld (1923-4) distinguished between two types of equinus deformity. He noted that contracture of the gastrocnemius caused a deformity which could not be corrected passively when the knee was fully extended, but which could be when the knee was flexed 90 degrees. A deformity which could not be corrected, regardless of the position of the knee, was considered to be due to a contracture of both the gastrocnemius and soleus. By releasing both heads of origin of the gastrocnemius, allowing them to slide distal to the knee joint, and re-attaching them there, not only did he convert a two-joint muscle into a one-joint one, but he corrected the equinus. He also, on occasion, did a selective neurectomy of some of the motor branches of the gastrocnemius to further weaken it. He did not record the results of this procedure.

197

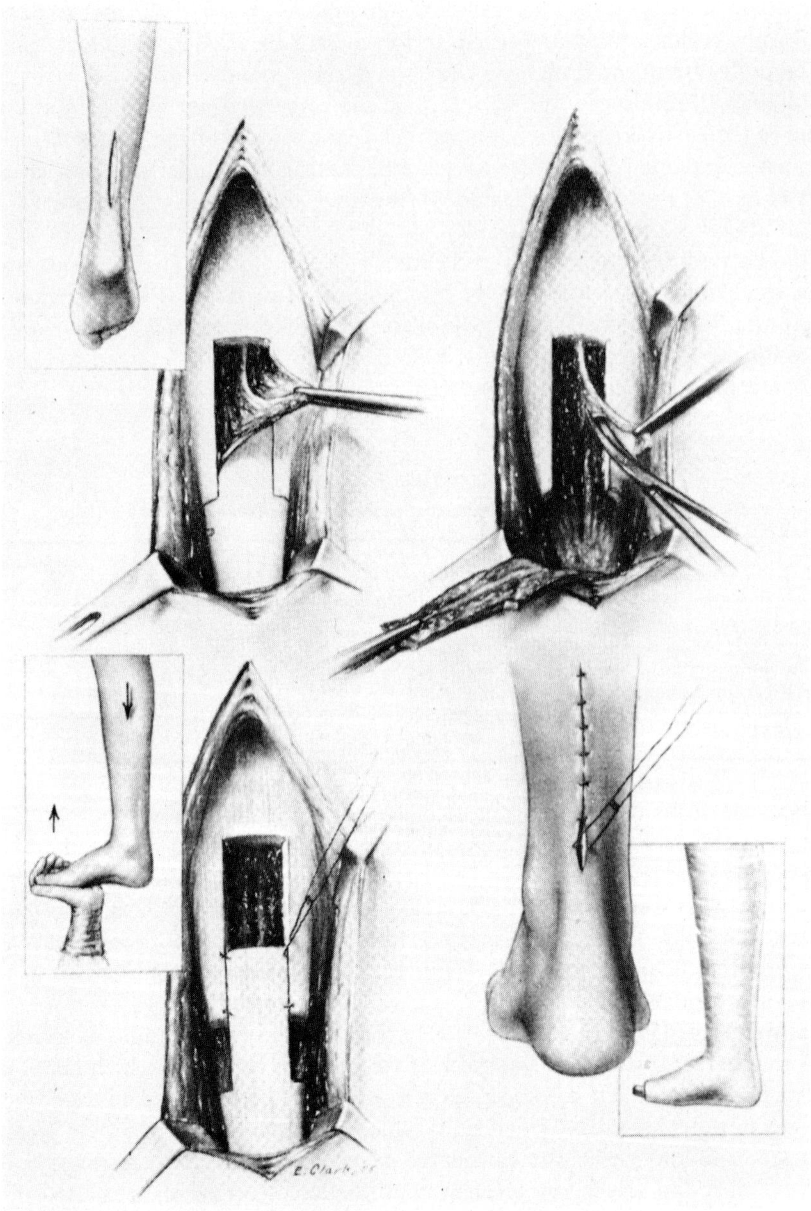

Fig. 3. Baker's 'tongue in groove' lengthening of the gastrocnemius aponeurosis. (From Baker 1956.)

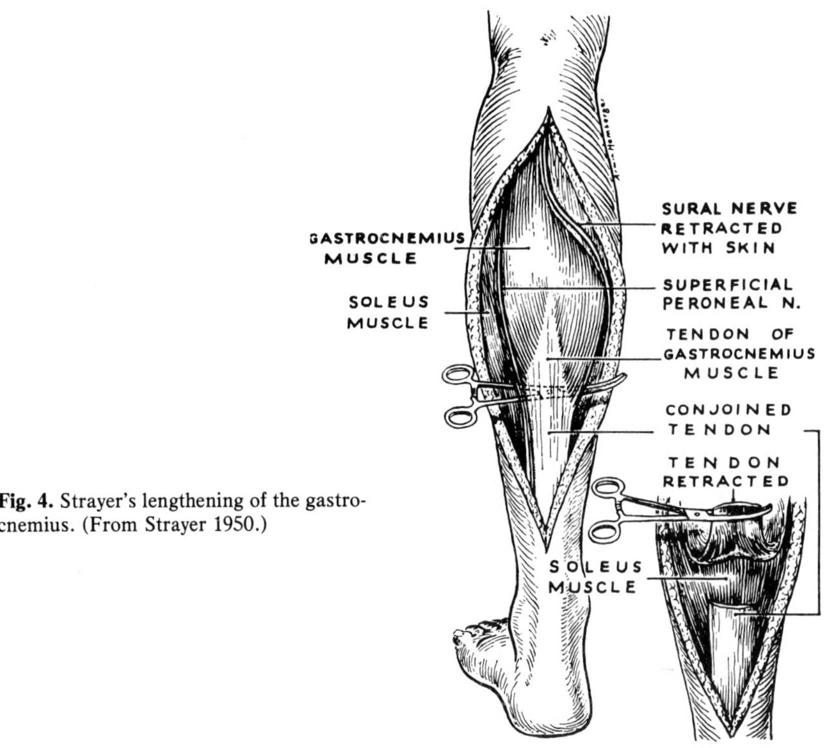

Fig. 4. Strayer's lengthening of the gastro-cnemius. (From Strayer 1950.)

Soon afterwards, Green and McDermott (1942) (Fig. 5), as well as Baker (1954, 1956) (Fig. 6), described a similar procedure for the correction of equinus. As noted in Table II, the results of Green's procedure were not always superior (Banks and Green 1958). Green believes that the procedure may be used for mild cases of equinus, especially when the hamstrings are being lengthened, but that it should not be considered as the primary procedure for the correction of this deformity (Banks and Green 1958).

TABLE II

Results obtained from Green's fractional lengthening of the gastrocnemius origin. (From Banks and Green 1958.)

| | *Results at follow-up* | | | | |
Total	Excellent	Good	Fair	Poor	No follow-up
19	0	8	7	4	0

All but three with hamstring lengthening
All but five with neurectomy of one head of gastrocnemius.

| | *Rating of Improvement* | | | | |
Total	+ + + +	+ + +	+ +	+	0
19	0	6	6	7	0

199

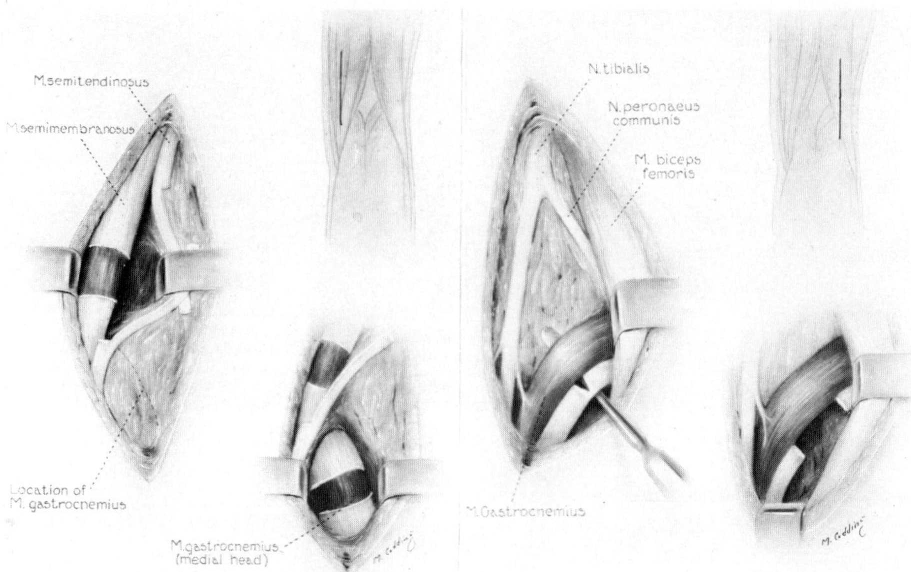

Fig. 5a. Green's fractional lengthening of the medial head of the gastrocnemius performed at the time of hamstring lengthening. (From Banks and Green 1958.)

Fig. 5b. Green's fractional lengthening of the lateral head of the gastrocnemius. Only the tendinous portion of the medial and lateral heads of the gastrocnemius are sectioned. (From Banks and Green 1958.)

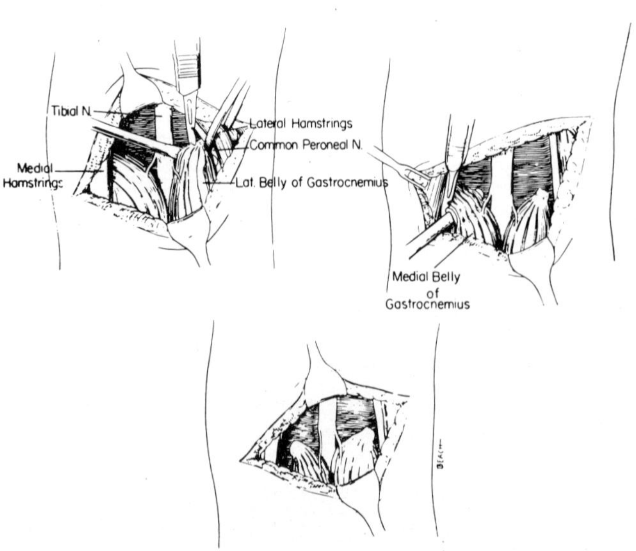

Fig. 6. Baker's recession of the origin of the gastrocnemius. (From Baker 1954.)

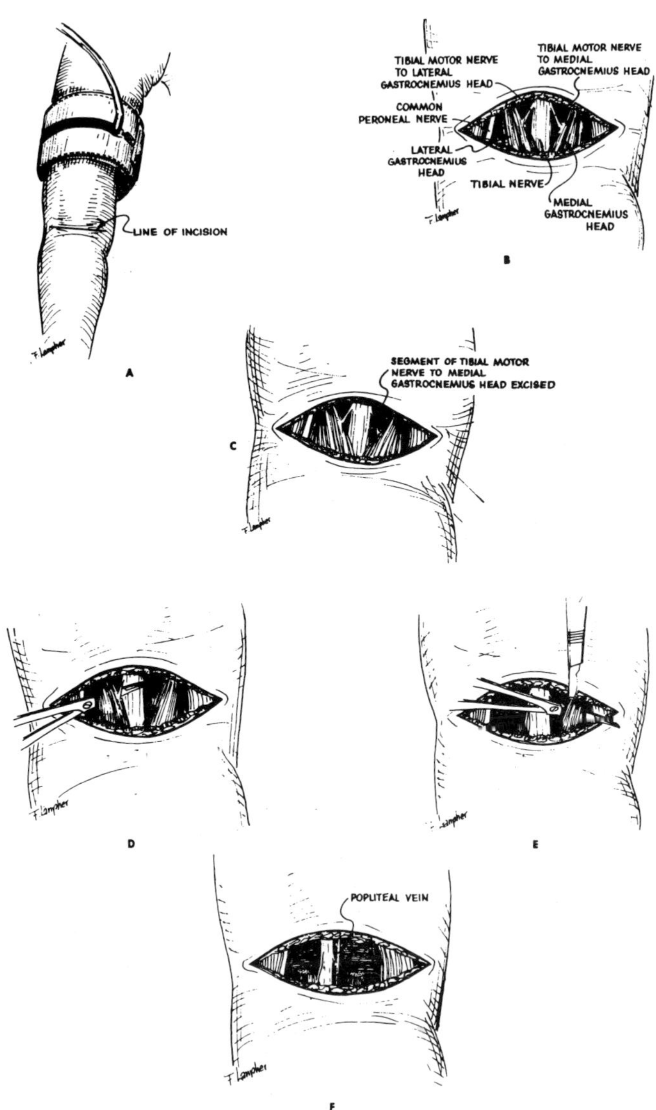

Fig. 7*a* (*top*) **and** 7*b* (*bottom*). Recession of the medial and lateral heads of the gastrocnemius, as performed by Silver and Simon. (From Silver and Simon 1959.)

In 1959, however, Silver and Simon reported the results of 110 gastrocnemius recession operations (with tibial neurectomy) performed between 1947 and 1958, of which only five were failures (Fig. 7). They used this procedure only when the gastrocnemius was the primary deforming factor. Post-operatively, casts were worn for only six weeks, after which time all types of immobilization were discontinued. Recently, these authors have reported that equinus has recurred in 5 per cent of a group of 200 such procedures performed over a 20-year period (Silver 1969).

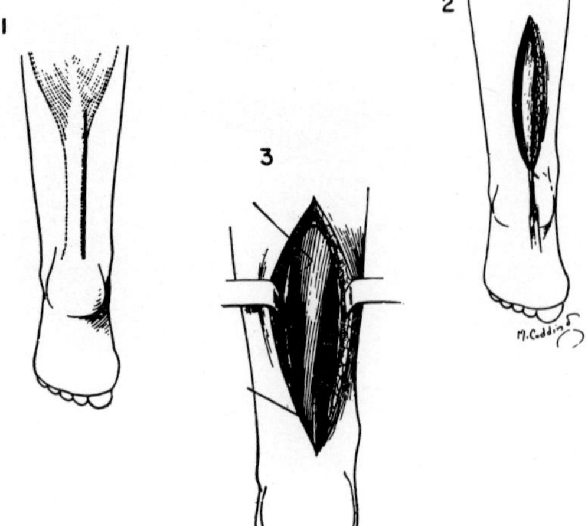

Fig. 8a. Sliding lengthening of the heel cord. The skin incision is medial in position. The incision of the subcutaneous tissues is carried directly through the tendon sheath so that the sheath can be reconstructed effectively. The rotation of the fibers is carefully identified so that one half can be divided above and one half below this rotation.

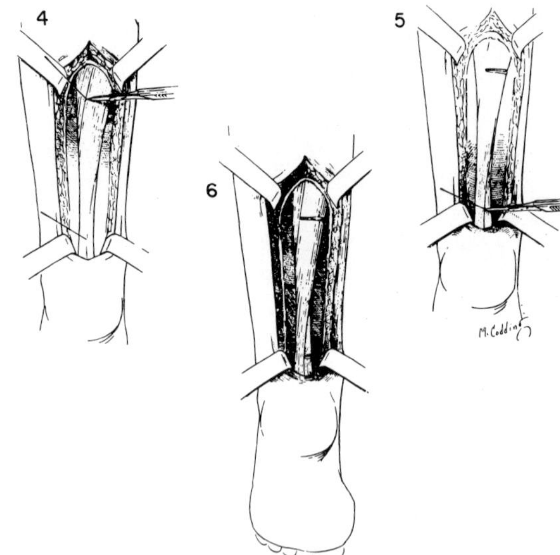

Fig. 8b. The tendon is then incised at two levels, observing the rotation of the fibers. A third incision mid-way between the others is occasionally indicated. (From Banks and Green 1958.)

Equinus has also been corrected by a Z or sliding lengthening of the tendo achilles. The Z lengthening, while effective, requires more dissection and repair than the sliding lengthening (Fig. 8), which has been used by Green since 1940 (Banks and Green 1958), and was described by White in 1943.

The sliding lengthening of the heel cord (Fig. 8) has for over 30 years been the preferred technique for the correction of equinus in cerebral palsy at the Children's Hospital Medical Center, Boston (Banks and Green 1958). Fortunately, the heel cord is made up of two groups of fibers, with a rotation, as seen in Figure 8a. After the surgeon has identified this rotation, the medial two-thirds of the fibers are cut proximally and the anterior two-thirds distally (Fig. 8b). If the foot is then passively

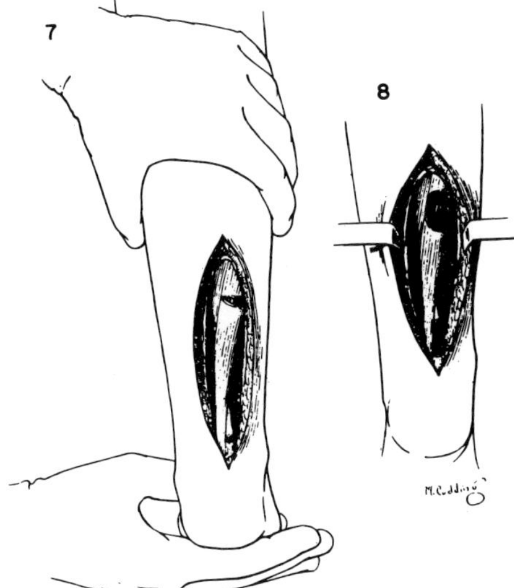

Fig. 8c. Passive dorsiflexion results in a sliding lengthening, with so firm a continuity of the heel cord that sutures are seldom used.

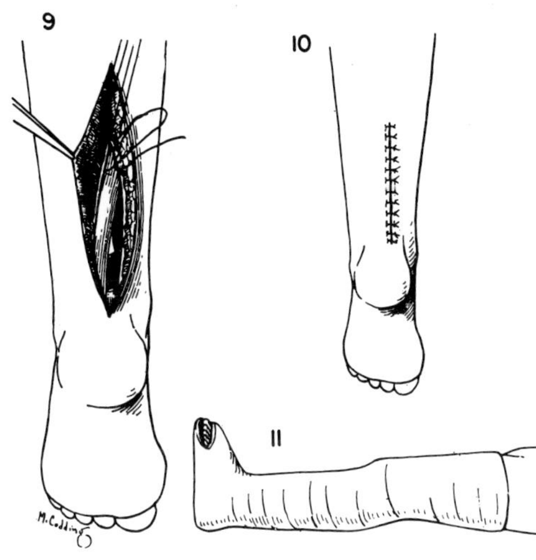

Fig. 8d. The sheath must be closed over the lengthened tendon. The limb is immobilized with a toe-to-groin cast, with the knee in extension and the foot in neutral dorsiflexion. (From Banks and Green 1958.)

dorsiflexed, a sliding lengthening in continuity is obtained (Fig. 8c). A long leg cast is then applied, with the foot held at neutral dorsiflexion and the knee in full extension (Fig. 8d).

To obtain a good result (Fig. 10), post-operative care must be very carefully supervised Banks and Green 1958). The case is bivalved and lined early so it can be used as a removable unit (Fig. 9). Active dorsiflexion and plantar flexion accompanied by knee exercises, are usually begun about one week post-operatively. Except for three exercise sessions daily, the patient is kept permanently in his bivalved, removable cast for six weeks. Night-time use of the cast then continues for several years. Indeed, it is not unusual to use such a cast at night for the remainder of the growth period in the young.

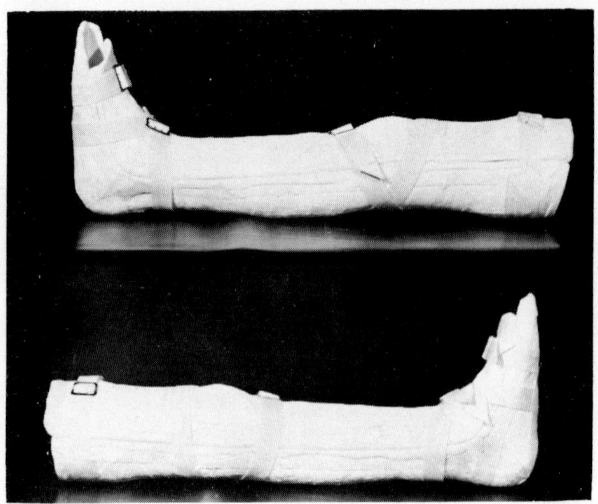

Fig. 9. Bivalved removable cast used pre-operatively to prevent deformity. It is used post-operatively to maintain correction. (From Banks and Green 1958.)

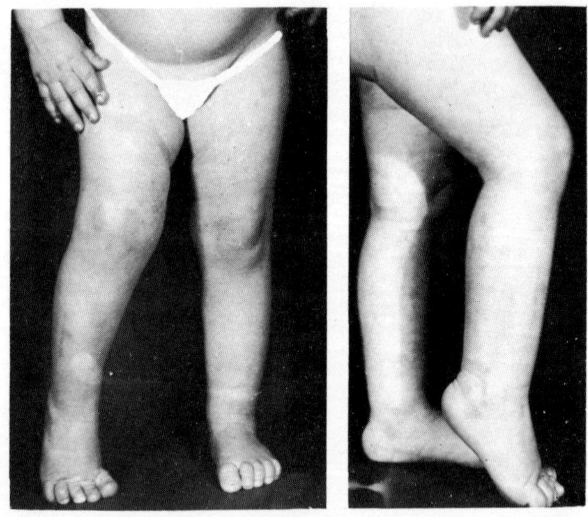

Fig. 10*a*. Patient B.H., age two years, right hemiplegia. Marked contracture of right heel cord. No previous treatment. (From Banks and Green 1958.)

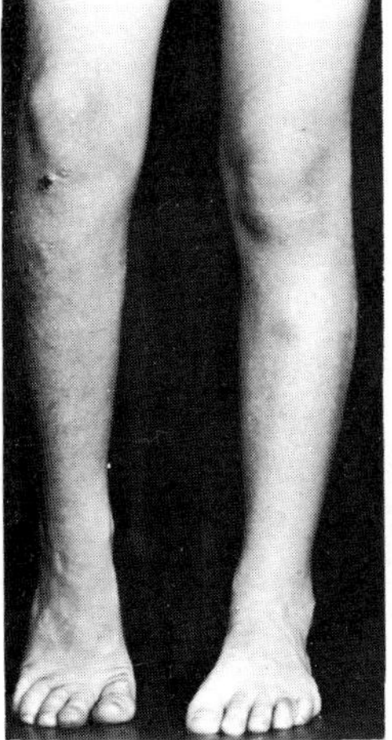 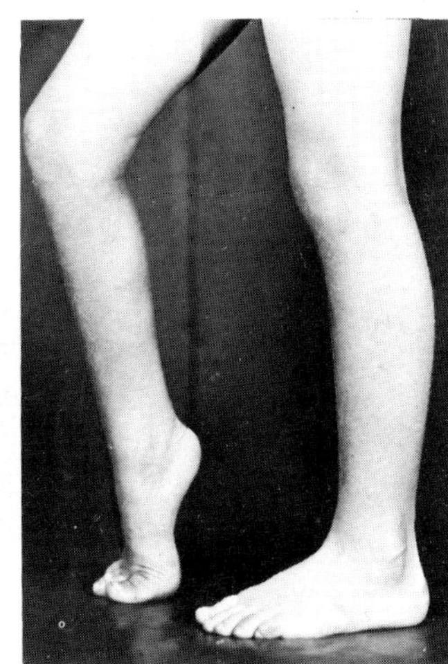

Fig. 10*b*. Patient B.H. aged seven years. Persistent equinus deformity noted just before heel-cord lengthening on 29th May 1941. (From Banks and Green 1958.)

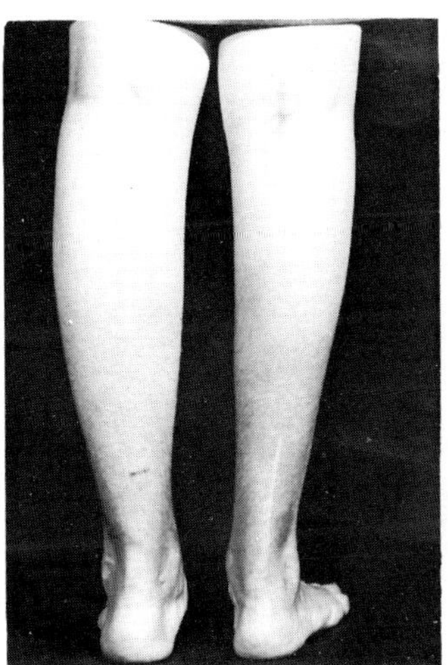 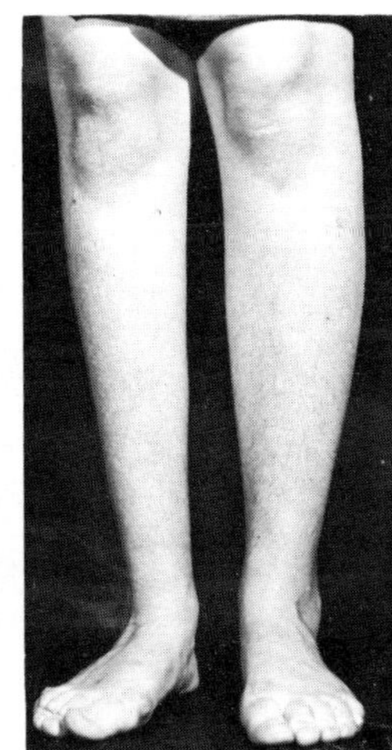

Fig. 10*c*. Patient B.H., aged twenty-one years, fourteen years post-operatively. Equinus deformity well corrected. (From Banks and Green 1958.)

Fig. 10*d*. Patient B.H., aged twenty-one years, fourteen years post-operatively. Phantom views (double exposures) showing active dorsiflexion to a right angle. (From Banks and Green 1958.)

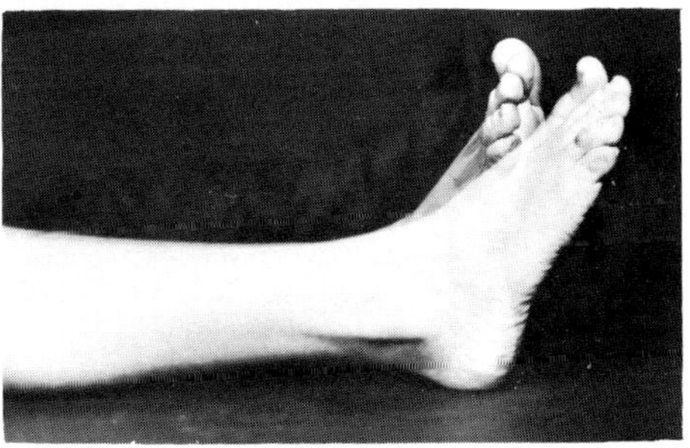

No passive stretch is applied to the heel cord until three weeks after the operation. At six weeks, standing is begun under supervision, at first with parallel bars and then with crutches. When satisfactory 'balance' has been developed, gait training is allowed. Crutches are used for at least six months to develop a good gait pattern. Some quadriplegic patients may need crutches indefinitely. Braces are not used post-operatively, unless there is difficulty in developing strength of the dorsi-flexors.

The long-term results are recorded in Table III (Banks and Green 1958), which shows that a good or excellent result on long-term follow-up (more than ten years) was obtained in seven out of every ten patients. Poor long-term results were usually associated with poor follow-up, poor co-operation on the part of the patient and family, poor choice of patient, and failure to maintain correction. Calcaneus was due to over-correction and failure of protection.

TABLE III
Results obtained from lengthening of heel cord (total operations 164). (From Banks and Green 1958.)

Results of long-term follow-up	*No. of cases*	*Per cent*
Excellent	22	13.4
Good	92	56.1
Fair	34	20.8
Poor	14	8.5
Not rated	2	1.2

		Rating of improvement				
Total	$++++$	$+++$	$++$	$+$	0	Not evaluated
164	29	55	57	8	13	2

Equinovalgus

Varying degrees of valgus are noted in approximately nine out of ten patients with equinus. In patients with mild equinovalgus, the valgus may respond well to conservative management of the equinus, combined with arch support. Where the equinus is significant, but the valgus mild, heel cord lengthening and arch supports post-operatively are successful. Marked degrees of equinovalgus require correction not only of the equinus, but also of the displacement of the os calcis beneath the talus (Fig. 12).

Years ago, equinovalgus was corrected at the end of the growing period by triple arthrodesis. So much bone needed to be removed to correct the equinus portion of the deformity, that the patient was left with a foot short in both height and length. The malleoli often impinged on the shoe edges. When the exaggerated stretch reflex of the triceps surae was not weakened, especially in the presence of

206

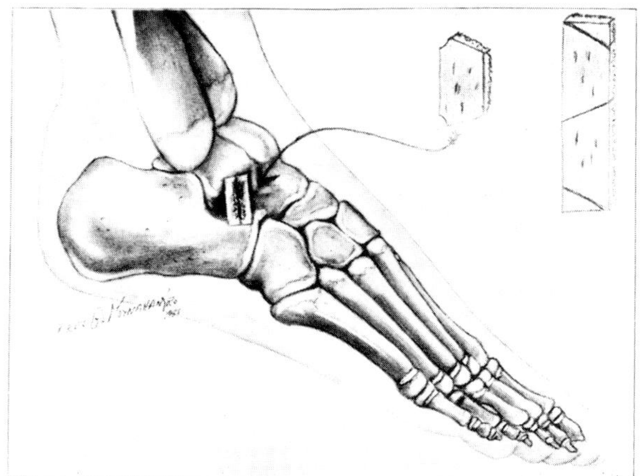

Fig. 11. Grice subtalar arthrodesis, using autogenous bone obtained from the tibia. (From Grice 1952.)

contracted hamstrings, the foot often yielded in the middle creating a 'rocker-bottom' deformity. If a triple arthrodesis is necessary, then it should be used to correct only valgus or varus, and not equinus. The latter deformity should be corrected by the appropriate soft tissue procedure.

In 1952, Grice reported on the use of subtalar arthrodesis (Fig. 11) in children, for the correction of valgus after poliomyelitis. He recognized the value of this procedure in cerebral palsy, particularly when significant equinus was corrected by heel cord lengthening. This procedure should not be perfomed unless roentgenograms have been taken which show that the os calcis can be passively repositioned under the talus, and from which it is possible to detect any valgus tilt of the talus in the ankle mortise, which should be allowed for if over correction is to be avoided (see Chapter 4).

Between 1951 and 1967 at the Children's Hospital Medical Center in Boston, 72 valgus feet in 44 patients with cerebral palsy were treated by subtalar arthrodesis. At a subsequent long-term follow-up examination (length of follow-up from 1 to 17 years), forty-three excellent (Fig. 12), fifteen good, eight fair and six poor feet were observed (Banks *et al.* 1968). The most significant complication was over correction, five feet showing minor and three severe degrees of varus.

Similar results using subtalar arthrodesis to treat valgus deformity in patients with cerebral palsy have been obtained by Baker and his colleagues (Baker 1956, 1964; Baker and Dodelin 1958) in 56 feet, Mortens et al. (1962) in 27 feet and Keats and Kouten (1968) in 63 feet. These experiences show that significant valgus can be corrected by subtalar arthrodesis in children, and that by the use of this procedure the need for triple arthrodesis at the end of the growth period can be avoided. Equinus should be corrected at the time of surgery by heel cord lengthening. Over correction should be carefully avoided. In most instances, post-operative immobilization is necessary for three months for the arthrodesis to heal.

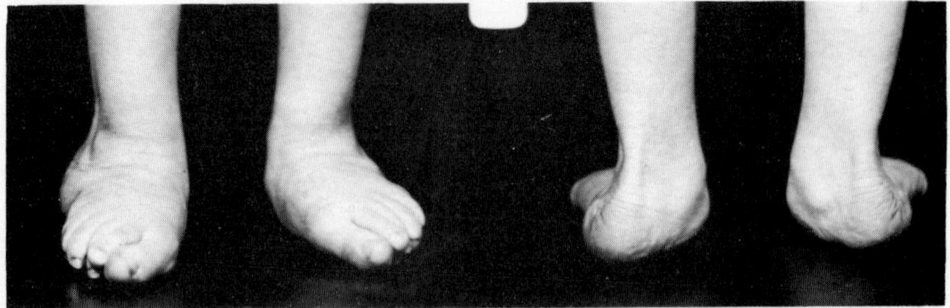

Fig. 12a. Patient D.L., aged three years three months. Spastic quadriplegia. Note severe valgus foot deformities in stance (1st March 1957). (From Banks and Panagakos 1967.)

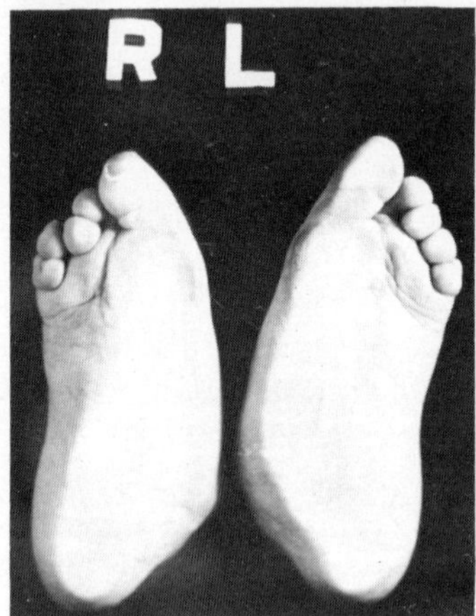

Fig. 12b. Patient D.L. Plantar view of severe valgus feet. (From Banks and Panagakos 1967.)

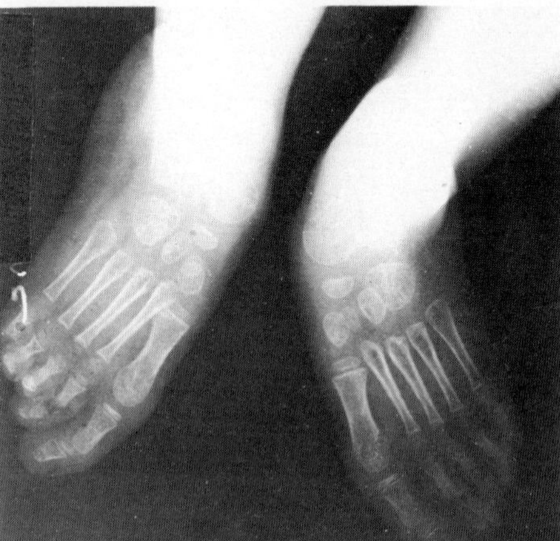

Fig. 12c. Patient D.L. Weight-bearing roentgenograms of feet pre-operatively (1st March 1957). (From Banks and Panagakos 1967.)

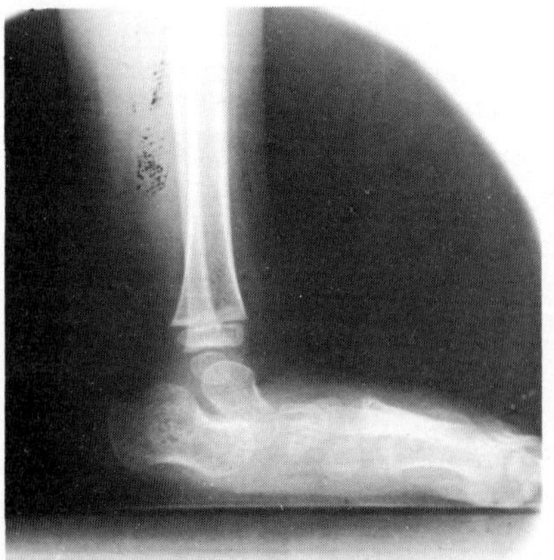

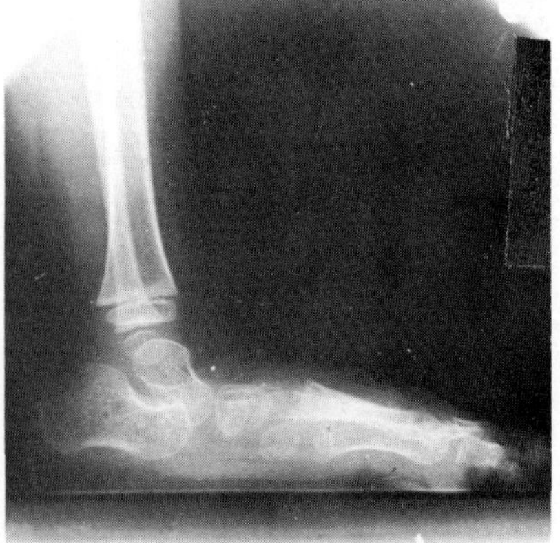

Fig. 12d. Patient D.L. Weight-bearing roentgenograms of feet pre-operatively (1st March 1957). (From Banks and Panagakos 1967.)

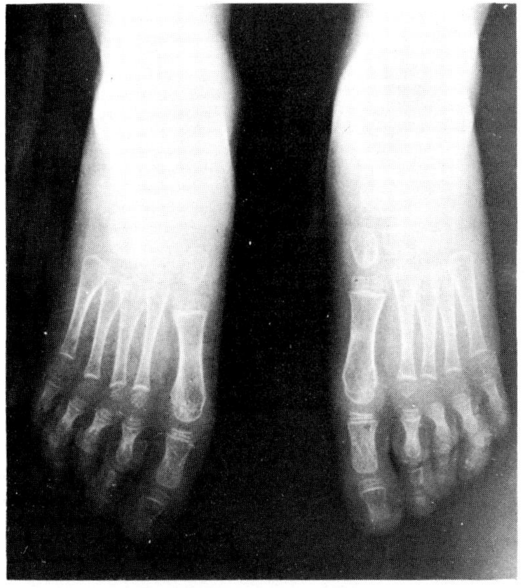 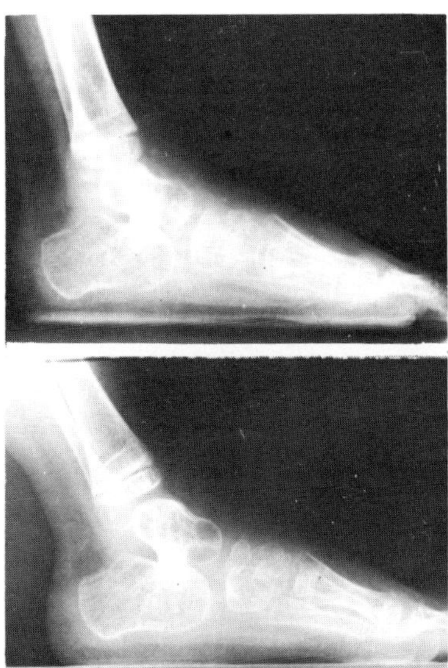

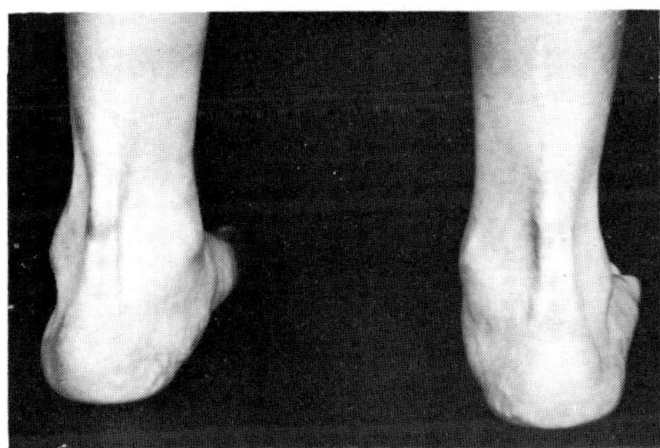 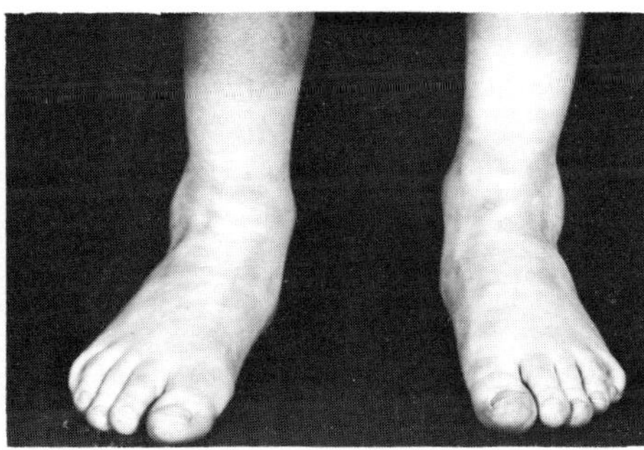

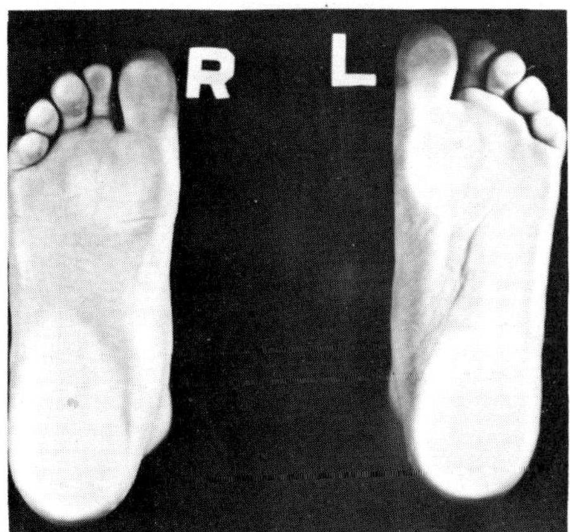

Figs. 12e (*top left*) and **12f** (*top right*). Patient D.L. Weight-bearing roentgenograms of feet eight months after bilateral heel cord lengthening and subtalar bone block arthrodesis. Note incorporation of talo-calcaneal bone graft. (From Banks and Panagakos 1967.)

Fig. 12g (*centre pictures*). Patient D.L. Weight-bearing photographs of feet three years six months post-operatively. (From Banks and Panagakos 1967.)

Fig. 12h (*left*). Patient D.L. Plantar views of feet when weight-bearing, three years six months post-operatively. (From Banks and Panagakos 1967.)

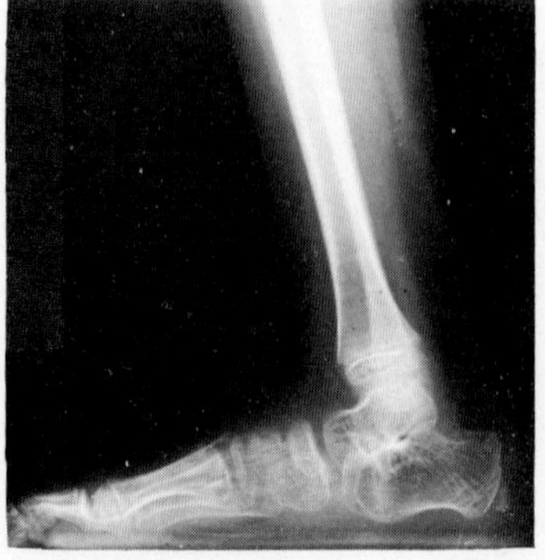

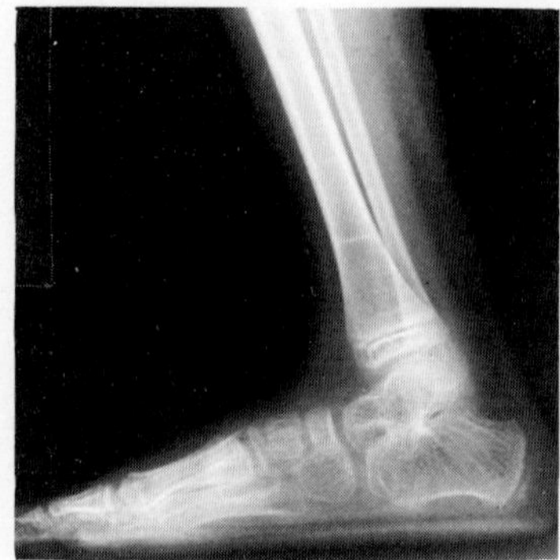

Fig. 12*i* (*left*). Patient D.L. Weight-bearing roentgenograms taken three years six months post-operatively. (From Banks and Panagakos 1967.)

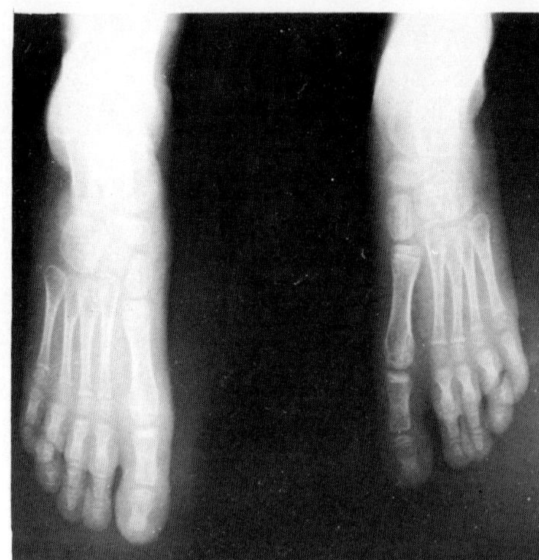

Fig. 12*j* (*above*). Patient D.L. Weight-bearing roentgenograms taken three years six months post-operatively. (From Banks and Panagakos 1967.)

Batchelor (1965—unpublished data) has achieved subtalar arthrodesis by the use of a fibular graft, which was inserted through the neck of the talus, across the sinus tarsi, and into the os calcis. Two small series of cases have been reported (Brown 1968, Seymour and Evans 1968). Problems with fractures of the graft have been reported.

Baker (1964) and Bassett and Baker (1966) reported a horizontal osteotomy through the base of the posterior articular process of the calcaneus, with lateral wedging grafts to correct valgus (Fig. 13). Of 31 feet treated by this osteotomy, two developed moderate varus due to over correction, eight had persisting mild valgus and 21 had satisfactory alignment. The average duration of follow-up in this series was two years.

Silver *et al.* (1967) and Silver (1969) have used the calcaneal osteotomy popularized by Dwyer (1960) in 75 cases, with excellent results (Fig. 14). However, this procedure sometimes creates a compensatory deformity which serves to mask the true site of deformity above (*i.e.* talus or subtalar joint).

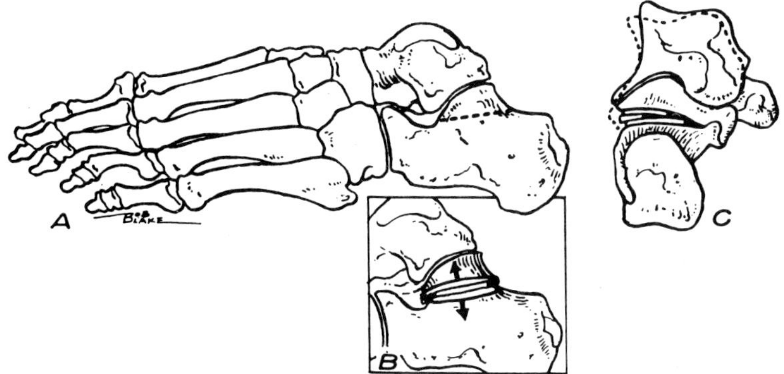

Fig. 13. Baker's horizontal osteotomy through the base of the posterior articular process of the calcaneus with lateral wedge grafts. (From Baker and Hill 1964.)

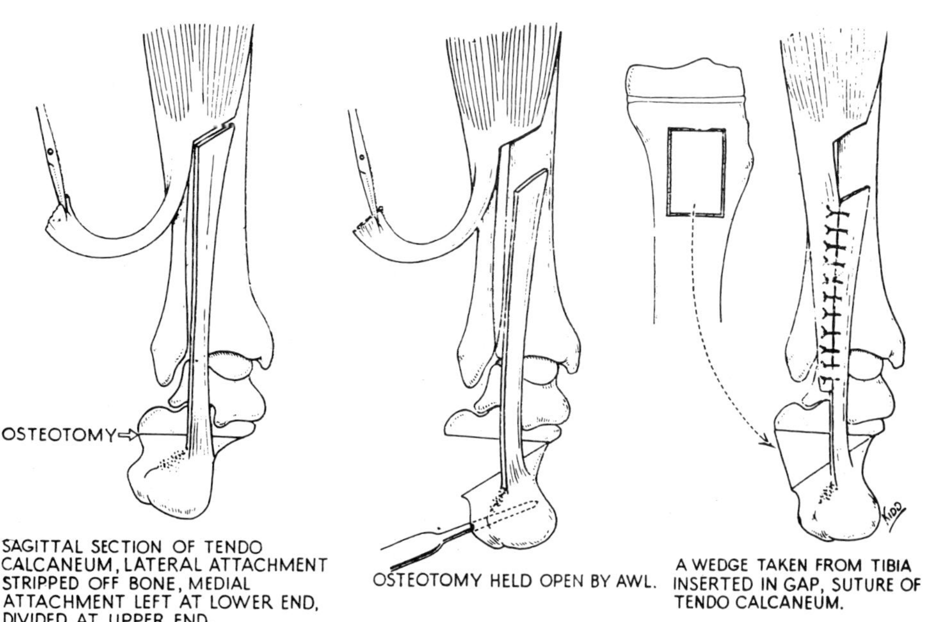

Fig. 14. Dwyer's correction of equinovalgus, by Z lengthening of the tendo achilles and osteotomy of the os calcis. For correction of quinovarus, Dwyer's osteotomy is made in the opposite direction. (From Dwyer 1960.)

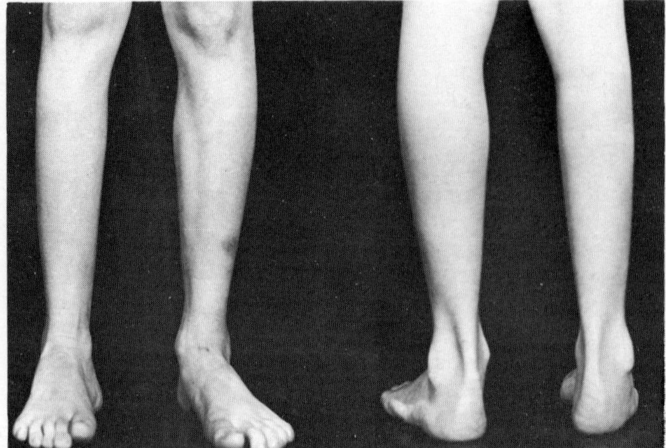

Fig. 15*a*. Patient G.L., aged eight years. Note varus, forefoot adduction and equinus (18th December 1961). (From Banks and Panagakos 1967.)

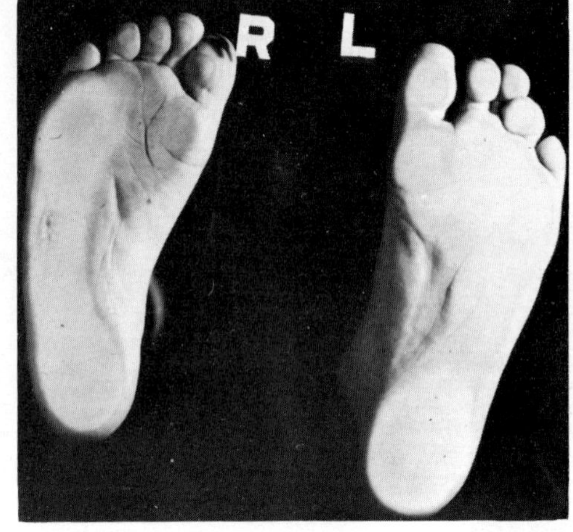

Fig. 15*b*. Patient G.L., aged eight years. Weight-bearing views taken on 18th December 1961. Note varus and forefoot adduction. (From Banks and Panagakos 1967.)

Equinovarus

Equinovarus (Figs. 15 and 16) is a much less common deformity in cerebral palsy than equinovalgus. When mild degrees of deformity are present, the following procedures are helpful: appropriate exercises for the heel cord, and for stretching the foot into eversion and forefoot abduction, bracing, outer heel and outer sole wedges, outflare shoes, and night support. Where the condition is more severe, difficult to control and progressive, surgical correction is necessary. Significant degrees of equinus should be corrected by re-establishing the length of the gastrocnemius, by the procedure with which the surgeon is best acquainted. The posterior tibial tendon also needs attention in severe equinovarus. It has been treated by re-routing anteriorly (Baker 1964, Bassett and Baker 1966), by tenotomy (Duncan 1960), by transplantation through the interosseous membrane to the dorsum of the foot, and by lengthening (Banks and Panagakos 1967). Obviously, any fixed equinus deformity must be corrected first.

Equinovarus has been managed at the Children's Hospital Medical Center in Boston by lengthening of the heel cord and the posterior tibial with good results

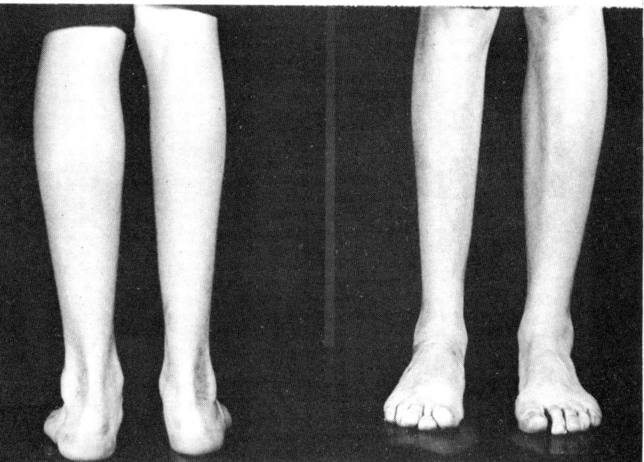

Fig. 15c. Patient G.L. Note correction of deformity observed five years after posterior tibial lengthening and heel cord lengthening on the right side. (From Banks and Panagakos 1967.)

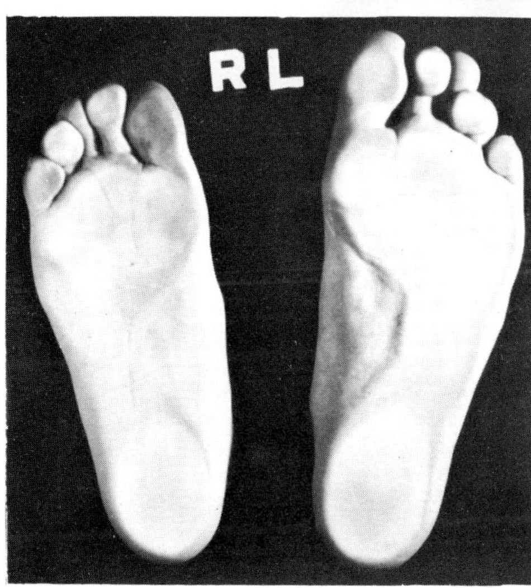

Fig. 15d. Patient G.L. Plantar views of feet obtained five years after surgery on the right side, Note correction of varus and forefoot adduction. (From Banks and Panagakos 1967.)

(Banks and Panagakos 1967) (Fig. 15). Tenotomy has been avoided, because of the possibility of a valgus foot developing during the growth period. Transplants of the posterior tibial through the interosseous membrane to the dorsum of the foot have been done in a few instances with only moderate success. It is questionable whether this muscle will perform under these circumstances.

Anterior re-routing of the posterior tibial tendon is reported by Baker as producing excellent results in 27 feet followed from six months to two years and four months (Baker 1964, Bassett and Baker 1966).

Where bony deformity is significant, these soft tissue procedures (correction of equinus and lengthening of the posterior tibial) will not be completely effective, and a triple arthrodesis is necessary (Fig. 16). A calcaneal wedge osteotomy has also been used successfully by Dwyer (1963) and Silver (Silver *et al.* 1967, Silver 1969) for this problem.

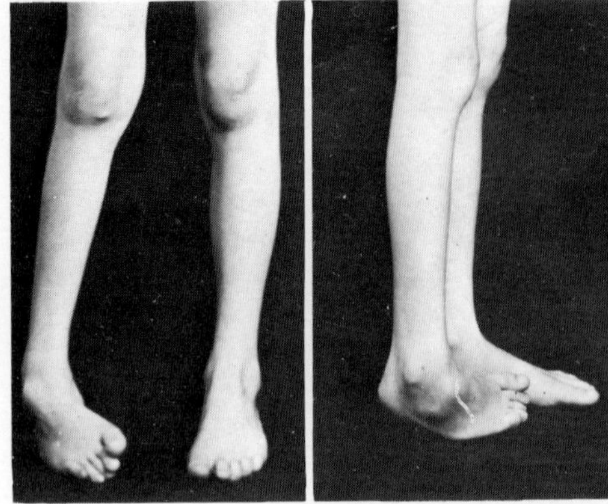

Fig. 16a. Patient P.B., aged seven years. Right hemiplegia. Equinovarus right foot, with marked adduction, prior to heel cord lengthening. (From Banks and Green 1958.)

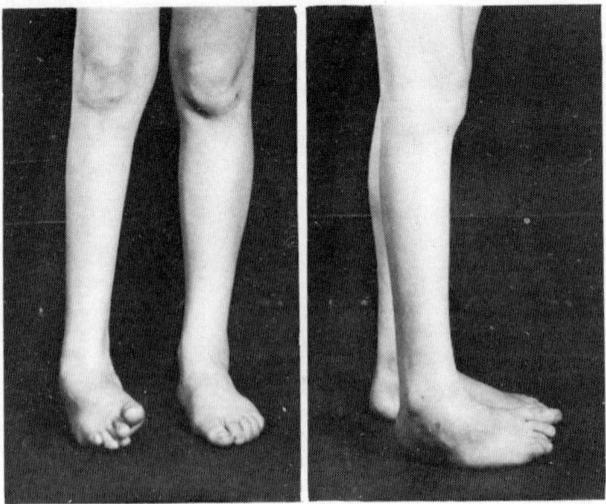

Fig. 16b. Patient P.B., aged nine years. Equinus deformity corrected, but varus and adduction persist after heel cord lengthening. Pre-operative pictures taken just prior to triple arthrodesis. (From Banks and Green 1958.)

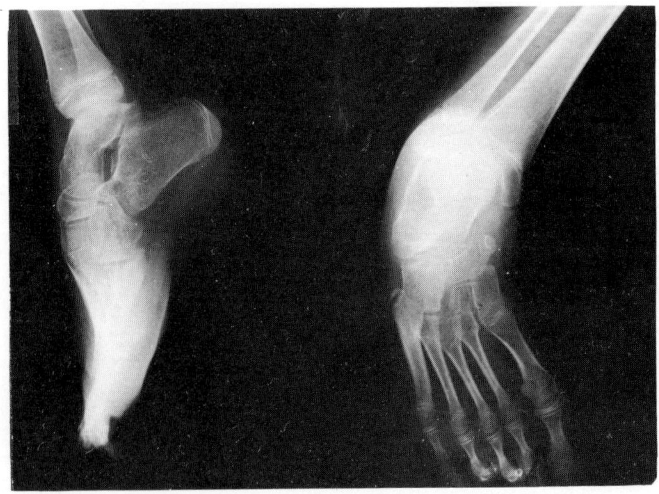

Fig. 16c. Patient P.B., aged nine years. Pre-operative X-rays taken in 1946. (From Banks and Green 1958.)

214

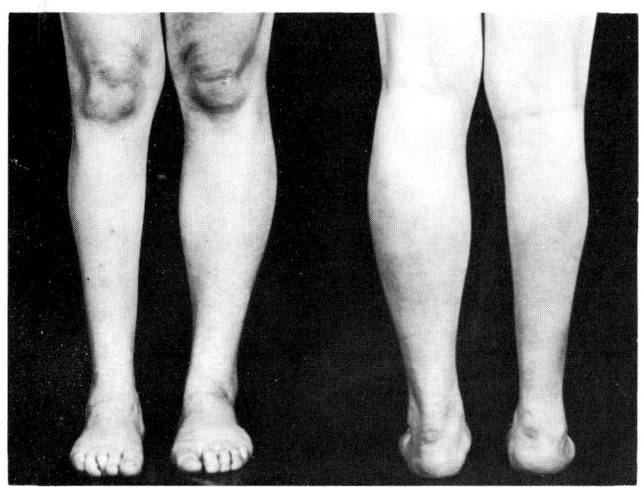

Fig. 16*d*. Patient P.B., aged nineteen years, eleven years after heel cord lengthening and nine years after triple arthrodesis. (From Banks and Green 1958.)

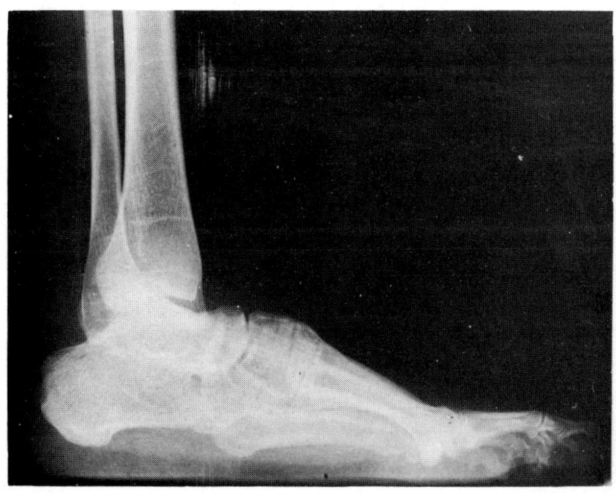

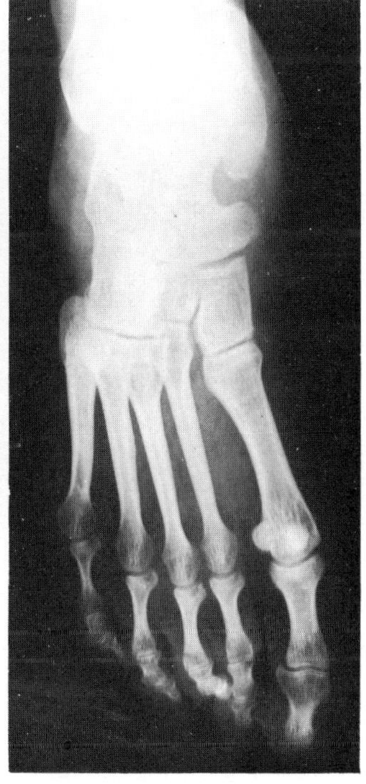

Fig. 16*e* (*above*). Patient P.B. Post-operative X-ray taken in 1955. (From Banks and Green 1958.)

Fig. 16*f* (*right*). Patient P.B. Post-operative X-ray taken in 1955. (From Banks and Green 1958.)

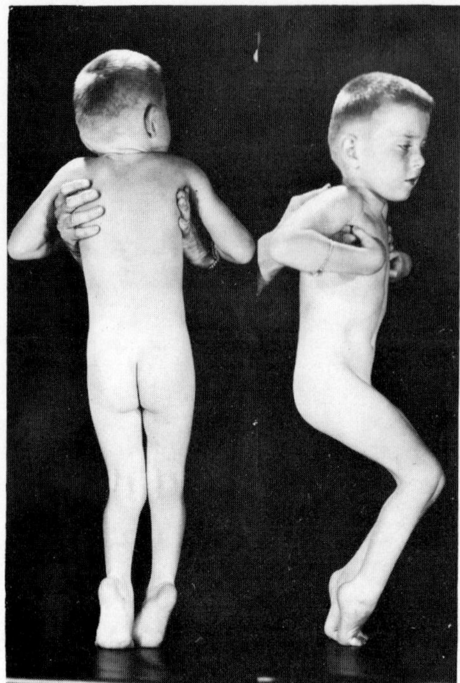
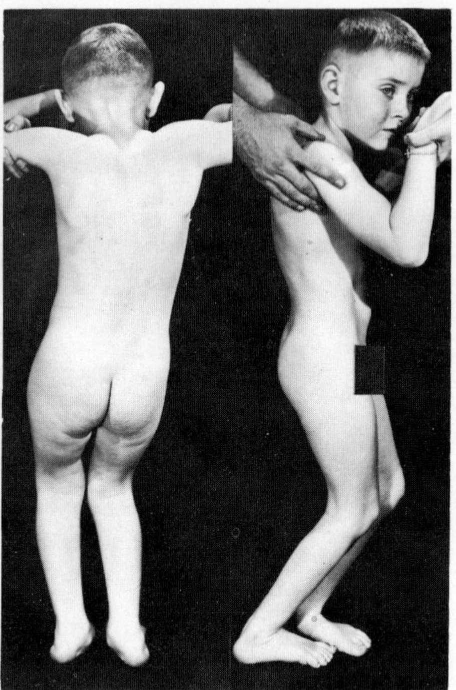

Fig. 17a. Patient T.H., aged five years. Note severe equinus and hip and knee flexion deformities.

Fig. 17b. Patient T.H. Note severe calcaneo-valgus, with hip and knee flexion deformity, two years after heel cord lengthening.

Tendon Transplantation

Tendon transplantation must be used very carefully in the foot of the patient with cerebral palsy. If equinovalgus is treated by correction of the equinus and transplantation of the peroneals anteriorly, post-operatively an apparently weak or 'absent' anterior tibial will often recover function and cause the opposite deformity. If equinovarus is treated by the correction of the equinus, a posterior tibial lengthening and an anterior tibial transplant laterally, significant valgus may result.

Calcaneus

Calcaneus deformity of the foot is usually secondary to over correction in heel-cord lengthening. Under these circumstances, protection, active exercises and night support are usually successful in reversing the deformity.

Where heel cord lengthening is done in the presence of significant hip and knee flexion deformities which are not corrected, the patient will walk with his feet in dorsiflexion and will develop a significant calcaneo-valgus deformity (Fig. 17). Obviously the treatment here is the prevention of the deformity by adequate correction of the hip and knee flexion deformity. Where calcaneo-valgus is allowed to persist during the growing period, the ankle mortise will develop a valgus contour

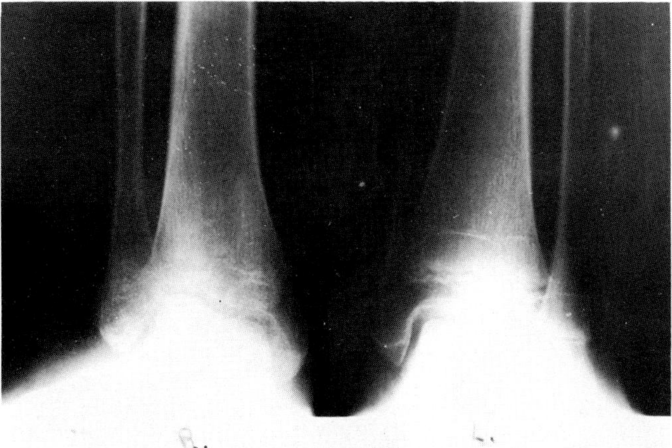

Fig. 18. Patient M.B. Note valgus contour on weight-bearing of ankle mortise on the right side, five years after heel cord lengthening, without correction of significant knee flexion deformities. Patient has severe calcaneovalgus foot deformity.

(Fig. 18). Not only will the hip and knee flexion deformities then need to be corrected, but a supramalleolar osteotomy may be necessary.

Hallux Valgus and Toe Deformities

Where equinovalgus has not been treated, a significant hallux valgus may develop (Fig. 19). This may be treated by any one of the many procedures available for correcting hallux valgus. The author prefers correction of the significant equinovalgus and the McBride procedure (1928, 1935), with or without an osteotomy of the first metatarsal as indicated (Fig. 20). The correction of pronation of the foot will diminish

Spastic hammer toes which do not respond to adequate shoe and metatarsal support may be treated by transplant of the extensor tendons to the metatarsal necks and arthrodesis of the appropriate interphalangeal joint. Flexor tenotomy may be necessary. Burman (1938) has recommended neurectomy of the motor branch of the lateral plantar nerve and of the twig to the interossei in the fouth interosseous space, plantar capsulotomy of the first metartarso-phalangeal joint, and a division of the flexor hallucis brevis.

Summary

The most common foot deformity in cerebral palsy is equinus. The triceps surae have received surgical attention at all levels to achieve lengthening in many related and unrelated ways. It probably makes little difference how the length of the muscle is re-established and how its stretch reflex is weakened, as long as the patient is carefully chosen, the procedure is done well, and the post-operative care is prolonged and detailed. The most common cause of failure is a lack of or inadequate use of night support during the growing period leading to a recurrence. One can

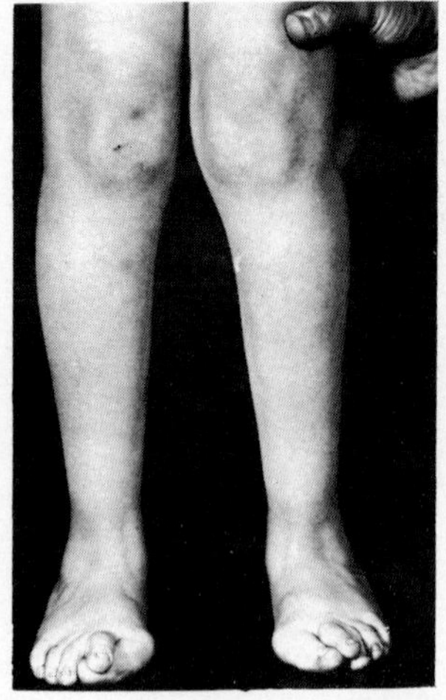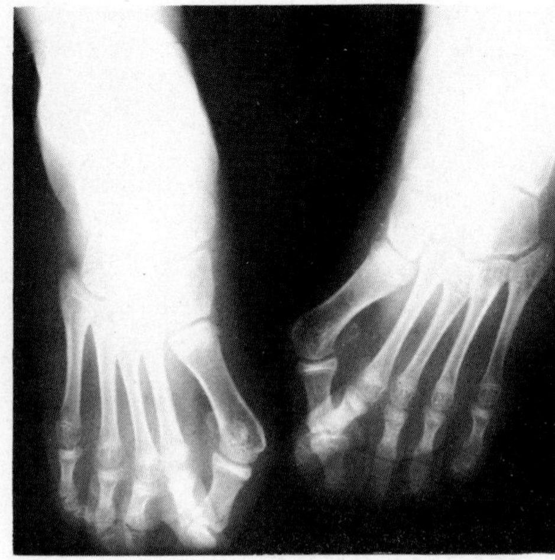

Fig. 19*a*. (*left*). Patient D.B. aged fourteen years. Note severe hallux valgus and overlapping toes (picture taken on 24th April 1967). Severe equinovalgus had been corrected bilaterally five years previously by subtalar arthrodesis and heel cord lengthening.

Fig. 19*b* (*right*). Patient D.B. Weight-bearing, antero-posterior roentgenograms of feet taken on 22nd April 1967. Note severe hallux valgus, with adduction of the first metatarsal.

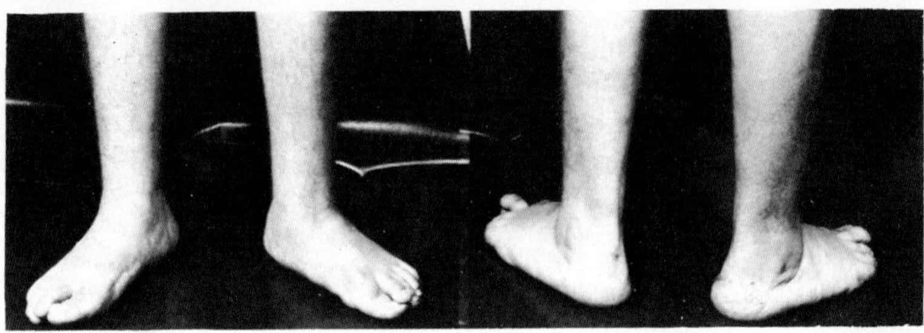

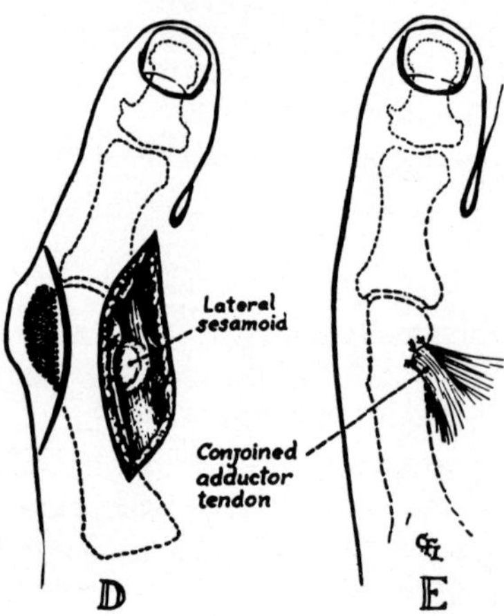

Fig. 19*c* (*above*). Patient D.B. Weight-bearing views of feet, one year after correction of hallux valgus by McBride procedure and osteotomy of the base of the first metatarsal.

Fig. 20 (*left*). The McBride Procedure for the correction of hallux valgus. Medial exostosis at the distal end of the first metatarsal is excised, the conjoined adductor tendon is transplanted to the neck of the first metatarsal, and the medial capsule is reefed. (Reprinted with permission from Edmonson 1963; redrawn from McBride 1935.)

expect an unsatisfactory result from any procedure used to correct equinus, if post-operative care is inadequate. It is well worth remembering that the patient is spastic no matter what procedure is performed, and that the deformity will recur unless efforts are made to prevent recurrence. In Boston, the procedure of choice has been the sliding lengthening of the heel cord. The results have certainly been satisfactory with long term follow-up.

Significant equinovalgus may be successfully managed by heel cord lengthening and subtalar arthrodesis. The subtalar arthrodesis should not be performed unless the equinus portion of the deformity is corrected either prior to or at the same time as the procedure to correct valgus. Over correction should be assiduously avoided.

Where equinovarus needs surgical correction and no significant bony deformity exists, heel cord and posterior tibial lengthening are recommended. If there is a significant bony deformity, an osteotomy of the os calcis or a triple arthrodesis may also be necessary.

A triple arthrodesis may be used to correct valgus or varus at the end of the growing period, but should not be used for equinus as well.

For recognition of pitfalls and complications in the management of foot and ankle problems in cerebral palsy, the reader is referred to Chapter 12.

REFERENCES

Baker, L. D. (1954) 'Triceps surae syndrome in cerebral palsy.' *Archives of Surgery,* **63,** 216.
—— (1956) 'A rational approach to the surgical needs of the cerebral palsy patient.' *Journal of Bone and Joint Surgery,* **38A,** 313.
—— Dodelin, R. A. (1958) 'Extra-articular arthrodesis of the subtaler joint (Grice procedure).' *Journal of the American Medical Association,* **168,** 1005.
—— Hill, L. M. (1964) 'Foot alignment in the cerebral palsy patient.' *Journal of Bone and Joint Surgery,* **46A,** 1.
Banks, H. H., Green, W. T. (1958) 'The correction of equinus deformity in cerebral palsy.' *Journal of Bone and Joint Surgery,* **40A,** 1359.
—— Panagakos, P. (1966) 'Orthopedic evaluation of the lower extremity in cerebral palsy.' *Clinical Orthopedics and Related Research,* **47,** 117.
—— —— (1967) 'The role of the orthopedic surgeon in cerebral palsy.' *Pediatric Clinics of North America,* **14,** 495.
—— —— Green, W. T. (1968) 'The correction of severe foot valgus in cerebral palsy.'
Bassett, F. H., Baker, L. D. (1966) 'Equinus deformity in cerebral palsy.' *in.* Adams, J. P. (Ed.) *Current Practice in Orthopedic Surgery, Vol 3.* St. Louis: C. V. Mosby Co.
Brown, A. (1968) 'A simple method of fusion of the subtalar joint in children.' *Journal of Bone and Joint Surgery,* **50B,** 369.
Burman, M. S. (1938) 'Spastic intrinsic muscle imbalance of the foot.' *Journal of Bone and Joint Surgery,* **20,** 145.
Delpech, J. M. (1823) 'Tenotomie du tendon d'Achille.' *in Chirugie Clinique de Montpellier, ou Observations et Réflexions Tirées des Travaux de Chirurgie Clinique de cette ecole.* Paris: Gabon. p. 181.
Duncan, W. R. (1960) 'Tonic reflexes of the foot.' *Journal of Bone and Joint Surgery,* **42A,** 859.
Dwyer, F. C. (1960) 'Osteotomy of the calcaneum in the treatment of grossly everted feet with special reference to cerebral palsy.' *in Proceedings of the 8th Congress of Orthopedic Surgeons and Trauma, New York, September, 1960.* Brussels: Imprimerie Medicale et Scientifique.
—— (1963) 'The treatment of relapsed club foot by the insertion of a wedge into the calcaneum.' *Journal of Bone and Joint Surgery,* **45B,** 67.

Edmonson, A. S. (1963) 'Postural deformities.' *in* Crenshaw, A. H. (Ed.) *Campbell's Operative Orthopaedics, 4th edn.* St. Louis: C. V. Mosby Co. p. 1601.

Eggers, G. W. N. (1952) 'Transplantation of hamstring tendons to femoral condyles in order to improve hip extension and to decrease knee flexion in cerebral spastic paralysis.' *Journal of Bone and Joint Surgery,* **34A,** 827.

Green, W. T., McDermott, L. J. (1942) 'Operative treatment for cerebral palsy of the spastic type.' *Journal of the American Medical Association,* **118,** 434.

Grice, D. S. (1952) 'Extra-articular arthrodesis of the subastragalar joint for correction of paralytic flat feet in children.' *Journal of Bone and Joint Surgery.* **34A,** 927.

Ingram, A. J. (1963) 'Miscellaneous affections of the nervous system.' *in* Crenshaw, A. H. (Ed.) *Campbell's Operative Orthopedics, 4th edn.* St. Louis: C. V. Mosby Co. p. 1601.

Keats, S., Kouten, J. (1968) 'Early surgical correction of the planovalgus foot in cerebral palsy.' *Clinical Orthopedics and Related Research,* **61,** 223.

McBride, R. D. (1928) 'A conservative operation for bunions.' *Journal of Bone and Joint Surgery,* **10,** 735.

—— (1935) 'The conservative operation for "bunions".' *Journal of the American Medical Association,* **105,** 1164.

Mortens, J., Moller, M., Salmonsen, L. (1962) 'Early operation for stabilizing spastic talipes equinovalgus by Grice's extra-articular subtaler arthrodesis.' *Acta Orthopaedica Scandinavica,* **32,** 485.

Phelps, W. M. (1951) 'Treatment of paralytic disorders exclusive of poliomyelitis.' *in* Bancroft, F. W., Marble, J. B. (Eds.) *Surgical Treatment of the Motor-Skeletal System.* Philadelphia: Lippincott.

—— (1957) 'Long-term results of orthopedic surgery in cerebral palsy.' *Journal of Bone and Joint Surgery,* **39A,** 53.

Seymour, N., Evans, D. K. (1968) 'A modification of the Grice subtalar arthrodesis.' *Journal of Bone and Joint Surgery,* **50B,** 372.

Silfverskiöld, M. (1923-4) 'Reduction of the uncrossed two-joints muscles of the leg to one-joint muscles in spastic conditions.' *Acta Chirurgica Scandinavica,* **56,** 315.

Silver, C. M. (1969) *Data presented to the American Academy for Cerebral Palsy, December, 1969.*

—— Simon, S. D. (1959) 'Gastrocnemius-muscle recession for spastic equinus deformity in cerebral palsy.' *Journal of Bone and Joint Surgery,* **41A,** 1021.

—— —— Spindell, H. M., Litchman, M., Scala, M. (1967) 'Calcaneal osteotomy for valgus and varus deformities of the foot in cerebral palsy.' *Journal of Bone and Joint Surgery,* **49A,** 232.

Stoffel, A. (1913) 'The treatment of spastic contractures.' *American Journal of Orthopedic Surgery,* **10,** 611.

Strayer, L. M. (1950) 'Recession of the gastrocnemius.' *Journal of Bone and Joint Surgery,* **32A,** 671.

—— (1958) 'Gastrocnemius recession.' *Journal of Bone and Joint Surgery,* **40A,** 1019.

Strohmeyer, G. F. (1838) *Beiträge zur operativen Orthopädik öder Erfahrungen über die subcutane Durchschneidung verkürzter Muskeln und deren Sehnen.* Hanover: Helwing.

Vulpius, O., Stoffel, A. (1913) *Orthopädische Operationslehre, Ed. I.* Stuttgart: F. Enke, p. 29.

White, J. W. (1943) 'Torsion of the Achilles tendon.' *Archives of Surgery,* **46,** 784.

CHAPTER 11

The Upper Extremity in Cerebral Palsy

J. LEONARD GOLDNER

Introduction

During the past twenty years, upper extremity surgery has become firmly established as an aid in the management of patients with cerebral palsy. Although surgery cannot be expected to make a functionally poor limb perfect, a marked and measurable improvement in comparison with the pre-operative condition can usually be demonstrated. The major reasons for selecting surgical treatment are to effect improvement in the performance of daily living activities, to increase the speed of hand and forearm movement, and to produce cosmetic improvement. The goals are limited, but a reasonable degree of success can be guaranteed, provided that patient selection is made in a precise way. If pre-operative assessment is thorough and accurate, if the operative procedures are carried out with care and caution, and if post-operative care is well planned and executed, surgery of the upper extremity will be helpful to certain patients with neuromuscular dysfunction due to cerebral pathology.

From the outset, the patient, the members of his family and the surgeon must all have modest and realistic expectations as regards the results that can be obtained by surgical treatment. A hand whose function is influenced by a brain that has been so seriously affected by hypoxia that permanent damage has occurred, will usually never be a dominant hand. Nevertheless, the affected hand will be of greater value to the patient if he or she can use it to grasp, to assist in holding large objects or to hold something such as a packet of papers while the uninvolved hand is used to perform some more complicated task (Fig. 1). Likewise, if the fingers can be opened

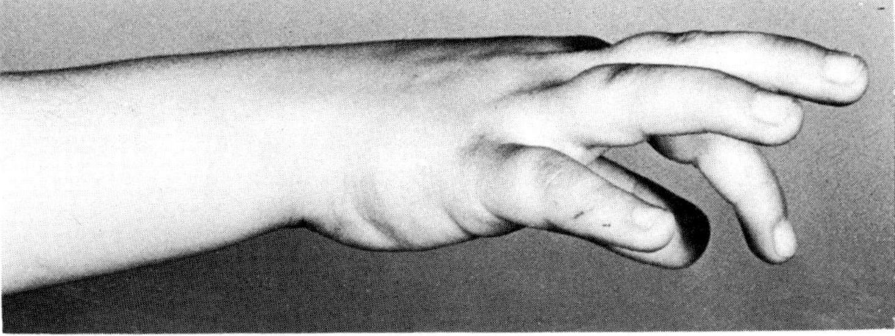

Fig. 1. This patient can voluntarily extend the ulnar three digits as well as the thumb, but the index finger cannot be extended readily. In the spastic hemiplegic patient, this digit frequently lags in extension, because of contracture of the flexor digitorum sublimis of the index finger and because of moderate weakness of the extensor digitorum communis and extensor indicis proprius and moderate spasticity of the first dorsal interosseus. Treatment directed towards the thumb and index finger will improve potential use of this hand.

voluntarily while the wrist joint is at zero degrees or in slight extension, the hand will be stronger and more useful as a grasping unit than if the wrist has to be in full flexion for finger extension to be achieved (Fig. 2). An involved hand may be of only minor use while the thumb is in the palm, but able to perform a much wider range of functions if the thumb is treated surgically so that it remains out of the palm (Fig. 3).

Even though the appearance of the extremity will not normally be the primary reason for surgical treatment, the child or adult with a tightly clenched fist, a flexed wrist joint and a thumb which is permanently in the palm will be delighted if treatment leaves him or her with fingers that extend actively, a hand and wrist joint in the neutral position and an elbow that does not remain constantly in the flexed position.

The goals must be realistic and in keeping with the patient's neuromuscular potential. The surgeon must avoid both optimism and pessimism when discussing the problem with the patient and the family.

Assessment and Evaluation

Motor Condition and Diagnostic Classification

The patient is classified as having a spastic, athetoid, ataxic or mixed form of cerebral palsy (see Chapter 4). This entails reflex testing, the elicitation of stretch reflex, and testing for clonus. The condition is designated as mild, moderate or severe.

The degree of control of individual muscles is determined by standard muscle testing procedures and observation. The examiner asks the patient to move a particular muscle against resistance, and the muscle is palpated during voluntary motion. The examiner rates the muscle as normal, good, fair, or poor. Though not as accurate in patients affected by cerebral palsy as it is in patients affected by flaccid paresis or paralysis, when used by an experienced examiner this method of estimating muscle strength is adequate for determining whether or not a particular muscle should be used as a motor for tendon transfer.

The patient is asked to pass objects of different sizes back and forth from one hand to the other, and voluntary control of the extremity is observed. The patient should be encouraged to use visual assistance in performing these actions. By watching the patient as he grasps and releases objects of varying size, the examiner can assess finger closing, hand opening, wrist elevation, wrist flexion and thumb control. After asking the patient to attempt voluntary pronation and supination, the examiner tests these movements passively. The major joints of the extremity (the shoulder, elbow, wrist and fingers) are tested for muscle and tendon contractures, tightness, hyper-relaxation and range of active and passive motion (Fig. 2).

Muscle testing should be concerned not only with attempts to rate individual muscles, but also with the rating of groups of muscles, such as the extensor digitorum communis, the wrist extensors and the wrist flexors. A description of joint motion is important, because joint postures can have a tenodesis effect, and the principle of tenodesis is essential in assessing the strength and voluntary or involuntary action of a particular muscle group. For example, it may be that the extensor muscle mass does not function voluntarily, but that, when the patient grasps an object, the extensor

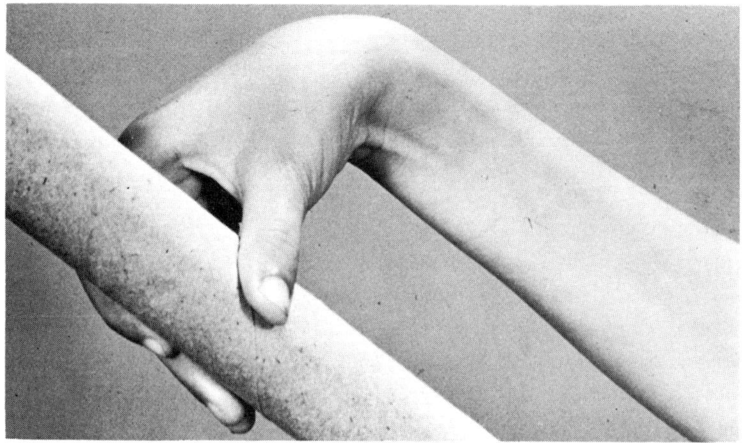

Fig. 2. Spastic hemiplegia, in which the wrist and finger extensors are weak, and the wrist flexors are moderately contracted and strong. Grasp is weakened by flexion of the wrist, because increased tension of the extensor tendons prevents full finger and thumb flexion. This hand provides a hook and a weak grasp sufficiently strong to hold a lightweight large object. Surgical treatment was directed towards reinforcing the wrist, finger and thumb extensors, and diminishing spasticity of the wrist flexors, without weakening them completely. Thumb abduction was improved by arthrodesis of the metacarpo-phalangeal joint, and reinforcement of the abductor pollicis longus. A release of elbow flexion contracture was done at the same operation.

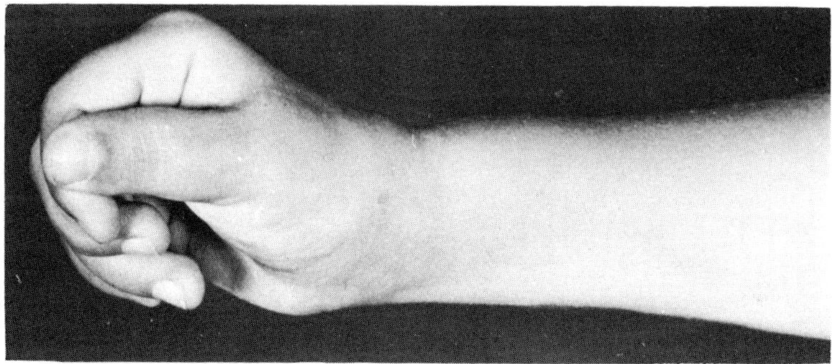

Fig. 3. Post-operative flexion of the hand of a six-year-old patient with spastic hemiplegia. During voluntary flexion of the fingers, tension of the extensor digitorum communis muscles and the extensor of the wrist results in increased elevation of the hand through about 15 degrees. This principle of tenodesis depends on active flexion of the digits increasing the tension of the wrist extensors, and upon active flexion of the wrist tendons increasing tension on the finger extensors. This principle provides automatic opening of the fingers and closing of the fingers. Thumb action follows the same pattern. As the wrist is flexed, the thumb extends by pull of the brachioradialis and the shortened abductor and extensor pollicis brevis. As the wrist elevates, the thumb participates in a thumb-to-side pinch. Arthrodesis of the metacarpo-phalangeal joint diminishes the thumb-in-palm deformity. The thumb-to-side pinch is stronger in the patient with hemiplegia than the tip-to-tip pinch.

223

tendons stand out and the forearm muscles are palpable and maintain fair resistance. In such a patient, it would not be desirable to move a tendon from the flexor surface to the extensor surface.

In young children, when muscle testing is difficult, muscle strength and co-ordination and joint function can be determined by observing hand activities while the child is playing. Conclusions about motor function can be made by observing patterns of grasp and release when the child holds objects of varying size and transfers them from one hand to the other. However, although observations of functional patterns during such activities are helpful in making a total assessment (Figs. 5a, b and c), they cannot replace individual muscle testing.

To assess the extent and severity of joint contractures, the examiner determines the degree of resistance to passive movement and the range of active motion of the involved part. These observations are of help in making decisions concerning soft tissue release and the correction of contractures.

In certain patients, complete correction of the joint contracture is impossible, because the deformity has been present for such a long time, and the forces involved in causing the contracture are so great, that, apart from capsular contracture, molding of the articular surfaces has occurred. Partial correction can, however, be obtained by surgical release and appropriate splinting (Figs. 4a, b and c).

Sensory Determination

Sensation is rated according to the patient's ability to recognise the shape, size

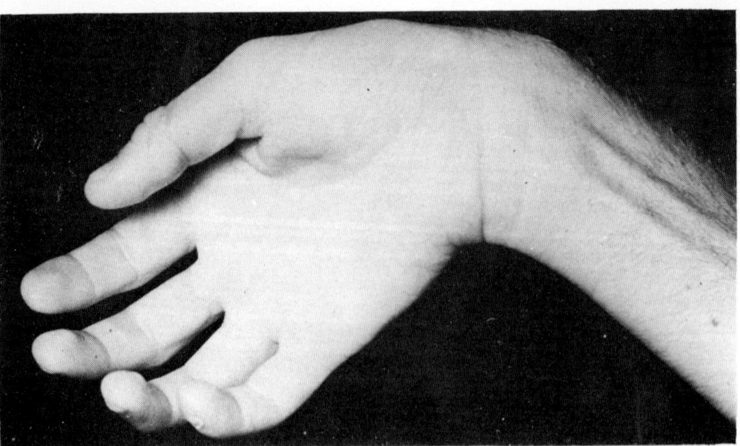

Fig. 4a. The hand of a sixteen-year-old boy with spastic hemiplegia and moderate athetosis. Stereognosis was fair, and muscle strength was adequate for voluntary flexion and extension of the digits. However, excessive ulnar deviation interfered with the rapidity of function. The ulnar deformity was progressive during growth, but became stationary when maximum growth was reached. In cerebral palsy, the primary condition is non-progressive, but the deformities change as the child grows and develops. In this patient, the ulnar deviation was maintaining the thumb out of the palm, but the degree of deviation was excessive, and treatment was directed at diminishing it.

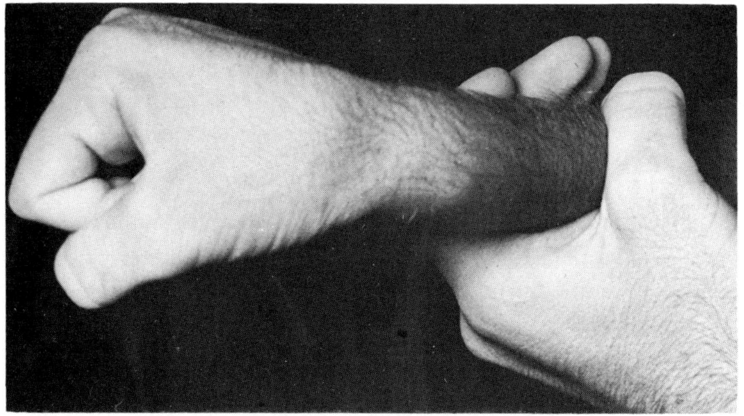

Fig. 4*b*. Same patient as in Figure 4*a*. Post-operatively, flexion of the thumb and fingers could be accomplished with the wrist at neutral. The hand was more stable in pronation than in supination. The operation consisted of the transfer of the extensor carpi ulnaris from the fifth metacarpal insertion to the third metacarpal. This single procedure was sufficient to eliminate the excessive ulnar deviation and strengthen elevation of the hand. The extensor carpi ulnaris can function as an ulnar deviator or dorsiflexor. This patient also had a flexion contracture of the elbow, which was released at the same time as the hand surgery was done.

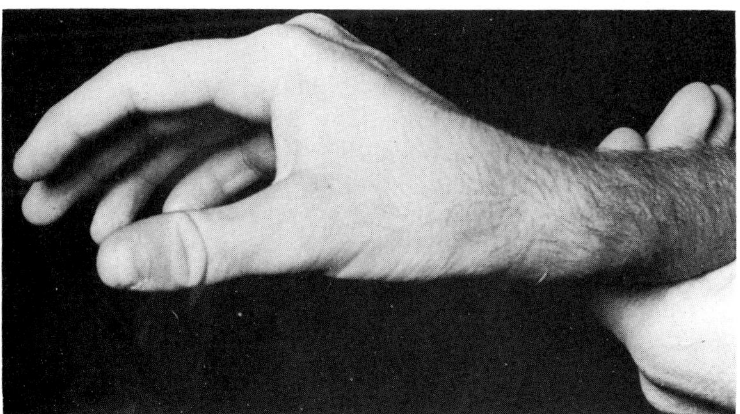

Fig. 4*c*. Same patient as in Figure 4*a*. Post-operatively, extension of the fingers and thumb was possible, even with the hand at 20 degrees of dorsiflexion. This position diminishes finger extension. When the metacarpals are elevated to 0 degrees or are in slight flexion, the fingers and thumb extend farther than when the hand is dorsiflexed. The decrease in ulnar deviation deformity provided a stronger grip. In this picture, the patient is holding the extremity with his opposite hand because of moderate athetosis. Many patients with a moderate athetosis show improvement in hand function after upper extremity surgery.

and consistence of objects. The speed of action is important, but should not be compared to that of a normal hand. An uncomplicated sensory test is to have the patient hold both hands overhead, close his eyes, and attempt to recognize objects placed in each hand by the examiner. The examiner asks the patient if the object is large or small, rough or smooth, square or round, and the consistence of the surfaces. The patient names the object if possible. If the patient is hemiplegic, the examiner, after testing the involved hand, places the object in the uninvolved hand, and repeats the questions. This allows a quick comparison between the two hands. If the patient replies in error when the involved hand is tested, and correctly when the uninvolved hand is tested, it is reasonable to assume that proprioception in the involved hand is diminished or absent.

A more accurate and more complete assessment of sensation can be made by performing each test procedure at least ten times in order to eliminate chance.

Most patients with cerebral palsy have satisfactory epicritic sensation, but many show deficits in proprioception, such as poor two-point discrimination and an inability to recognize the size and shape of objects. If sensation in all of these categories is good or normal, then surgical treatment is more likely to succeed, whereas poor or absent proprioception seems to correlate fairly closely with poor surgical results.

Nevertheless, an operation on the hand of a patient with cerebral palsy is not contra-indicated merely because certain sensory characteristics are abnormal or absent. If the patient has good visual acuity, reasonable motivation and a desire to become independent, he will need a hand that will grasp and release with relative ease, even though this hand may not compare in efficiency with a normal hand.

Emotional and Intellectual Maturity

Emotional and intellectual maturity can be determined by the use of various standard psychological tests. The results should be interpreted by an individual trained in analyzing the intellectual capabilities of patients with cerebral palsy.

From a brief session with the patient, the examiner can learn much about the child's desire to improve hand function, his attention span, and his ability to co-operate with his physician and therapist.

The child's behaviour patterns, ability to co-operate, motivation and intelligence quotient (I.Q.) are all likely to affect the results of an operation, and should be considered when the decision to operate is being taken. However, even if a patient's rating on one or more of these characteristics is poor, the decision to operate may be justified if reasonable functional improvement can be expected. The patient in a training school or a permanent care institution, with a hand that is flexed and an elbow which is flexed with a fixed contracture, will appreciate having the deformities diminished or eliminated, that, even if the extremity is used only a few times a day for carrying objects and assisting in certain activities of daily living, the operative procedures will have been justified.

Thus, although psychological testing is desirable before surgery is initiated, the results of the psychological tests will not necessarily determine whether or not surgical treatment is indicated. There is no absolute contra-indication to surgery in an otherwise healthy patient with cerebral palsy, provided that the preliminary assessment on which the decision to operate is based has been thorough and complete, and that the neuromuscular improvements expected are reasonable. The final decision will depend upon the likelihood of surgical treatment providing appreciable improvement in function, co-ordination and appearance (Figs. 5a, b and c).

Attitudes and Expectations

The expectations of the patient's family and friends are discussed at the outset of the examination. As soon as a plan of treatment has been outlined, many parents visualize a normal hand in place of the deformed hand, and only when the limitations of treatment are repeatedly explained to them do they recognize these.

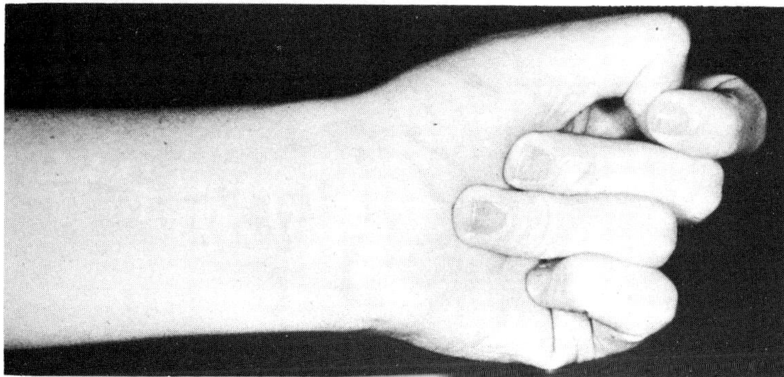

Fig. 5a. This the hand of an 18-year-old girl with spastic hemiplegia and a prominent athetoid component. The distal joint of the thumb was constantly pulled over by the spastic flexor pollicis longus. In the adult, arthrodesis of this joint is an acceptable solution to the deformed thumb tip. In this patient, the long and ring fingers showed a flexed position when the wrist was elevated. Lengthening or transfer of the flexores digitorum sublimes tendons was necessary to allow smoother opening and closing of the fingers. Previously, a transfer of the flexor carpi ulnaris to the wrist had been done; this had resulted in an improvement of hand elevation but not of finger function.

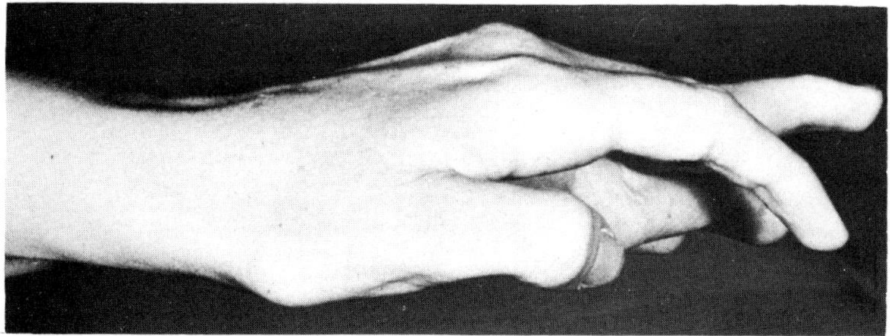

Fig. 5b. Same patient as in Figure 5a. When the patient held the forearm in a pronated position and the wrist in a few degrees of dorsiflexion, she could voluntarily extend the fingers, but the distal joint of the thumb remained in flexion. The treatment planned and carried out for improvement of the thumb deformity included: (1) lengthening of the flexor pollicis longus tendon at the wrist; (2) arthrodesis of the distal interphalangeal joint of the thumb; and (3) lengthening of two flexor digitorum sublimes tendons.

227

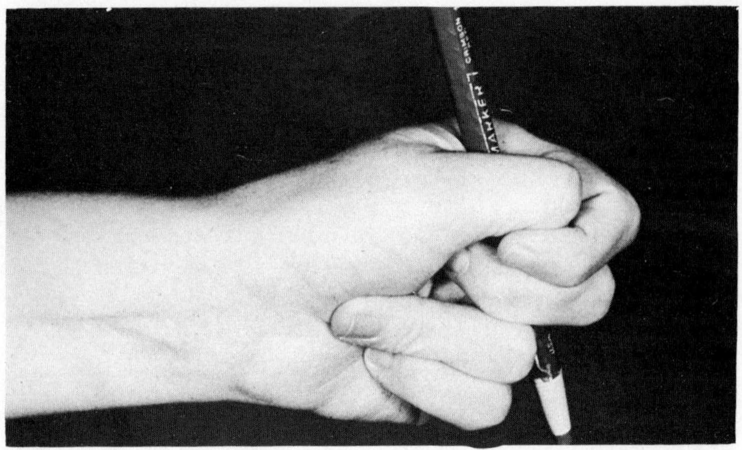

Fig. 5*c*. Same patient as in Figures 5*a* and 5*b*. Pre-operative picture, showing patient's efforts to hold a pencil. The pathological reflex of the thumb resulted in hyperflexion of the distal joint. The index and long fingers could not be controlled adequately to provide a thumb-finger pinch. After the thumb web had been released, the distal joint of the thumb arthrodesed, and two flexor sublimes tendons lengthened, a three digit pinch around the pencil was possible.

ACCOUNT OF SERIES OF UPPER EXTREMITY OPERATIONS PERFORMED
ON CEREBRAL PALSIED PATIENTS BETWEEN 1950 AND 1970

Clinical Material: Selection and Classification

Between 1950 and 1970, over one hundred patients with cerebral palsy involving the upper extremity were treated surgically at the Duke Medical Center and the North Carolina Cerebral Palsy Hospital. In the majority of these patients, the primary diagnosis was spastic hemiplegia. Several, however, also manifested an element of athetosis, but this additional problem was not in itself considered to be a contra-indication to surgical treatment.

The operative procedures were planned in groups, and several operations were performed simultaneously. The conclusions drawn here concerning the patterns of diagnosis and the results of treatment have been arrived at after observing the patients for periods ranging from two to twenty years.

The patients were selected for surgical treatment after careful assessment, on the basis of the criteria described earlier in this chapter.

Patients with predominantly spastic conditions were operated upon without hesitation if a reasonable degree of improvement could be predicted. Those with spasticity and a minor degree of athetosis were managed in a similar way. The patients with a predominance of athetosis, who had greater difficulty in carrying out co-ordinated movements of the fingers and wrist, were rarely submitted to upper extremity surgery. Efforts in such patients were usually directed towards stereotactic brain surgery, in the hope of controlling the severe deformities.

Pattern Classification

By classifying the patients' hands according to the pattern of deformtiy, the examiner is able to make an immediate diagnostic and prognostic evaluation. Emphasis should be placed on both assets and deficiencies, this approach being helpful in the determination of whether or not reasonable hand balance can be established.

The pattern classification is made after consideration of motor power, joint deformity, contracture, sensation and function (see above).

Pattern I. The hand shows good grasp and release, but the thumb is kept in the palm; proprioceptive sensation is poor, and the patient seldom uses the hand (Fig. 6). The appearance of the extremity is satisfactory, apart from mild elbow flexion. These patients will benefit from early training in visual cues and from being encouraged to use the extremity to help in carrying out activities of daily living. If proprioceptive sensation should happen to be good, hand function in these patients is usually excellent.

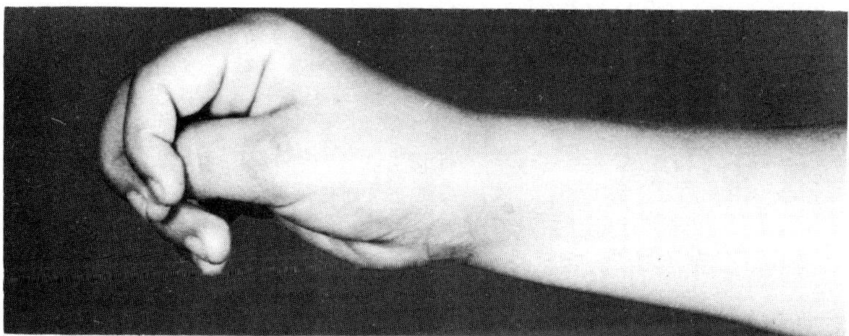

Fig. 6. The hand of a 6-year-old child with spastic hemiplegia. As the fingers are flexed, the thumb crosses into the palm, because of a persistent primitive reflex. This thumb activity is pathological. Flexion occurs at the metacarpo-phalangeal joint and the distal phalangeal joint due to spasticity or contracture of the adductor and the flexor pollicis longus. The interossei hold the first and second metacarpals together. If the extensor muscles are of adequate strength, the thumb can be pulled out of the palm when the patient flexes the wrist slightly and activates the digit extensors. Operative treatment can improve this condition.

Pattern II. The hand and fingers are maintained in flexion, with the thumb in the palm. Active extension of the wrist, fingers and thumb is limited or absent. The wrist extends as the fingers are forcibly flexed round an object. The fingers extend as the wrist is flexed (see Figs. 5a, b and c). Hand function is limited, but is often surprisingly good considering the limited motor power and the diminished proprioceptive sensation. Surgical treatment can provide moderate improvement in these patients. If the patient has good proprioception, then surgical treatment will be even more helpful.

Pattern III. There is a severe flexion deformity of the hand at the wrist joint, but passive finger extension is possible when the wrist is flexed. The thumb is held in the palm. Proprioceptive sensation can be poor, fair or good. Potentially, the hand is of some functional use, but this potential will not be realised until the contractures are diminished and the grasp and release mechanism is improved. Adequate muscle motors are present on the flexor surface for use as extensors (see Figs. *4a, b* and *c*).

Within each of these three patterns, the level of neuromuscular control and joint status are reasonably constant from patient to patient, but the degree of sensory impairment may vary considerably. Epicritic sensation is usually present, the patient being able to recognise hot, cold, sharp and dull without difficulty. Proprioceptive sensation may, however, be profoundly impaired, because of cortical involvement. After gross testing has been completed and the degree of proprioception determined, an opinion as to the potential ultimate use of the hand in two-handed activities can be given with greater certainty.

Pattern IV. The hand is maintained in a position of extension. Wrist flexion is limited because of weakness of the flexor muscles. The wrist extensor muscles are active, although the finger extensors may be weak. The thumb is in the palm, and release of the digits and thumb is slow because of the position of extension and because of a limited amount of extensor tenodesis (Figs. *7b* and *7c*). Sensation may be good, fair or poor. This condition is most frequently seen in patients with post-traumatic hemiplegia who were born with normal musculo-skeletal function, rather than in patients with congenital cerebral palsy.

Pattern V. Both the wrist and the fingers show a severe flexion deformity, and the thumb is held firmly in the palm. There are no active wrist or finger extensor muscles. Flexor strength is weak, and elbow contracture is severe. Proprioceptive sensation is poor (Fig. 8). The patient uses the forearm and the back of the hand for supporting objects. Neither large nor small items can be placed in the palm with certainty. The extremity can be improved greatly in appearance and moderately in function, by elbow release, stabilization of the wrist and straightening of the fingers. Active flexion and extension of the digits cannot be expected.

Following pattern classification, each of the patients was submitted to detailed muscle testing and sensory examination. The plan of treatment and the likely prognosis were then forthcoming in a logical way.

Classification of Patients Selected for Treatment

For analysis, those patients who had operative procedures on the upper extremities were classified into four groups. Groups I, II and III were composed primarily of patients with spastic cerebral palsy, although in a few cases a minimal degree of other neurological deficits was present. Group IV was composed of patients with mixed types of cerebral palsy.

Group I. The hands of Group I patients are minimally involved and show a reasonable range of active motion of the fingers, the wrist and the thumb. The wrist can be dorsiflexed to neutral, and the metacarpo-phalangeal joints can be extended, while the hand is held at neutral or in slight dorsiflexion. Active grasp and release are possible, and the hand can be used for some actions. The main deficits are delayed speed, minimal dexterity and slow co-ordination. Functional improvement can be achieved by tendon lengthening and minimal joint stabilization. Elbow release improves appearance and function.

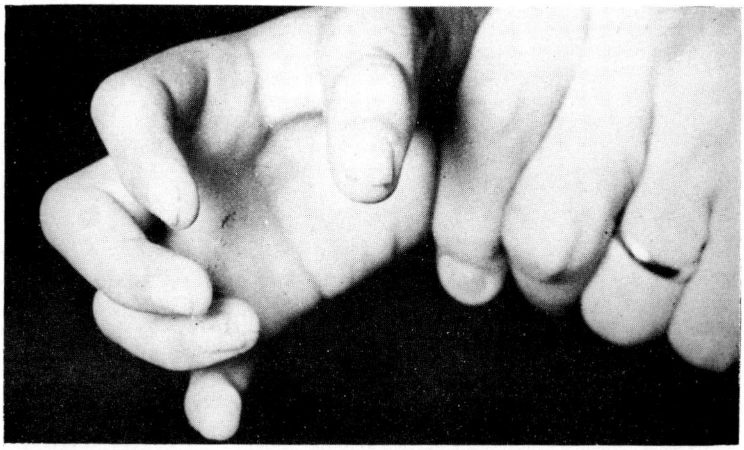

Fig. 7a. This is the hand of an eight-year-old boy with spastic hemiplegia. Stereognosis was good, and his intelligence quotient was 90. The wrist was held in 20 degrees of flexion, and the hand could not be elevated voluntarily to neutral. The fingers could be flexed and extended voluntarily. Grasp was of fair strength, but release was slow, because of weakness of the wrist extensor muscles. The operative plan comprised (1) transfer of the flexor carpi ulnaris through the interosseous membrane to the extensor carpi radialis brevis; and (2) reinforcement of the abductor pollicis longus with the brachioradialis, and plication of the abductor pollicis longus.

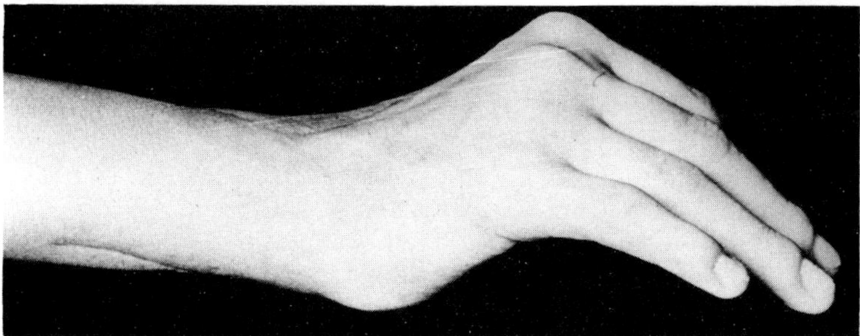

Fig. 7b. Same patient as in Figure 7a. Post-operative picture showing condition of the hand after transfer of the wrist flexor tendon to the wrist extensor tendon. Immediately after the operation, the wrist had been in flexion, but after several months the strength of extension had improved to the point where the hand was held persistently in excessive dorsiflexion. This over-correction had occurred because the flexor carpi ulnaris was too strong a muscle to transfer, and the inherent strength of the wrist extensors was slightly better than had been realized. Excessive dorsiflexion was a handicap because finger flexion was slow and incomplete. Excessive dorsiflexion is just as much a handicap as excessive volar flexion.

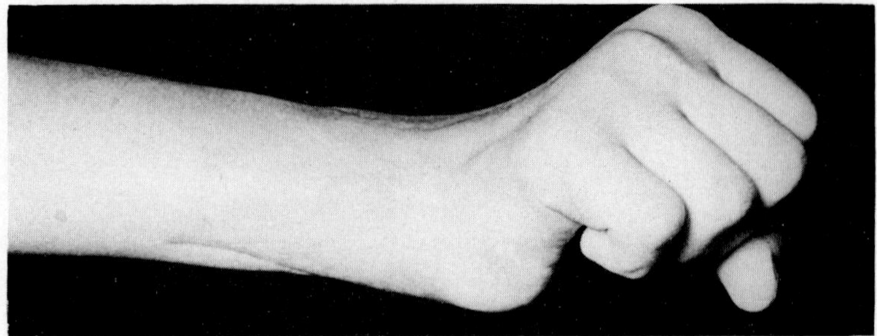

Fig. 7c. Same patient as in Figure 7a. Post-operatively, the patient could flex his fingers when the wrist was elevated. Finger flexion automatically increased wrist dorsiflexion. The grip was strong and helpful, but rapid extension of the fingers was prevented by the excessive dorsiflexion of the hand. Wrist flexion was difficult to achieve. When the hand was placed in a cast and held at 10 degrees of flexion and 5 degrees of ulnar deviation, finger flexion and extension could be performed rapidly and with great ease. It was therefore decided to perform a radius-carpal wrist arthrodesis, which was done without affecting the radial epiphysis. Wrist arthrodesis is useful when active flexion and extension of the fingers can be done quickly and are controlled by voluntary motion and not by tenodesis. It is essential that an operation for wrist arthrodesis should be preceded by a trial period of immobilization in a cast and then in a brace.

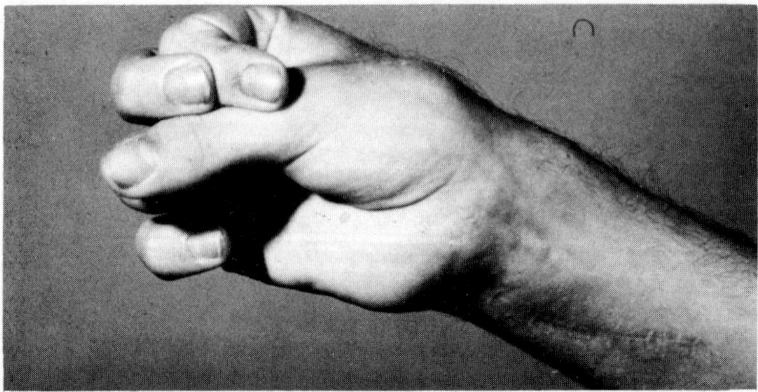

Fig. 8. This is the hand of a 16-year-old male with spastic hemiplegia and athetosis secondary to a head injury that had occurred when he was 12 years old. Tendon transfer has been carried out to improve wrist and finger control. Post-operatively, the thumb continued to flex at the metacarpo-phalangeal joint, because of spasticity of the flexor pollicis brevis and the adductor pollicis, and because of weakness of the abductor pollicis and the extensor pollicis brevis. Treatment had included release of the thumb web by lengthening the adductor, release of the origins of the interossei in the web, transfer of a flexor sublimis to the extensor pollicis longus, and plication of the abductor pollicis longus and tendon transfer to reinforce it. These surgical procedures can be done in patients with athetosis, and improvement has been observed.

Group II. The hands of Group II patients are characterised by a flexor/extensor imbalance. The wrist, fingers and thumb flexors show mild contractures. Weakness of the extensor muscles prevents wrist elevation above neutral. Voluntary extension of the fingers is weak because of diminished strength of the extensor digitorum communis. The thumb tends to remain in the palm when the hand is in extension, but moves away from the palm when the wrist is in flexion. The patients in this group utilize the hand as a stabilizer and to assist in some two-handed actions. Hand strength is weak, and activity is slow (see Fig. 2). Moderate functional improvement and modest cosmetic alteration are reasonable goals after surgical treatment on the hands of these patients.

Group III. The extremities of patients in this group are particularly severely involved. The flexors overbalance the extensors. The fingers can be opened only when the wrist is in full flexion (Fig. 9). The hand and the extremity are unsightly. Cosmetic improvement is the primary goal of surgical treatment, although it is also possible that after treatment the hand will be of slight assistance to the patient in carrying out two-handed activities.

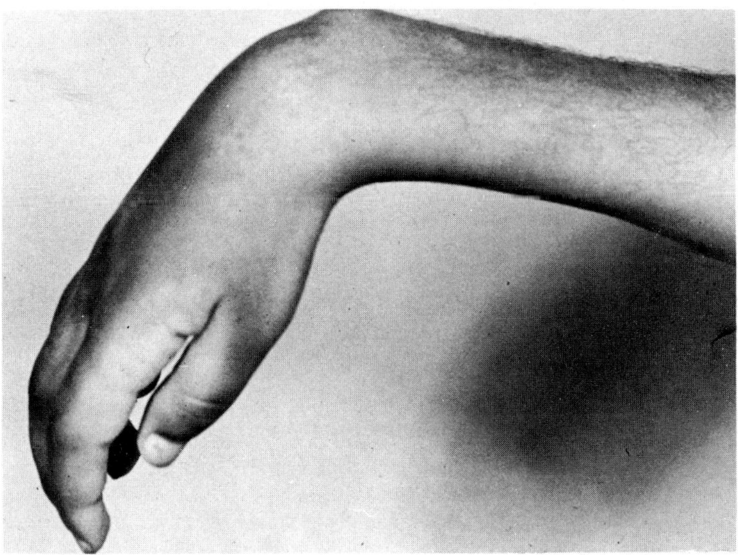

Fig. 9. Hand of a patient with tetraparesis, with severe involvement of one upper extremity. The wrist was constantly held in acute flexion, and the flexor muscles were contracted. There was no voluntary active extension of the wrist, fingers or thumb. The wrist flexors were very weak. In this position, the fingers are passively extended by tension of the extensor digitorum communis; the thumb is likewise extended by tension of the extensor pollicis longus and abductor pollicis longus. Muscle testing can be carried out using several different maneuvers. Observations of muscle strength must be accompanied by palpation of the muscle bellies. Occasionally, an extremity in this position will demonstrate active wrist extensors, but only after a period of immobilization and nerve block. With the wrist in acute flexion, the extensors become stretched and inactive, and release or transfer of the flexors is necessary before the extensor becomes reasonably functional. In the patient illustrated here, flexor tendon lengthening, proximal row carpalectomy, and transfer of one flexor to a wrist extensor, were sufficient to hold the hand up and provide improvement in the performance of gross activities.

Group IV. The hands of patients in this group are both spastic and athetoid, but although the prognosis is less good than for Groups, I, II and III, some improvement can be expected after surgical treatment.

Patients with predominant syndrome of hemiballismus or athetosis were not selected for surgical treatment, although a few mainly athetoid patients were classified anatomically in Group II, and had operations on the thumb and tendons about the wrist as a secondary form of treatment.

Other patients who had athetoid upper extremities, but in whom the athetosis was not severe enough to warrant stereotactic surgery, and who desired an extremity with less tension, improved co-ordination and a more normal appearance, did undergo various operative procedure (Figs. 10*a* and 10*b*). Multiple operative procedures on the extremities of such patients are well tolerated, and can be expected to produce reasonable improvement, although extensive tendon surgery, with multiple tendon transfers, usually results in a flexion deformity of the wrist being changed into an extension deformity (Figs. 10*a* and 10*b*). However, a localized metacarpophalangeal joint fusion, an isolated tendon transfer and lengthening of a contracted flexor digitorum sublimis, followed by protective bracing, can provide a reasonably favourable result.

Results

The assessment of the results of surgical treatment in patients with such widely differing upper extremity deformities is less straightforward than it is in patients with a paralytic hand or a hand that has been affected by trauma. The following five main factors require consideration in making the assessment:

 (i) improvement in the ability to carry out activities of daily living;

 (ii) improvement in co-ordination and speed of movement;

 (iii) increase in endurance and strength;

 (iv) increase in dexterity;

 (v) improvement in appearance.

An important part of the post-operative assessment involved questioning the patients themselves about hand function. Each patient was asked whether the hand was used for new activities or was used more rapidly in doing old activities. The hand was then classified as improved, unimproved or worse. Cosmetic improvement was rated highly by the patients, and on its own was considered by many as being sufficient grounds for calling the operation a success. However, in the assessment of the results, this aspect of alteration was considered separately from functional improvement.

The attempt to improve hand function and appearance in a patient with cerebral palsy may necessarily involve secondary operative procedures and supplementary splinting. The need for such procedures does not indicate failure or a lack of improvement.

The results for each of the four pre-operative groups are described separately.

Group I. The patients in this group usually showed functional improvement. They were able to extend the hand more rapidly, to grasp objects more strongly, to receive objects more quickly and to hold objects more firmly than pre-operatively,

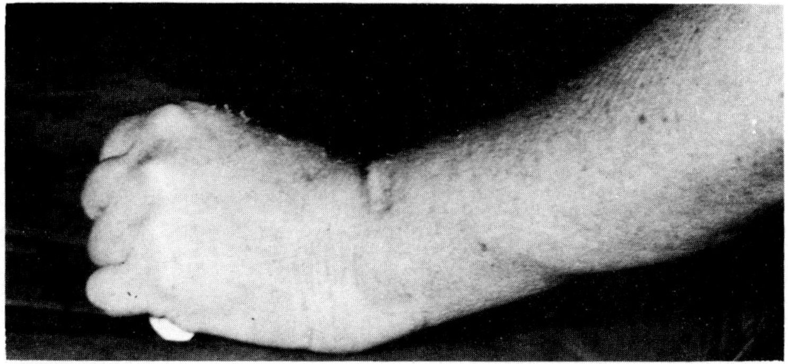

Fig. 10a. This is the hand of a patient with primary athetosis and a degree of spasticity involving the upper extremity. A position of severe flexion has been transformed into one of extension. Finger extension was limited when the patient was tense, but could be performed if she was allowed a reasonable amount of time. In this picture she is holding an object in her hands which she has grasped voluntarily, but she is having difficulty in releasing it because of wrist dorsiflexion and increased tension.

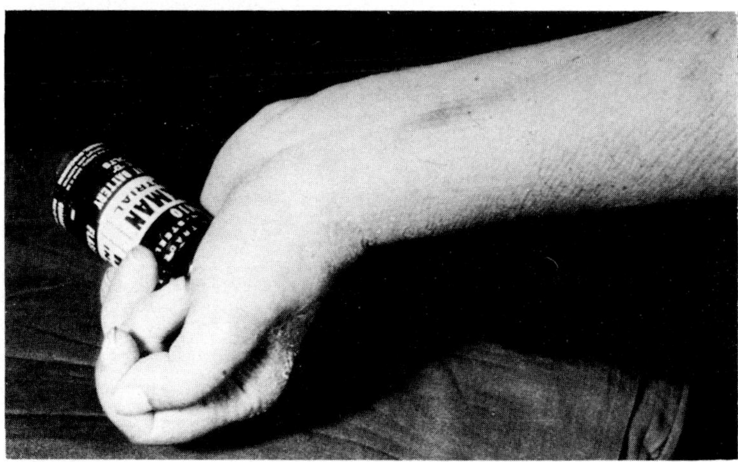

Fig. 10b. Same patient as in Figure 10a. With the forearm in supination, dorsiflexion of the wrist was even more severe, and digit release was even more difficult. Placement of an object in the hand when the forearm was in supination was done with greater difficulty than when the forearm was in pronation. Operative procedures have been performed on the athetoid hand with reasonable success. Joint arthrodesis, tendon lengthening and an occasional transfer are reasonable considerations in such cases. The pre-operative analysis of muscle power, voluntary action, and sensation is particularly important in athetoid patients. Patients with severe athetosis who have great difficulty in controlling the extremity are best managed by central nervous system surgery.

because of the alteration in the position of the wrist and fingers and because of the improvement in muscle balance. The patients with long-standing deformities did not necessarily show any dramatic change in their ability to carry out activities of daily living, but the hand did show increased speed of action, greater dexterity and greater independence than before treatment.

Group II. Post-operatively, patients in this group showed improvement in grasp, voluntary finger extension and hand elevation. Tension of the finger flexors and wrist flexors was diminished. These patients usually had only hook function pre-operatively, but after the operation they were able to grasp even large objects and release them voluntarily when the wrist was at neutral. Those patients without even a 'hook' pre-operatively did have one after the operation.

Group III. Pre-operatively, these patients had a severely flexed wrist, severely flexed fingers and a relatively functionless extremity. Surgical treatment, which included flexor tendon lengthening, carpalectomy, wrist arthrodesis and release of the flexed fingers, produced a straight wrist, elongated forearm, thumb out of the palm and moderate passive extension of the fingers. Elbow flexion deformity was also diminished, and the appearance of the extremity was improved.

Group IV. Modest improvement secured if athetosis was not severe. However, not all the pathological aspects of deformity in this group were improved by surgical treatment. Persistent involuntary movement continued, dexterity remained slow, and involuntary finger flexion continued to interfere with release when the wrist was elevated.

Results of Surgical Treatment Correlated with Other Findings at Pre-operative Assessment

Other factors, such as hand sensation, intelligence, motivation, the patient's age at the time of the treatment and the training program after treatment were all considered in relation to the outcome of the surgical treatment. The most important correlations are reported below.

Sensory Status

Many of the patients were given a formal multimodality sensory examination, while others were given a sensory examination which placed emphasis on the texture of objects and the recognition of form and shape. These tests were repeated a number of times for accuracy. Of all the tests given, those for detecting the presence or absence of stereognosis are the most effective for differentiating between patients whose hands are and are not affected by cerebral damage. With a high level of motivation and adaptability, patients who do not have good stereognosis can achieve good hand use, but only through making greater use of visual cues than would be necessary for patients with good stereognosis.

Group I. Several of the patients in this group had only slight deformity but inadequate stereognosis, whereas others with more serious deformities showed great skill in recognizing the size and shape of objects. The latter generally made better and more frequent use of the hand post-operatively, although the diminished stereognosis of the former did not preclude good hand use.

In Group II, less then half of the patients showed good stereognosis, and in the others stereognosis was inadequate or difficult to measure. Thus, improvement in this group did not correlate directly with the presence or absence of stereognosis.

In Group III, where the physical defects were greater, the patients with recognizable stereognosis did only slightly better functionally than those without stereognosis.

Group IV. These patients were usually incapable of responding to the sensory examination, yet some improvement in their ability to perform activities of daily living were observed following such procedures as wrist arthrodesis or the release of elbow contracture.

Astereognosis is not a contra-indication to surgical treatment of the upper extremity in cerebral palsy. Functional improvement can be obtained, even in patients who are unable to recognize the physical characteristics of an object without using visual cues.

Intelligence Quotient

Following formal psychological testing using a number of standard examinations, including tests of social maturity and IQ tests, the patients were divided into three groups.

(a) Those designated as normal, with an IQ of more than 90.
(b) Those designated as 'mildly retarded', with an IQ of between 70 and 90.
(c) Those considered to be 'severely retarded', who had IQs of less than 70.

Group I. These patients were usually improved by surgical treatment, whatever their IQs. If the pre-operative condition of the extremity had been assessed correctly, and if the right surgical technique had been employed, improvement was almost certain, even in the presence of mild or severe mental retardation.

Group II. Of the patients in this group who showed improvement after surgical treatment, some were 'normal' and some were intellectually retarded. Improvement was *not* noticeably more frequent in the patients with a higher intelligence quotient.

Correlation Between the Results of Surgical Treatment and the Presence of Both Severe Mental Retardation and Sensory Deficits

A small number of the patients submitted to surgery had estimated IQs of below 70 and absent stereognosis. In more than half of these patients, some degree of functional improvement was noted.

Group II patients who were mentally retarded and showed a lack of stereognosis usually showed mild to moderate improvement following tendon transfers or tendon lengthening.

Group III patients showed modest improvement after either wrist arthrodesis or carpal resection and arthrodesis, with or without flexor tenotomy of several tendons.

Thus, a combination of a severe motor deficit, mental retardation and sensory deficiency did not contra-indicate an operation, provided that the patient was ambulatory and utilized the shoulder and elbow for certain activities of daily living.

Discussion of Those Patients Whose Condition Remained Unchanged after Surgical Treatment

None of the patients in *Group I* who underwent surgery of the upper extremity were left unchanged or worse off post-operatively. The patients in *Group II* showed greater variation in the degree of improvement. Some showed evidence of an error in assessment, in that tendon transfers had been performed when the muscle motors used were not strong enough to warrant the transfer. Occasionally, a technical failure resulted in a tendon insertion pulling out prior to healing. In general, however, patients in Group II showed some degree of post-operative improvement, and technical failures were rare.

Group III patients usually showed some cosmetic improvement, a slight functional improvement, and, unexpectedly, in a few cases, a slight improvement in grasp and release.

Whatever group they were in, patients with both athetosis and spasticity were more likely to regress to their former condition or show no improvement at all than those patients who were purely spastic. Treatment in patients with athetosis and spasticity was directed towards joint stabilization and release of contractures, taking care to avoid over-correction as a result of tendon transfer.

In a few patients the condition of the extremity was unimproved or even worsened by operative treatment. However, any deterioration that occurred usually took place in patients going through periods of rapid growth, and was not irreparable. In one patient, release of contractures and tendon lengthenings at five years produced a satisfactory hand balance, which lasted for approximately four years. A growth spurt resulted in a recurrence of the flexion deformity at the wrist and adduction deformity of the thumb which had been present prior to the operation. Proximal carpalectomy, additional tendon lengthenings, and tendon re-inforcement of the thumb with an active motor, resulted in a noticeable improvement in function and appearance.

Two patients showed a change in hand position from severe flexion to excessive extension, after transfer of flexor tendons to extensor tendons. Initial assessment of the potential strength of the extensors had been inaccurate, and determination of the active strength of the wrist flexors incorrect. Additional surgery was needed, for when the hand was in extension, excessive tension on the finger flexors prevented the patient from voluntarily opening the fingers. Arthrodesis of the wrist in a position of flexion and slight ulnar deviation resulted in a balance of tension between the flexors and extensors, and a reasonable grasp and release (Fig. 11).

On the basis of the results described, it seems that the prognosis of treatment depends upon the amount of voluntary motor strength, and whether or not it is possible to maintain a mobile wrist, while correcting a 'thumb in the palm' deformity and establishing a satisfactory grasp and release. Factors such as the patient's age, motivation, vision and stereognosis are all important, and must be assessed before operation, but a deficiency in any one of these, or even in more than one, does not necessarily contra-indicate surgical treatment.

Finally, it would appear that patients with a purely spastic form of cerebral palsy have hand conditions that are more consistently predictable in their response to

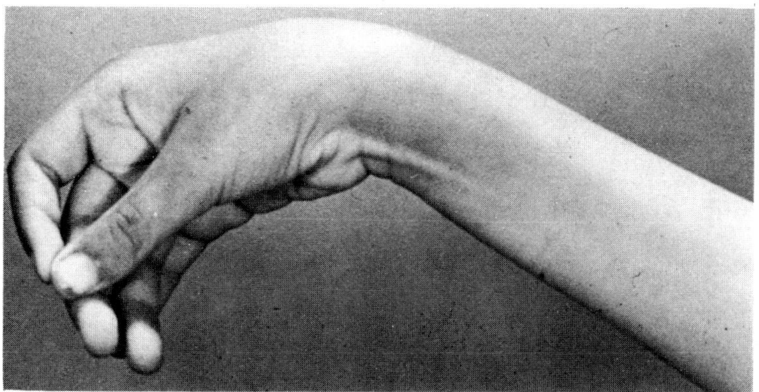

Fig. 11. This is the hand of a patient with spastic hemiplegia. The pre-operative position was one of acute flexion with the thumb in the palm. The operation consisted of (1) arthrodesis of the metacarpo-phalangeal joint of the thumb, (2) reinforcement of the extensor pollicis longus, and (3) transfer of the flexor carpi ulnaris to the extensor carpi radialis brevis. The surgery resulted in dorsiflexion, because of over-activity of the tendon transfer and improved strength of the wrist extensor muscles. Subsequently, the wrist was arthrodesed in a position of 10 degrees of wrist flexion and 10 degrees of ulnar deviation. This provides an automatic initiation of extension, and does not weaken flexion sufficiently to cause the hand to be held in dorsiflexion.

surgical treatment than do patients with combined spasticity and athetosis. Patients with athetosis alone show less functional improvement and the results of surgery are usually not predictable.

A majority of patients with cerebral palsy are not considered as candidates for surgical treatment. This is because of the degree of adaptation they already show to the motor deficit and their limited potential for improvement, rather than because they have a poor rating on such measurable parameters as intellect, stereognosis, motivation and training.

There is no justification for leaving an ambulatory patient with hemiplegia due to cerebral palsy to try to lead a normal life with an extremity that is flexed at the elbow and wrist, and with a hand whose function is impeded by permanently clenched fingers and a 'thumb in the palm' deformity. Functional and cosmetic improvements are desirable, and both can often be obtained by surgical treatment.

Important Considerations in the Treatment of the Upper Extremity in Cerebral Palsy

The following list has been drawn up on the basis of 25 years experience in treating the upper extremity of patients with cerebral palsy.
(1) The patient should be encouraged to make maximum use of the affected hand in performing activities of daily living. Minimal splinting during the daytime encourages the patient to do this. Night splinting is justifiable and probably helpful.
(2) Manual muscle testing can be done with reasonable accuracy and is an essential part of of the assessment of the upper extremity prior to a decision to carry out operative procedures.

(3) Tendon lengthening in the child aged three or four years is reliable.
(4) After proper assessment, it is possible to predict whether or not tendon transfer will be effective.
(5) Flexor tendons, if transferred, will function as extensors; extensor tendons, if transferred, will function as active voluntary flexors.
(6) A flexible wrist should be maintained until all other efforts at treatment have been tried. Arthrodesis of the wrist is usually the last step in the management of the involved upper extremity. If arthrodesis is indicated, a position of 0 degrees or a few degrees of flexion is desirable.
(7) A 'thumb in the palm' deformity can be corrected or improved.
(8) Hypermobile interphalangeal joints can be corrected by surgical procedures.
(9) A pronated position is more useful and desirable than a supinated position, if the latter can only be obtained at the expense of voluntary pronation.
(10) Elbow muscle/tendon lengthening and release will diminish elbow contracture and improve over-all use of the extremity. This correction should be done early, but it does not replace localized surgery of the wrist, fingers and thumb.

DESCRIPTION OF OPERATIVE PROCEDURES USED IN UPPER
EXTREMITY SURGICAL RECONSTRUCTION IN PATIENTS WITH
CEREBRAL PALSY

In this section, a number of upper extremity surgical procedures are described in detail. Each of the operations described has been performed with successful results many times by the author. However, other surgeons may prefer variations of these procedures, and certain technical details may have to be altered to take account of individual problems.

The operations will be considered under 16 headings.
(1) Arthrodesis of the metacarpo-phalangeal joint of the thumb.
(2) Arthrodesis of the distal interphalangeal joint of the thumb.
(3) Arthrodesis of the wrist joint.
(4) Extensor pollicis longus: re-routing and/or addition of motor.
(5) Correction of adductor contracture.
(6) Transfer of the extensor carpi radialis longus to the extensor digitorum communis.
(7) Transfer of flexor carpi ulnaris to finger or wrist extensors.
(8) Tenotomy or myotomy of pronator radii teres.
(9) Surgical correction of interphalangeal joint hyperextension.
(10) Extensor carpi ulnaris transfer.
(11) Shortening and/or reinforcement of both abductor pollicis longus and extensor pollicis brevis.
(12) Abductor pollicis longus and extensor pollicis brevis as a check rein or pulley.
(13) Shortening of abductor pollicis longus and extensor pollicis brevis proximal to the annular ligament of the distal radius.
(14) Transfer of the flexores digitorum sublimes.

(15) Tendon lengthening of the wrist flexors and/or finger flexors.
(16) Elbow flexor release.

(1) Arthrodesis of the Metacarpo-phalangeal Joint of the Thumb

Indications

(1) Arthrodesis of the metacarpo-phalangeal joint of the thumb is indicated in the young child or adult when the joint is hypermobile in both flexion and extension. If the patient has a 'thumb in the palm' deformity, tendon and muscle release about the first metacarpal and reinforcement of the abductor pollicis longus will allow abduction and extension of the first metacarpal. If excessive flexion at the metacarpo-phalangeal joint is allowed to persist, the proximal and distal phalanges may migrate towards the palm. Arthrodesis will diminish this tendency.

(2) If the thumb adductor is moderately spastic and if fibrosis occurs as the child grows, then the first metacarpal will tend to migrate towards the second metacarpal; in this situation, hyper-extension of the proximal phalanx, if it occurs, will aggravate the deformity and result in a prominent metacarpal head in the palm.

Arthrodesis of the metacarpo-phalangeal joint obviates both the above problems. However, arthrodesis alone, without release of contractures and diminution of spasticity, and without reinforcement of the abductor and extensor muscles, will not in itself eliminate a 'thumb in the palm' deformity.

Arthrodesis of the thumb can be successfully performed in children as young as four years old or in patients of 30 years or even older. Damage to the epiphyseal line of the proximal end of the proximal phalanx can be avoided by smooth fixation pins. There have been no problems related to growth disturbance or angulation, even in cases where the fusion has been perfomed in a young child.

Contra-indications

Arthrodesis is not necessary when the metacarpo-phalangeal joint is stable in both flexion and extension. If the thumb shows only slight limitation of movement in both flexion and extension, and if the metacarpo-phalangeal joint is stable, then arthrodesis is not indicated.

Thumb instability can be managed in other ways, such as volar capsulorraphy. This procedure is useful, provided that a flexion deformity does not occur.

Operative Procedure

Through a mid-lateral incision on the radial or ulnar side, and with a sharp dissection down to the fibers of the extensor mechanism, the lateral band is isolated and reflected toward the dorsum of the thumb. An incision is then made in the capsule and collateral ligaments, and the soft tissue is cut away from the periphery of the joint. The joint is dislocated manually. A small sharp rongeur is used to remove the cartilaginous surface of the metacarpal head, taking very little subchondral bone. The rongeur is used also to remove the articular surface from the proximal end of the phalanx. The epiphyses of the metacarpal and the phalanx, if present, are left unharmed. The ulnar or radial collateral ligament is usually left intact as an aid to internal fixation. The joint is secured in position for arthrodesis—usually in a position of

10 degrees flexion and 10 degrees internal rotation, which allows the thumb to be brought easily to the radial side of the index finger. Fine Kirschner wires are then inserted across the bone fragments, using a flexible shaft electric drill (wire sizes 0.06 and 0.04 in). As many wires are used as are necessary to obtain stability. The wires are allowed to cross the epiphyseal plate if necessary; these wires are left long under the skin, and are removed at about four to six weeks. Wires that do not cross the epiphysis are left in place until firm union occurs. Small chips of bone from the Bone Bank or from the thumb are used to fill crevices after fixation. The capsule is closed with 4-0 polyester suture for additional internal fixation, and a plaster cast is applied from the tip of the thumb to, and including, the wrist. The cast should be left on for six weeks. After the cast is removed, activity is limited, and the pins are left in place until they project under the skin and cause pain, or until firm union has occurred.

(2) Arthrodesis of the Distal Interphalangeal Joint of the Thumb

Indications

This procedure is carried out when the thumb shows a hypermobile distal phalanx in extension, and a tendency to radial and ulnar deviation, a situation seen occasionally both in adults and in children. In addition, if the flexor pollicis longus has been lengthened or is not functioning, the tendency to hyperextension can be diminished by arthrodesis of this joint.

Contra-indications

Contra-indications are (1) a distal joint that is well controlled by an active flexor pollicis longus and an active extensor pollicis longus, and (2) a joint that can be voluntarily controlled by the patient when the wrist is moderately flexed or hyper-extended.

Operative Procedure

Through a dorsal incision, the central portion of which follows a skin crease, and the lateral limbs of which extend towards the radial and the ulnar side of the thumb, the joint is opened. The extensor tendon is then sectioned as far distally as possible and folded proximally. The collateral ligaments are sectioned partially. With the distal joint in flexion, the digit is placed over an anvil. With a small osteotome, the articular cartilage is removed, maintaining the contour of the distal end of the proximal phalanx and the proximal end of the distal phalanx. About three quarters of the articular surface is removed this way, and then the volar segment is removed with a small rongeur to avoid damaging the distal nerves and the flexor tendons. The entire articular surfaces are then roughened with a rongeur. The phalanges are positioned, and small chips of bone, either removed from the articulation or taken from the Bone Bank, are packed in the crevices of the joint. A central fixation pin is placed across the joint for impaction and for easy correction of rotation. Cross-fixation pins are then placed across the arthrodesis site. These can be placed direct or initiated in a retrograde manner. The articular surfaces are compressed by forcing the phalanges together manually. The extensor tendon is used for partial internal fixation. The tendon is plicated and sutured with non-absorbable polyester suture. Plaster is added around the thumb and the wrist and immobilization maintained for six to eight weeks, depending on the patient's age and the stability of the fixation of the fragments.

(3) Arthrodesis of the Wrist Joint

Indications

Arthrodesis of the wrist joint is the exception rather than the rule. It is considered, in the growing child, when motor power is weak and the potential for active flexion and extension of the fingers is limited or absent. The arthrodesis can be done without damaging the distal epiphysis. Carpalectomy is necessary, occasionally, if the deformity is ancient and severe.

The adult with active function of the extensor digitorum communis and active intrinsic function when the wrist is held at 5 to 10 degrees of flexion, and who is able to actively flex and voluntarily extend the fingers, can be treated by arthrodesis of the radio-carpal joint. Arthrodesis is particularly indicated when there is a tendency to 30 to 40 degrees flexion deformity of the joint, in spite of a prior tendon transfer.

Arthrodesis of the wrist should also be considered when, following tendon transfers, a hand which was originally in flexion assumes a position of hypertension. The hand should be positioned in neutral or 10 degrees of flexion, and, if the patient has voluntary grasp and release in spite of the fixed wrist, then arthrodesis should be considered.

Under no circumstances should arthrodesis be done until a trial of wrist fixation has been carried out using a plaster cast, and until the patient has had an opportunity to carry out activities of daily living when the wrist is not moveable. All tendon transfers should precede wrist arthrodesis.

Contra-indications

Wrist arthrodesis is contra-indicated (1) in a patient who requires wrist flexion in order to obtain finger extension; (2) if wrist extension is necessary for closure of the fingers; (3) if the hand is held immobile in a neutral or slightly flexed position and the patient cannot voluntarily open the digits completely or close them completely; (4) if tendon transfers (*i.e.,* moving extensors to flexors or flexors to extensors) are planned, wrist arthrodesis prior to or too soon after tendon transfer eliminates the mobility necessary to re-educate the muscle tendon unit in a new position, and usually leads to failure of the transfer; (5) if there is an incomplete range of flexion or extension of the digit.

The decision to stabilize the wrist depends ultimately upon the efficiency of finger grasp and release and the efficiency of thumb function. A review of over 200 cerebral palsied patients with involvement of the upper extremity, many of whom both young and old had multiple operative procedures, has shown that arthrodesis of the wrist was done in only 10 per cent. Wrist arthrodesis was usually the last procedure considered, and was utilized only as a last resort.

Procedure

In the adult, when the epiphyses are closed, wrist arthrodesis may be done in the usual way. Through a dorsal S-incision or straight incision, the extensor tendons and the deep dorsal carpal ligament are reflected in one mass towards the ulnar side, and the thumb extensor is reflected towards the radial side. The wrist joint is opened, and the cartilage is removed from the distal end of the radius and from the carpal bones. If the arthrodesis is being done for a fixed contracture, it may be necessary to remove the proximal carpal row, including primarily the scaphoid and the lunate bones. A dorsal flap of bone and periosteum is elevated down to and including the second and third metacarpals. The radius is then split, and a rib graft from the Bone Bank or a graft from the ilium is inserted into the radius and wedged into the metacarpals. Bone chips are then placed around the graft and in the crevices in the carpal area. The ulna is not included in the fusion, nor are the greater or lesser multangular bones. If spasticity is present, two large 3/32 pins should be inserted across the area of arthrodesis. These pins should cross at the fusion site. Another method of pin fixation is done by drilling a pin through the base of the third metacarpal, through the carpal bones and into the distal radius. A long arm plaster cast is applied, with the elbow held at right angles, and the hand in the predetermined position, which is usually neutral or a few degrees of flexion and slight ulnar deviation.

If the contracture is not severe and only moderate limitation of motion is desired, the distal radius can be fused to the proximal row of the carpals, leaving the midcarpal and the carpal-metacarpal area intact. Some of the local bone removed can be re-inserted as a graft, and bone can be added from the Bank to fill the crevices. Crossed fixation pins are desirable here also, since the surface area of fusion is not large.

If wrist arthodesis is to be done in a ten- or eleven-year-old child, it is usually necessary to include the second and third metacarpals, and follow the same technique as described for the radial-carpal fusion. The distal radial epiphysis is not disturbed.

(4) Extensor Pollicis Longus: Re-routing and/or Addition of Motor

Indications

Re-routing of the extensor pollicis longus, by taking it out of the fibro-osseus tunnel and re-directing it subcutaneously towards the radial side of the wrist, is one of the multiple operative procedures used to release the thumb web and keep the thumb out of the palm.

Reinforcement of the extensor pollicis longus by the addition of a flexor digitorum sublimis or the brachioradialis is indicated in a patient with a 'thumb in the palm' deformity when no active thumb extensor power is detectable.

Contra-indications

The adding of a motor to the re-routed extensor pollicis longus is contra-indicated (1) when there is an active extensor pollicis longus, (2) when the metacarpo-phalangeal joint tends to hyperextend and has not yet been stabilized, and (3) when the first metacarpal is in flexion and the distal phalanx is in hyperextension. The tendon to be reinforced in this instance is the abductor pollicis longus and not the extensor pollicis longus, *i.e.,* the abductor pollicis longus is reinforced and the extensor pollicis longus is repositioned but not reinforced.

Occasionally, the extensor pollicis longus is left in its usual course, but is reinforced, along with the abductor pollicis longus. Additional surgery to the thumb, such as arthrodesis of the metacarpo-phalangeal joint and lengthening of the flexor pollicis longus, will then allow abduction and external rotation, without leading to excessive repositioning of the thumb towards the volar surface.

Occasionally, the flexor digitorum sublimis is transferred through the interosseous membrane and sutured directly to the extensor pollicis longus, which is left in its usual course. The procedure selected depends on the ultimate position of the thumb desired.

Procedure

(a) Re-routing of the thumb extensor may be done by making a slight S-shaped incision from the metacarpal-phalangeal joint of the thumb to about 4 cm proximal to the radio-carpal joint. The extensor tendon is freed proximally from the annular ligament, and split distally up to the point where it inserts into the dorsal hood of the thumb. It is then moved in a volar direction; the thumb is rotated internally and abducted, and the tendon is held in place by suturing it into the subcutaneous tissue with 3-0 polyester suture over an area of about two inches. The incision should be made so that the scar is not directly over the new course of the extensor. Plaster is needed to hold the thumb in this position for approximately three weeks. If the extensor is very tight, it can be lengthened at the level of the radial styloid, and the increase in length will allow it to remain towards the volar aspect. Occasionally, with a very loose carpometacarpal joint, more security is needed than can be provided by subcutaneous tissue; this can be obtained by tenotomizing the extensor pollicis brevis at the level of the radial styloid, pulling the distal end of the short extensor around the long extensor, and re-suturing the short extensor to its own muscle belly. This will provide a pulley, and aid as a holding agent for the long extensor.

(b) If the extensor pollicis longus is not an active muscle, the flexor carpi radialis or a flexor digitorum sublimis can be used as a motor. The extensor tendon is severed at its musculotendinous junction through a straight radial incision over the anatomical 'snuff box'. If the flexor carpi radialis is to be used, it is detached at the wrist level, pulled out about four inches proximal to the wrist joint, and attached so that a smooth union is obtained at the level of the volar aspect of the radial side of the styloid. The suture line should be far enough proximal to avoid impingement on the radial styloid. The tension should be of such a degree that, when the wrist is held in neutral, the thumb can be passively moved to a point opposite the index finger and can be extended at least one inch radial to the index finger. It should be possible to adduct the thumb to within half an inch of the palm.

If a sublimis tendon is used, it may be pulled out and severed at the wrist, and the muscle belly utilized in the same way as the wrist flexor. If wrist arthrodesis is not planned for the future, it is better to use the sublimis, provided that the digit is strong enough.

(c) Transfer of the brachioradialis to the thumb extensor. Through a radial incision, the brachioradialis is identified and released from its insertion into the radius. The incision is carried proximally to the junction of the upper musculotendinous segment, to allow adequate excursion. The thumb extensor is then sectioned at its musculotendinous junction, and the extensor tendon is re-routed and sutured to the brachioradialis by interweaving the tendon ends and using several 2-0 polyester sutures for fixation.

(5) Correction of Thumb Adductor Contracture

Indications

(1) Release and lengthening of the thumb adductor are indicated in a patient with palpable and visible spasticity of the adductor muscle. The tendon is lengthened at its insertion, and the muscle belly is released from its origin. Motor supply is not damaged.

(2) The first dorsal interosseous is released from the first and second metacarpals if spasticity and contracture are evident and if the distance between the first and second metacarpals can only be increased to a limited extent by passive manipulation or is impossible to enlarge by voluntary action.

(3) The muscles in the thumb web space must be assessed whenever there is a 'thumb in the palm' deformity.

(4) The flexor pollicis longus acts as an adductor, and may require lengthening as part of the release of the adduction deformity.

Contra-indications

Release of the adductor and first dorsal interosseous muscles is contra-indicated (1) when prior surgery has already weakened the thumb and opened the web space; (2) when the patient has voluntary control of the thumb, which can be adducted, extended and flexed; and (3) when there is no visible and palpable spasticity of the adductor and no 'thumb in the palm' deformity.

Procedure

An adductor contracture with spasticity usually requires fusion of the meta-carpo-phalangeal joint of the thumb and re-routing of the extensor, as already described; in addition it is usually necessary to release the first dorsal interosseous from the first and second metacarpals and lengthen the adductor tendon. Destruction of the motor branch of the ulnar nerve is not advisable or necessary under normal circumstances. If the contracture is severe, the origin of the adductor can be released from the third metacarpal through the web space. Only in rare instances is an incision in the palm necessary to relieve the adduction deformity.

(6) Transfer of the Extensor Carpi Radialis Longus to the Extensor Digitorum Communis

Indications

Transfer of the extensor carpi radialis to the extensor digitorum communis may be necessary if the patient has active voluntary wrist extension which is reinforced by active flexion of the fingers, and if, with the wrist in the neutral position, he or she cannot extend the digits at the metacarpo-phalangeal joints—a finding which indicates weakness or absence of strength in the extensor digitorum communis muscle. If the extensor carpi radialis is available and strong, and if it is not needed to reinforce the extensor pollicis longus, it can be transferred to the ulnar side of the wrist and into the extensor digitorum communis. This pattern is unusual, however, and is more frequently seen in patients who have had brain damage secondary to trauma, than in those with developmental cerebral palsy.

Contra-indications

This transfer is contra-indicated (1) if the extensor carpi radialis longus is not of normal strength, (2) if the extensor carpi radialis longus is needed for the extensor pollicis substitute and (3) if the flexor digitorum sublimis or the flexor carpi ulnaris is available and can be spared.

Excessive dorsiflexion strength due to transfer of a flexor to an extensor should be avoided if there are sufficient extensor muscles to make up the deficit of either the fingers or the thumb.

Procedure

Through a slightly curved dorsal incision, the insertion of the extensor carpi radialis longus is severed from the second metacarpal, and the tendon is pulled out about 5 centimeters proximal to the wrist joint. The superficial layer of the dorsal carpal ligament is excised, and the common extensor tendons are identified to the fingers. The distal end of the extensor carpi radialis longus tendon is then split in half, and one segment is threaded through the two extensors which control the index finger, the extensors to the long and ring fingers, and the two extensors to the little finger. This is done so that the tension on this transfer holds the metacarpo-phalangeal joints at zero degrees when the wrist is in neutral. Each extensor tendon is then sutured to the slip of the extensor carpi radialis longus. The remaining tendon is then used to reinforce the original transfer, either by tightening up any tendons that may be slack or by reinforcing the over-all transfer. This transfer, even though not necessarily synergistic, does give good action to the common extensors. In certain bizarre situations, such as weakness following trauma to the cervical cord with mixed paralysis and spasticity, this extensor carpi radialis longus tendon may be transferred to a paralyzed extensor pollicis longus or a weak flexor digitorum profundus, by passing the extensor through the interosseous membrane.

(7) Transfer of Flexor Carpi Ulnaris to Finger or Wrist Extensions

Indications

The flexor carpi ulnaris may act as a deforming muscle, and cause the hand to persist in flexion. If increased strength on the dorsum of the hand is necessary, the flexor carpi ulnaris can be transferred to the insertion of the extensor carpi radialis brevis. This will give active elevation of the hand. The flexor carpi radialis will continue to function on the volar surface, as will the palmaris longus. If the wrist extensors and the finger extensors are not normal, then over-correction because of the tendon transfer will not occur.

The flexor carpi ulnaris may be transferred to the extensor digitorum communis (a) if there is no extensor carpi radialis longus available for transfer, (b) if a brachioradialis is not available for transfer to the extensor communis, or (c) if the extensor carpi radialis brevis rates about 50 per cent of normal and the extensor digitorum communis rates trace to zero, in which case strengthening of the digitorum communis may be sufficient to restore balance of both the fingers and the wrist.

Contra-indications

(1) Flexor carpi ulnaris transfer to the wrist or finger extensors is not indicated when a combination of the extensor muscles rates fair (50 per cent) or better. In such a situation, transfer of a flexor to an extensor may cause excessive dorsiflexion. A weaker muscle, such as a flexor digitorum sublimis, may be sufficient to restore balance, if transferred to the extensor carpi radialis brevis.

(2) If there is no other available wrist flexor, then the flexor carpi ulnaris should not be transferred, or the patient will develop a dorsiflexion deformity.

(3) The flexed position of the wrist and hand may, paradoxically, be due to the action of the flexor digitorum sublimis; once the flexor digitorum sublimis and, possibly, one of the wrist flexors, are lengthened, the existing wrist and finger extensor muscles may be sufficient to elevate the hand and eliminate the flexed position. Careful testing of the extremity, after nerve block and preliminary immobilization, is necessary to determine this.

If supination is necessary and if the tendency to pronation is severe, the flexor carpi ulnaris is transferred around the ulnar border. If straight elevation of the hand or fingers is desired, then the flexor carpi ulnaris is transferred through the interosseous membrane.

Procedure

(a) Transfer of the flexor carpi ulnaris to the extensor digitorum communis through the interosseous membrane. Through a slightly curved volar incision, in line with a radial border of the pisiform, the extensor carpi ulnaris tendon is isolated and dissected back to the musculotendinous junction. The muscle fibers usually extend down to the insertion, and it is necessary to excise a segment of muscle about 3×2 cm to give a tendon for transfer. The ulnar nerve and artery are identified, isolated with a rubber dam, and retracted towards the radial side. The sublimis and profundus tendon mass is retracted to the radial side, and the pronator quadratus is identified. An incision about $7\frac{1}{2}$ centimeters long is made along the radial aspect of the ulna, with small transverse cuts in order to open the interosseous space. To spread the soft tissue a hemostat is forced through the dorsal surface, where it is projected to tent the skin. An incision is then made on the dorsum of the wrist, the extensor tendons are identified and retracted, usually to the radial side. The opening on the dorsum is elongated for about three centimeters, and the flexor carpi ulnaris is pulled through to the dorsum. The dorsal carpal ligament is opened, and the flexor carpi ulnaris is inserted into the common extensor tendon as far distally as possible, with the wrist held in the neutral position and the metacarpo-phalangeal joints at zero degrees.

(b) The flexor carpi ulnaris, if needed for a wrist extensor and supinator, may be passed around the ulnar aspect of the wrist and sutured into the extensor carpi radialis brevis. The extensor brevis is the major dorsiflexor of the hand, and it is desirable to use it as the point of anchor rather than the extensor carpi radialis longus. The flexor carpi ulnaris is usually short, and there is difficulty in pulling it to the wrist extensor. The insertion of the extensor carpi radialis brevis is allowed to remain attached distally, and is used as a graft to the flexor carpi ulnaris. If wrist extension is needed and supination is not necessary, the flexor carpi ulnaris can be passed through the interosseous membrane and sutured to the wrist extensor.

(8) Tenotomy or Myotomy of Pronator Radii Teres
Indications

(1) Tenotomy or myotomy of the pronator radii teres is indicated when the patient has a fixed contracture of the forearm which is not correctable by active or passive manipulation. It is also indicated if the patient desires improved supination and notices difficulties in carrying out activities of daily living. Transfer of the insertion through the interosseous membrane to the dorsal surface of the radius has been done occasionally to diminish pronation and in an attempt to strengthen supination.

(2) Release of the pronator muscle origin is done in order to decrease elbow flexion deformity and diminish pronation contracture.

Contra-indications

(1) Myotomy or tenotomy of the pronator is not indicated where the range of supination is sufficient to allow the patient to direct the palm of the hand upwards, and where the patient is able to carry out activities of daily living with the hand and forearm in the mid or pronated position.

(2) When there is no elbow contracture and the activities of daily living are carried out with ease, there is no reason to release the pronator, even though the forearm cannot be fully supinated.

Procedure

Tenotomy or myotomy of the pronator radii teres may be done readily through a straight incision at the junction of the upper and middle third of the forearm. The pronator tendon is identified at its insertion into the radius, and a 2 cm section is excised. If the muscle is extremely spastic, it is probably desirable to make a straight incision in the forearm, identify the muscle belly, and excise the mid-section of the muscle. This is seldom necessary, however. The pronator quadratus can be excised at the wrist if the pronation is severe. In many instances, however, the pronator quadratus should be left in place, particularly if a flexor tendon is being passed through the interosseous membrane. This tends to give a good protective barrier for the tendon to pass between the bones.

(9) Surgical Correction of Interphalangeal Joint Hyperextension
Indications

(1) When the interphalangeal joints can be hyperextended voluntarily or in-

voluntarily to a right angle, stabilization of these joints is indicated for both functional and cosmetic reasons.

(2) If the interphalangeal joints lock in hyperextension, and the patient cannot flex the interphalangeal joints until the opposite hand is used to displace the phalanges distally, then surgical correction is indicated.

(3) If flexion strength is diminished because of persistent hyperextension of the proximal interphalangeal joints and flexion of the distal joints, then the interphalangeal joint deformity should be corrected.

Contra-indications

(1) If the interphalangeal joints lock in hyperextension but can be voluntarily unlocked and flexed, there is no reason to operate on these joints unless the patient has a particular need to have the appearance corrected.

(2) If the patient had voluntary control of the hyperextended interphalangeal joint using the flexor digitorum sublimis and profundus, and if locking does not occur, operative correction is not indicated.

Procedure

(a) A straight lateral incision is made on either side of the proximal interphalangeal joint. The retinaculum is identified and sectioned, and incised in line with the long axis of the finger. The retinaculum is elevated carefully, and the volar capsule is identified. The joint is entered, and the capsule is peeled off the distal end of the proximal phalanx, leaving enough periosteum and capsule proximally so that the flap can be moved towards the base of the digit as far as necessary. The same dissection is carried out on the opposite side of the digit. Three polyester sutures are used to anchor the flap to the phalanx. The retinaculum is then closed with 3-0 polyester suture. Advancing the dorsal leaf distally and moving the volar leaf proximally adds to the flexor tendency. The digits are immobilized in plaster in this position for three weeks, and then started on gentle active exercises. If intrinsic spasticity is present, it must be treated independently of the plicating procedure done on the interphalangeal joints. A separate dorsal incision is made over the proximal end of the proximal phalanx, and the oblique fibers of the lateral bands are excised from the common extensor tendon, leaving the transverse fibers intact.

(b) The hyperextension, if less severe, can be managed as follows. A lateral incision is made at the level of the proximal interphalangeal joint, and the neurovascular structures are identified and reflected towards the palm. The flexor tendon sheath is then identified, and the flexor digitorum sublimis and profundus are isolated at the level of the joint and retracted towards the volar surface. The retinaculum of the finger is not opened. The capsule is incised proximal to the joint, so that the distal end can be advanced proximally and shortened. The flexor digitorum sublimis insertion is identified, and one slip of the tendon is severed proximal to the joint. This slip is then sutured to the inferior fibers of the retinacular ligament of the finger and to the volar capsule. The chiasm of Camper of the sublimis is split, so that the proximal end of the tendon can be advanced and sutured over the distal end. A second mid-lateral incision is made on the opposite side of the finger, and the same procedure is carried out on that side. This provides shortening of the proximal joint to a position of about 10 degrees of flexion, firm fixation of the volar capsule, and a moderate advancement of the flexor sublimis.

(10) Extensor Carpi Ulnaris Transfer

Indications

(1) If the hand tends to deviate towards the ulnar side, and if the wrist extensors are not of sufficient strength to maintain a neutral position, the extensor carpi ulnaris tendon is detached and transferred to the base of the fourth metacarpal. This provides increased dorsiflexion and diminishes ulnar deviation.

(2) If the extensor carpi ulnaris is strong and overactive and the wrist extensors are weaker than in situation (1), the extensor carpi ulnaris may be transferred to the third metacarpal, so that a straight upward pull can be developed.

Procedure

A curved incision is made over the insertion of the extensor carpi ulnaris distal to the styloid process of the ulna. The tendon sheath is incised, and a tape is placed around the tendon for identification. A second incision is made about 5 cm proximal to the styloid process, and the musculotendinous junction is identified. The distal segment of the tendon is then incised, the tendon is delivered through the proximal incision, and a subcutaneous tunnel is passed from the proximal incision to the fourth or third metacarpal area. The extensor carpi ulnaris is inserted through a hole made in the base of the metacarpal or into the extensor carpi radialis brevis, depending on the existing balance of the hand. Before the tendon is inserted into bone, it can be split, allowing one half to go through the bone from the ulnar side and the other half to go through the bone from the radial side, thus permitting adjustment of tension. The tendon is fixed to itself, after passing through the bone, with 2-0 polyester sutures.

(11) Shortening and/or Reinforcement of Both Abductor Pollicis Longus and Extensor Pollicis Brevis

Indications

(1) A hand with the first metacarpal in flexion and a 'thumb in the palm' deformity always requires shortening of the abductor pollicis longus, and usually requires reinforcement of this muscle by an additional motor.

(2) The extensor pollicis brevis is shortened if there is a flexion deformity of the metacarpo-phalangeal joint, but not if there is a hyperextension deformity.

(3) If the abductor pollicis longus is analyzed as being less than a 50 per cent muscle, a motor should always be added at the same time as the shortening is carried out.

Contra-indications

(1) If the thumb is not in the palm, or if there is not a tendency to adduction or external rotation, the abductor pollicis longus does not have to be shortened.

(2) Shortening alone without reinforcement will usually not be successful in the

presence of a severe deformity of the first metacarpal.

(3) Shortening and reinforcement should not be done alone, but in conjunction with release of the adductor, lengthening of the flexor pollicis longus, and arthrodesis of the metacarpo-phalangeal joint of the thumb. These procedures should be done simultaneously, rather than one at a time.

Procedure

A curved dorsal incision is made, extending from the centre portion of the first metacarpal to about 7½ centimeters proximal to the styloid process of the radius. The incision is curved moderately over the 'snuff box'. Superficial branches of the radial nerve are identified and retracted, and the annular ligament covering the abductor pollicis longus and extensor pollicis brevis is incised. The tendons are elevated from their canal on a cloth tape; the largest ones are isolated, and a Z-lengthening is done. The proximal segment is then advanced distally, and anchored to the base of the metacarpal and the distal end of the lengthened tendon, using non-absorbable suture. Each individual tendon is then cut and advanced, and the tendon segments are sutured firmly into the periosteum of the metacarpal and to each other. The metacarpal is immobilized in extension and external rotation for four weeks. Any additional surgery to the web space, to the extensor pollicis longus or to the metacarpo-phalangeal joint is done in conjunction with the tenotomy and tendon shortening. If required, arthrodesis of the metacarpo-phalangeal joint should precede the tendon shortening, to avoid stress on the suture line. These several operative procedures can be done during the same period of anesthesia.

(12) Abductor Pollicis Longus and Extensor Pollicis Brevis as a Check Rein or Pulley

Indications

When a motor is transferred to the re-routed extensor pollicis longus and the metacarpal trapezium joint is loose, the motor from the volar surface to the extensor pollicis longus may cause the thumb to pull into opposition. If the transfer is placed proximal to and under the insertion of the abductor pollicis longus, excessive displacement of the extensor pollicis longus is not possible, and the opposition position will not occur.

Contra-indications

When there is no hypermobility of the base of the thumb, when the alignment of the extensor pollicis longus is directly parallel with the abductor pollicis longus, and when reinforcement of the extensor pollicis longus is done by the brachioradialis or by muscle passed through the interosseous membrane, a stabilizing pulley is not necessary.

Procedure

The operative procedure just described for the abductor pollicis longus and extensor pollicis brevis can be completed prior to transferring the extensor pollicis longus under the shortened tendons; in this way it is possible to prevent the thumb extensor and the motor transferred to it, such as the brachioradialis, from migrating too far towards the volar surface. The suture line of the tendon to be transferred to the extensor pollicis longus is placed about two centimeters proximal to the suture line of the abductor pollicis brevis to avoid adhesions.

(13)   Shortening of Abductor Pollicis Longus and Extensor Pollicis Brevis Proximal to the Annular Ligament of the Distal Radius

Indications

When reinforcement of the abductor pollicis longus and the extensor pollicis longus is necessary by another motor, or when the extensor pollicis longus is reinforced by a flexor digitorum sublimis, then secondary shortening and reinforcement of the abductor pollicis longus is necessary. This should be done at a point proximal to the annular ligament and not distal to the ligament. The deformity is usually not as severe as when the shortening is done distally and closer to the insertion.

Contra-indications

This procedure is contra-indicated when the abductor pollicis longus has good strength, when the thumb is not in the palm, and when the extensor pollicis longus does not have to be repositioned.

Procedure

The shortening of these two tendons at a point proximal to the annular ligament is done in conjunction with (a) transfer of the brachioradialis to either the extensor pollicis longus or extensor carpi radialis brevis, or (b) transfer of the flexor digitorum sublimis through the interosseous membrane to the extensor pollicis longus, in order to tighten up the first metacarpal. A slightly curved incision is made over the distal radius, so that the annular ligament can be incised. The abductor pollicis longus and extensor pollicis brevis are identified and severed obliquely just distal to the musculo-tendinous junction. The distal segments are inserted through a small opening in the proximal tendons, and the tension is increased sufficiently to hold the first metacarpal extended and externally rotated. The point of tenotomy and overlap is sutured with 3-0 polyester suture. The part is immobilized for about four weeks. If the metacarpo-phalangeal joint is hypermobile, it can be arthrodesed at the same time.

(14)   Transfer of the Flexores Digitorum Sublimes

Indications

One, two or three of the flexores digitorum sublimes tendons are transferred to other locations if the flexores digitorum profundi are strong and if the flexores sublimes are spastic or contracted. This is a more common deformity than is usually realized. One sublimis may be transferred to the extensor pollicis longus and another to the extensor carpi radialis brevis; alternatively, one sublimis may be transferred to the extensor digitorum communis.

In other instances, the flexores digitorum sublimes are transferred to the abductor pollicis longus or to the extensor carpi ulnaris.

Contra-indications

(1) When the strength of the flexores digitorum profundi is less than 50 per cent, the flexor digitorum sublimis should not be transferred, but should be lengthened and left in place to act across the proximal interphalangeal joint of the digit.

(2) The flexores digitorum sublimes should not be transferred if their strength is not equivalent to at least a 50 per cent muscle.

Procedure

The flexores digitorum sublimes of the long or ring fingers are identified through a curved incision on the volar aspect of the wrist. The hand is flexed, traction is applied to the individual tendon, and tenotomy is done as far distally in the wrist as possible, so that the actual point of severance of the tendon is at the mid-palmar level, but without requiring extension of the incision into the palm. The tendon is dissected proximally to a point where the muscle fibers can be identified. The median nerve is retracted, as are the flexores digitorum profundi, and the pronator quadratus is identified deep in the wrist region. A large opening is made in the pronator quadratus, using a curved hemostat, which is extended through the interosseous space to the extensor surface. A skin incision is made over the sub-cutaneous forceps, and the extensor tendons are retracted; a tendon passer is then inserted from the dorsum to the volar surface, in order to receive the sublimis tendon or tendons. The sublimis or sublimes can then be used to reinforce the extensor pollicis longus tendon, the extensor digitorum communis or the extensor carpi radialis brevis. In most instances, however, the extensor pollicis longus is removed from its surrounding canal and allowed to shift slightly towards the abductor pollicis longus.

(15) Tendon Lengthening of the Wrist Flexors and/or Finger Flexors

Indications

(1) The wrist flexors are lengthened if they are contracted or spastic and interfering with voluntary elevation of the hand.

(2) In the growing child, a spastic wrist flexor warrants lengthening, so that wrists and finger extensors can be maintained at maximum strength.

(3) If contracted, finger flexors, particularly the flexores digitorum sublimes, should be lengthened in the growing child.

Contra-indications

(1) Lengthening should not be done if the muscle is extremely weak and not shortened.

(2) Lenthening should not be done if the hand can be voluntarily elevated to at least neutral.

(3) Tendon lengthening should not be done if the grasp is weak and if another muscle is not available to reinforce the lengthened tendon.

Procedure

The wrist flexor tendons are exposed at the wrist on the volar surface by making a curved incision, with the distal segment extending from the insertion of the flexor carpi radialis, and the proximal portion directed towards the flexor carpi ulnaris in the form of an S. The flexor carpi radialis is lengthened about three centimeters proximal to its insertion, and the palmaris longus is lengthened at the same level. The wrist is then extended maximally and the digits are hyperextended at the metacarpophalangeal joints and the interphalangeal joints. If the proximal interphalangeal joint does not allow complete extension of a particular digit, then the flexor digitorum sublimis is lengthened by a coronal or step-cut incision at the musculotendinous junction and is resutured.

The flexores digitorum profundi are tested in the same manner, and any contracted tendons are lengthened in such a way that the digits are flexed to about 45 degrees when the wrist is in dorsiflexion. The flexor pollicis longus is tested in a similar way, and if necessary lengthened at its musculotendinous junction, in order to allow adequate extension of the distal phalanx when the wrist is elevated and the thumb is hyperextended. Over-lengthening should be avoided, as this will diminish flexion strength.

(16) Elbow Flexor Release

Indications

(1) A flexion deformity of the elbow due to contracture and/or spasticity can be managed by isolated lengthening of the biceps humerus, myotomy of the brachialis, and release of the origin of the wrist flexor muscles.

(2) All of these muscles are lengthened if the contracture is fixed and if it is progressive.

(3) The primary purpose of the lengthening is to correct contracture of the elbow, and, to a lesser extent, to limit wrist flexion deformity.

Contra-indications

(1) The forearm flexor origin should not be released if there is not a flexion deformity of the elbow. Tendon lengthenings are more selective and provide control of the wrist and digits.

(2) The forearm muscle should not be released if the individual muscle can be identified as being contracted, and if this contracture can be managed by lengthening at the musculotendinous junction. I prefer to lengthen the flexor carpi ulnaris and the flexor carpi radialis at the musculo tendinous junctions, because releasing these muscles at their origins tends to weaken the muscles considerably more and may affect the motor nerves.

(3) Contracture of the flexores digitorum sublimes, the flexores digitorum profundi and the flexor pollicis longus should not be managed by lengthening in the forearm or at the elbow area. Contractures of these muscles should be managed by lengthening at the musculotendinous junction.

(4) Myotomy of the pronator radii teres is not necessary if there is no elbow contracture and if there is no fixed deformity of the forearm.

Procedure

A curved incision is made just anterior to the medial epicondyle of the humerus.

Following isolation and retraction of the ulnar nerve, the muscle origin of the flexor carpi ulnaris is released from the medial epicondyle and from its attachment to the proximal ulna. The pronator radii teres muscle is released by sharp dissection, as is the flexor carpi radialis. The depth of the flexores digitorum profundi and flexores digitorum sublimes, and the contiguity of the motor branches of the ulnar and median nerves to these muscle masses, make it inadvisable to release them proximally if noticeable contracture exists. A distal lengthening is more physiological.

Elbow contractures are managed by lengthening of the biceps at the musculotendinous junction and by myotomy of the brachialis muscle. If the brachioradialis is strongly contracted and spastic, its muscle origin can be released from the lateral aspect of the humeral epicondyle. The ulnar nerve is then transferred anteriorly, and the elbow is immobilized towards extension.

BIBLIOGRAPHY

Abbott, L. C., Saunders, J. B. de C. M., Bost, F. C. (1942) 'Arthrodesis of the wrist with the use of grafts of cancellous bone.' *Journal of Bone and Joint Surgery,* **24,** 883.

Bobath, B., Finnie, N. (1958) 'Re-education of movement patterns in everyday life in the treatment of cerebral palsy.' *Occupational Therapy,* **21,** (6), 23.

Bobath, K. (1965) 'The motor deficit in patients with cerebral paresis.' *Paper presented to the Study Group on Orthopaedics and Physical Medicine in Cerebral Palsy, Bristol, September.*

—— (1959) 'The neuropathology of cerebral palsy and its importance in treatment and diagnosis.' *Cerebral Palsy Bulletin,* **1,** (8), 13.

Boyes, J. H. (1962) 'Selection of a donor muscle for tendon transfers.' *Journal of the Hospital for Joint Diseases,* **23,** (1) 1.

Bunnell, S. (1964) *Surgery of the Hand, 4th edn., edited by Boyes, J. H.* Philadelphia: Lippincott. p. 24.

Carroll, R. E., Craig, F. S. (1958) 'The treatment of cerebral palsy in the upper extremity.' *Bulletin, New York Orthopedic Hospital,* (December).

Cooper, W. (1952) 'Surgery of the upper extremity in spastic paralysis.' *Quarterly Review of Pediatrics,* **7,** 139.

Fiorentino, M. R. (1963) *Reflex Testing Methods for Evaluating CNS Development.* Springfield, Ill.: C. C. Thomas.

Gesell, A., Amatruda, C. S. (1947) *Developmental Diagnosis.* New York: Hoeber.

Goldner, J. L. (1955) 'Reconstructive surgery of the hand in cerebral palsy and spastic paralysis from injury to the spinal cord.' *Journal of Bone and Joint Surgery,* **37A,** 1141.

—— (1961) 'Upper extremity reconstructive surgery in cerebral palsy or similar conditions.' *American Academy of Orthopedic Surgeons, Instructional Course Lectures,* **18,** 169.

—— (1966) Reconstructive surgery of the upper extremity affected by cerebral palsy or brain or spinal cord trauma.' *Current Practice in Orthopedic Surgery,* **3,** 125.

—— (1971*a*) 'Outline of operative procedures for reconstruction of the upper extremity in cerebral palsy.' *in* Keats, S. (Ed.) *Operative Orthopedics in Cerebral Palsy.* Springfield, Ill.: C. C. Thomas, p. 71.

—— (1971*b*) Upper extremity surgery in cerebral palsy—assessment and operative procedure.' *in* Bleck, E. E., *Instructional Course, American Academy for Cerebral Palsy.*

—— Ferlic, D. C. (1966) 'Sensory status of the hand as related to reconstructive surgery of the upper extremity in cerebral palsy.' *Clinical Orthopedics and Related Research,* **46,** 87.

Green, W. T., Banks, H. D. (1962) 'Flexor carpi ulnaris transplant and its use in cerebral palsy.' *Journal of Bone and Joint Surgery,* **44A,** 1343.

Inglis, A. E., Cooper, W. (1966) 'Release of the flexor-pronator origin for flexion deformities of the hand and wrist in spastic paralysis. A study of eighteen cases.' *Journal of Bone and Joint Surgery,* **48A,** 847.

Jensen, G. D., Alderman, M. E. (1963) 'The prehensile grasp of spastic diplegia.' *Pediatrics,* **31,** 470.

Keats, S. (1965) 'Surgical treatment of the hand in cerebral palsy: correction of the thumb-in-palm and other deformities. Report of nineteen cases.' *Journal of Bone and Joint Surgery,* **47A,** 274.

Mortens, J. (1965) 'Orthopedic operations in the treatment of children with cerebral palsy.' *Danish Medical Bulletin,* **12,** 22.

Paine, R. (1965) 'Early recognition of cerebral palsy and prognostic signs.' *Instructional Course Lecture, American Academy for Cerebral Palsy.*

Pollock, G. A., Sharrard, W. J. W. (1958) 'Orthopaedic surgery in the treatment of cerebral palsy.' *in* Illingworth, R. S. (Ed.) *Recent Advances in Cerebral Palsy.* London: Churchill. p. 286.

Rushworth, G. (1960) 'Spasticity and rigidity—an experimental study and review.' *Journal of Neurology, Neurosurgery and Psychiatry,* **23,** 99.

Samilson, R. L. (1966) 'Principles of assessment of the upper limb in cerebral palsy.' *Clinical Orthopedics and Related Research,* **47,** 105.

—— Morris, J. M. (1964) 'Surgical improvement of the cerebral palsied upper limb—electromyographic studies and results in 128 operations.' *Journal of Bone and Joint Surgery,* **46A,** 1203.

Speed, J. S., Knight, R. A. (Eds.) (1956) *Campbell's Operative Orthopedics.* St Louis: C. V. Mosby.

Stamp, W. G. (1963) 'Bracing in cerebral palsy.' *Orthopedic Prostheses and Appliances,* (December).

Steindler, A. (1952) 'Pathokinetics of cerebral palsy.' American Academy of Orthopedic Surgeons, Instructional Course Lectures, **9,** 118.

Stelling, R. H., Meyer, L. C. (1959) 'Cerebral palsy, the upper extremity.' *Clinical Orthopedics and Related Research,* **14,** 70.

Swanson, A. B. (1960) 'Surgery of the hand in cerebral palsy and swan-neck deformity. *Journal of Bone and Joint Surgery,* **42A,** 951.

—— (1964) 'Considerations for surgery of the hand in cerebral palsy.' *Bulletin, Academy of Medicine of New Jersey,* **1,** 170.

—— (1968) 'Surgery of the hand in cerebral palsy and muscle origin release procedures.' *Surgical Clinics of North America,* **48,** 1129.

Tachdjian, M. O., Minear, W. L. (1958) 'Sensory disturbances in the hands of children with cerebral palsy.' *Journal of Bone and Joint Surgery,* **40A,** 85.

Zancolli, E. (1968) *The Structural and Dynamic Bases of Hand Surgery.* Philadelphia: Lippincott.

CHAPTER 12

Problems and Complications in Orthopaedic Management of Cerebral Palsy

ROBERT L. SAMILSON and M. MARK HOFFER

Because cerebral palsy represents a varying group of difficult and intriguing peripheral manifestations, we must not lose sight of the fact that associated defects directly related to cerebral malfunction may be just as important as the musculo-skeletal abnormalities.

Diagnosis

Problems in management of cerebral palsy will arise if we are treating the wrong disease. All spastic states should not be treated as cerebral palsy.

The prognosis for brain-injured children with acquired spasticity is different from that for cerebral palsied neonates. Seizures are far more frequent in the former, and, depending on the age of brain insult, a past experience of normal function and usage is imprinted in the brain. The first 24 months following brain injury is a dynamic, unpredictable neurological period. Temporary splinting and bracing are appropriate during this period. Cerebral-palsy type operations should be reserved for the period after the initial 24 months. Failure to heed this dictum may result in iatrogenic deformity (Figs. 1a and b).

Patients with progressive spastic syndromes (e.g. cerebral sclerosis) require

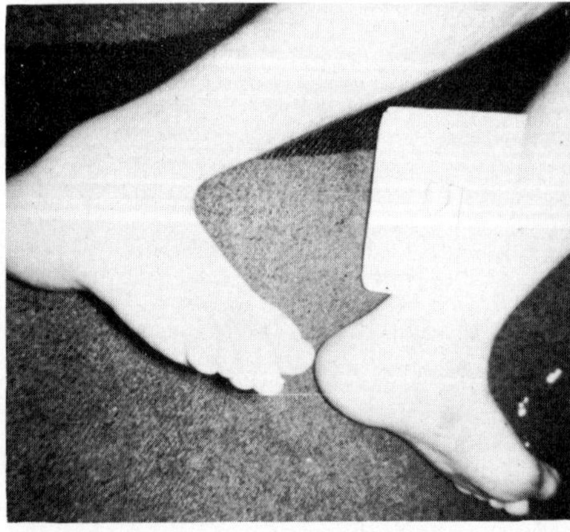

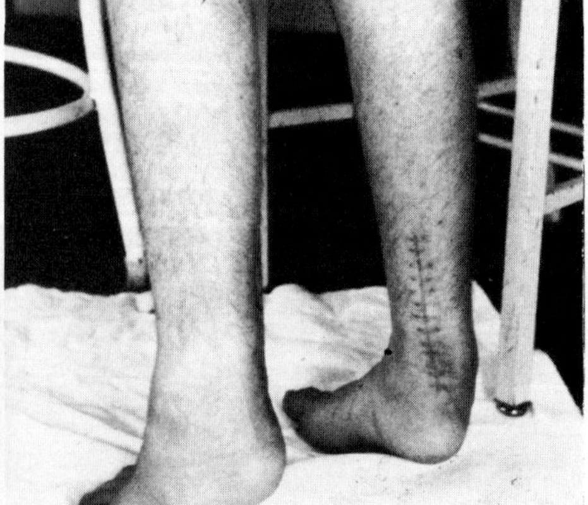

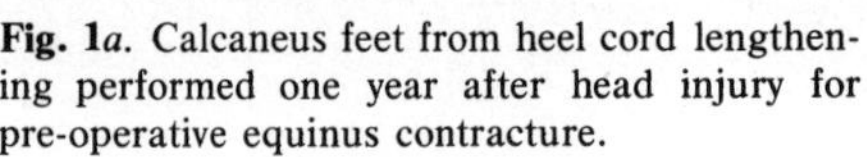

Fig. 1a. Calcaneus feet from heel cord lengthening performed one year after head injury for pre-operative equinus contracture.

Fig. 1b. Recurrence of equinus following heel cord lengthening performed six months after head injury for pre-operative equinus.

planning which takes account of the natural history of their progressive disease state (Fig. 2).

Metabolic diseases can cause spasticity, and some are better treated by drugs than by the surgeon. For years the self-mutilating children with Lesch-Nyhan syndrome were treated with total dental extractions and all manner of upper extremity restraints. Now it is recognized that these patients have hyperuricemia, and anti-gout medications often control their irritability and self-mutilation (Lesch and Nyhan 1964).

Mental retardation is present in association with cerebral palsy in about 50 per cent of patients (Paine and Oppé 1966). However, mental retardation may occur in patients with motor retardation, in the absence of cerebral palsy. The management of children with mental retardation is more difficult, and communication between health care personnel and the patient is of great importance. Small gains are often much appreciated by mentally retarded patients, and they should not be denied rational operative procedures (*i.e.* those designed to improve perineal care, prevent dislocated hips, or correct contractures which inhibit comfortable sitting or standing). More complicated procedures such as tendon transfers have a much poorer prognosis in the mentally retarded.

Beals (1971) has outlined a comprehensive differential diagnosis for cerebral palsy which is well worth reading. The reader is referred, as well, to Chapter 2 of this volume.

Evaluation

Treatment plans based on the erroneous evaluation of motor problems may result in complications. Beware of applying selective flail muscle tests to the spastic patterned patient. A muscle may be weak in a given posture, but in gait or after release of an antagonist that weak muscle may prove to have hidden strength. This

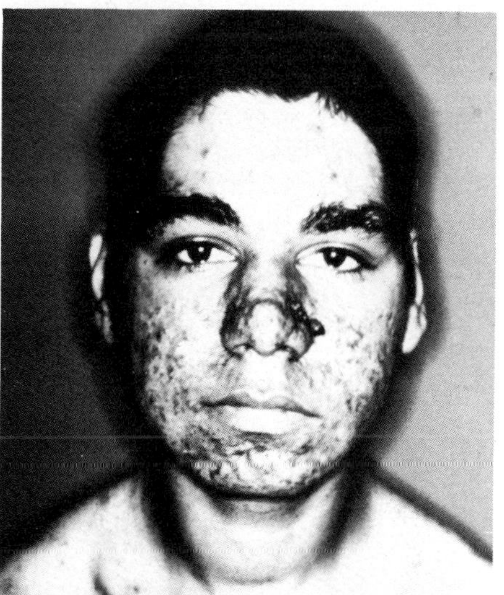

Fig. 2. Facies of tuberous sclerosis.

admonition is particularly true in rigidities associated with cerebral palsy, and explains the poor results in these states. It is also applicable in spastic states where spasticity is present in both agonist and antagonist.

Pre-operative antagonists should be evaluated in gait, in pattern, and in multiple positions. If there is doubt about the true nature of the antagonist, the operative plan should be reconsidered, and certainly should be less bold.

Sensory examination involving fine cortical modalities can avoid many problems in surgical and therapeutic programs for the upper extremity. Unfortunately, the paradox of upper extremity surgery in cerebral palsy is that the best functional results can be achieved in patients with selective control and good cortical sensation, but these patients have the least need. A useful dictum in cerebral palsy surgery is 'the enemy of good is better!'

Timing

Errors in timing and spacing of operative procedures may lead to problems. We have been unable to accomplish independent ambulation, for example, after the age of eight years. Thus procedures designed to promote ambulation after that age should be viewed cautiously.

In the first three or four years of life, it is often difficult to know exactly where the main problems will occur. For example, spasticity is rarely manifested early on, and during the early months many cerebral palsied patients are 'floppy infants'. Only after several years is their definitive neurological deficit manifest. Bracing and operative procedures in this early period (the first three to four years) should be directed only towards prevention, correction, and maintenance of correction of dangerous contractures. A subluxed hip should be treated vigorously, whereas heel cord lengthening may be inappropriate. The success of upper extremity surgery, as previously noted, depends on the degree of cortical sensation and selective control. This may be difficult to evaluate before five or six years of age, and surgery of the upper extremity in the younger child is not appropriate.

The performance of more than one procedure at the same time is an effective way of avoiding anesthetics and repeated hospitalizations. However, we must realize that it is most difficult to evaluate eventual 'muscle balance' pre-operatively, when multiple concurrent procedures are planned. It is far safer to do one thing at a time.

Consider 'patterns' in planning potential concurrent surgery. Primitive extensor pattern in the lower extremities often involves hip adductors, quadriceps, triceps surae and gluteus maximus. Primitive flexor pattern usually involves iliopsoas, hamstrings, ankle dorsiflexors and hip abductors. It is important to note that these are not absolutes, and patterns vary a great deal from patient to patient. In a child with a strong extensor thrust and extensor spasticity, one may be tempted to do adductor releases and heel cord lengthenings at the same time. However, if both adductors and triceps surae are insulted in one operative sitting, the patient may be overwhelmed by flexors and collapse, making it most difficult to get him or her walking in a reasonable period of time. Release of hip adductors *or* simple heel cord lengthening might effect the whole-extensor pattern. We feel that concurrent procedures are best done on either side of the pattern scale to maintain balance of powers (Table I).

Age is an important determinant in avoiding growth disturbance in arthrodesing operations (see Chapter 5).

TABLE I

Flexor pattern	*Extensor pattern*
Iliopsoas	Gluteus Maximus
Hamstrings	Quadriceps
Ankle Dorsiflexors	Triceps Surae
Hip Abductors	Hip Adductors

Goals

Some of the greatest failures in cerebral palsy therapy, bracing, and surgery are due to inappropriate goals. Foot surgery, for example, may be performed well with a superb operative result, a well-fitting post-operative brace, and excellent therapeutic follow-up. All of this may be to no avail in a patient who cannot walk because of a lack of neurological balance reactions or persistent neonatal reflexes. Procedures to keep the spine straight and the hips located and mobile are appropriate in any patient, because all patients should be able to be propped to sit. Procedures about the knee and feet should be done on patients who utilize their lower limbs for ambulation or transfer. Upper extremity procedures should be carried out only on patients who have an ability to co-operate and who have some selective control. Other surgical procedures in the upper extremities are appropriate for hygiene or cosmesis, but they should be presented as such to the patient and his family, or all will interpret the surgery as a complete failure.

Fractures in Cerebral Palsy

Dent (1970) has noted that patients on long-term anticonvulsants may suffer osteomalacia which leads to a propensity to fractures.

McIvor and Samilson (1966) studied the incidence of fractures in patients with cerebral palsy, and found that most occurred in severely involved spastic quadriplegics. Pre-existent contractures of contiguous joints was the factor most consistently associated with fracture, a finding which provides yet another reason for prevention and early correction of contractures. Closed treatment, modified according to the individual patient's needs, is most efficacious.

Pitfalls—the Upper Limb

Poor results occur with wrist fusion, where the operation is done in the absence of good finger extensors, or where tenodesis effect of a mobile wrist for grasp and release is unrecognised (Samilson and Green 1972) (Fig. 3). We prefer to cast the patient pre-operatively in the proposed arthrodesed position, and ascertain finger function in this new position before proceeding to surgery.

261

Proximal row carpectomy has been suggested in association with wrist fusion in the presence of very tight finger and wrist flexors. We prefer to do a preliminary flexor pronator release, and then cast the patient so that we can observe grasp and release in the proposed fused wrist position. If this is satisfactory, we then proceed to wrist arthrodesis. Unsuccessful flexor carpi ulnaris transfers to the radial wrist extensors may be salvaged by wrist fusion, provided that grasp and release in the fused position is adequate.

Flexor capri ulnaris transfer to radial wrist extensors (Figs. 4*a* and *b*) will fail, unless the wrist is mobile and grasp and release are possible. The transfer must have a direct line pull, and be inserted under proper tension. If too tight, the wrist will be tenodesed in a dorsiflexed position, and finger flexion will be weak (Fig. 5). Additionally, the transfer may pull out, if inserted under too much tension (Fig. 6). Transfer through the interosseous membrane may be temporarily successful, but, at long-term follow-up, excursion progressively diminishes and most results are unsatisfactory (Samilson and Green 1972). Unfortunately, in this instance, where the transfer is to the common finger extensors, poor results cannot be salvaged by wrist fusion, because weak finger extension persists, and release of grasp is impaired. Excessive weakness of finger extensors remains a most difficult problem, and, as yet, we have not found a satisfactory surgical solution.

Flexor carpi radialis transfer to long thumb extensor (Figs. 7*a* and *b*) (see Chapter 12) will fail if the transfer is made in a too volar direction; it may fail also

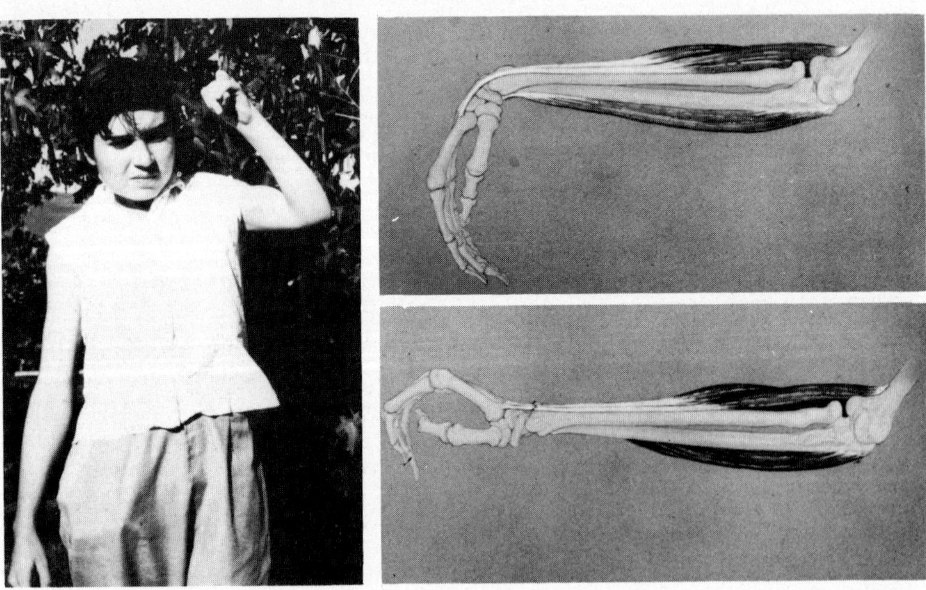

Fig. 3 (*left*). Wrist fusion in satisfactory position but poor functional result.

Fig. 4a (*top right*). Pre-operative diagram of flexor carpi ulnaris (volar) and radial wrist extensors (dorsal).

Fig. 4b (*bottom right*). Post-operative transfer of flexor carpi ulnaris to radial wrist extensors to improve wrist dorsiflexion and supination.

because the thumb adductor and/or flexor were tight, or because of failure to stabilize the thumb metacarpo-phalangeal joint. If both flexor carpi radialis and flexor carpi ulnaris are to be used for transfers, wrist fusion will probably be required because of resultant weakness in palmar flexion.

The flexed and adducted thumb with weak extensor and abductor presents a vexing problem (Fig. 8). Release of the thumb adductor, first dorsal interosseus and palmar brevis when tight is a prerequisite to other procedures on the thumb.

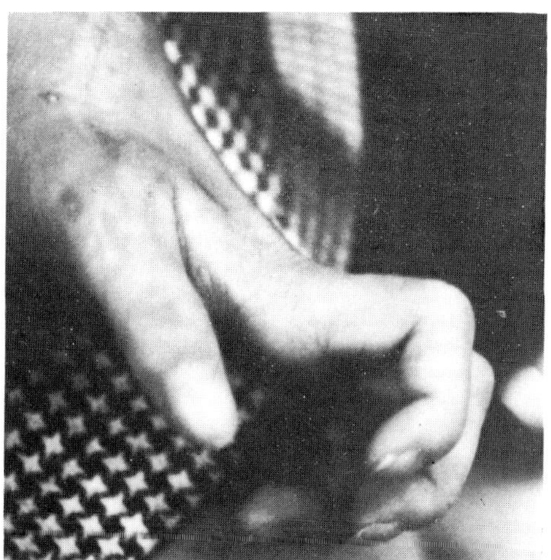

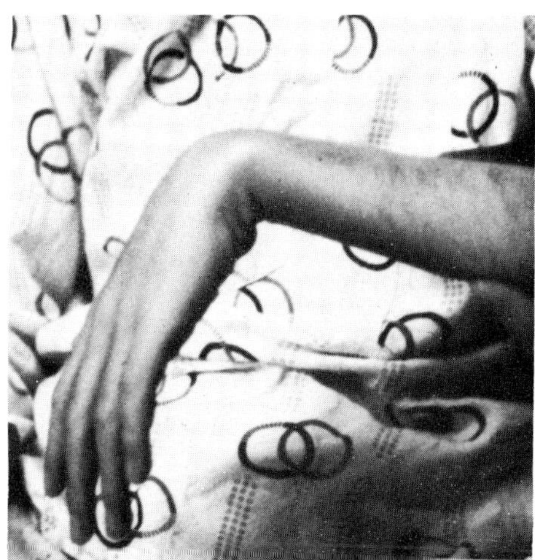

Fig. 5. Flexor carpi ulnaris transfer to radial wrist extensors, with transfer put in under excessive tension. Tenodesis in extension results in poor function.

Fig. 6. Flexor carpi ulnaris transfer to radial wrist extensors put in under excessive tension. Transfer pulled out with recurrent deformity.

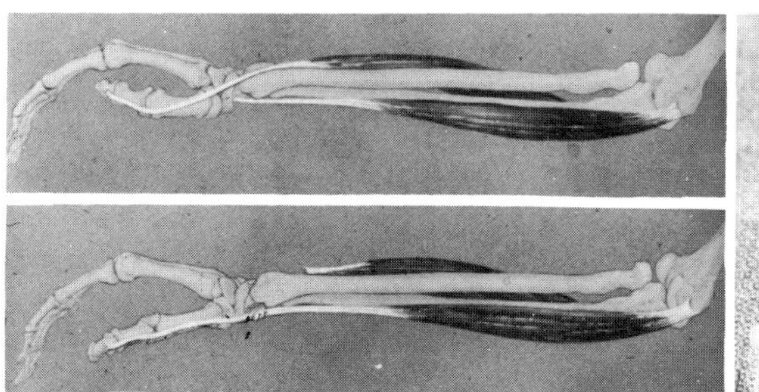

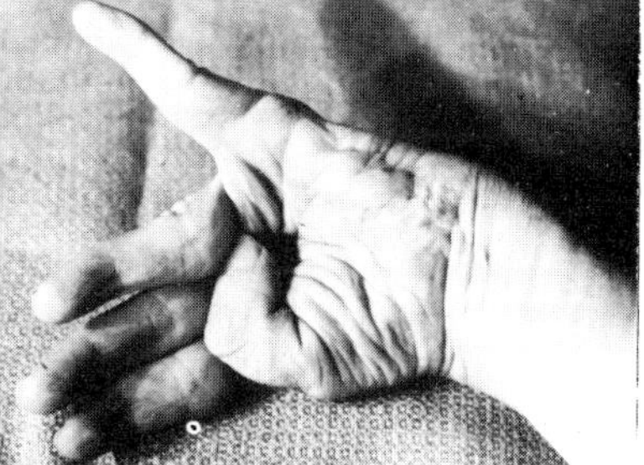

Fig. 7a (*top left*). Pre-operative flexor carpi ulnaris (volar) transfer to extensor pollicis longus (dorsal).
Fig. 7b (*bottom left*). Post-operative flexor carpi ulnaris transfer to extensor pollicis longus. Transfer should be made in line with long thumb abductor.
Fig. 8 (*right*). Thumb-clutched hand.

Addition of first carpo-metacarpal fusion to procedures designed to get the thumb out of the palm and to keep it there, seems to result in no significant improvement in function. Intermetacarpal bone block between the first and second metacarpals often fails because pinch requires some ability to adduct the thumb, and that ability is obviated by the bone block.

Elbow flexion releases have been uniformly unsuccessful, in our experience. Occasionally, in the presence of spastic elbow flexors without a fixed elbow flexion contracture, musculo-cutaneous neurectomy at the level of the coracoid has given satisfactory results, but it should never be done bilaterally, since loss of elbow flexion on both sides will prevent self-feeding. Following elbow flexion release, Bleck has occasionally noted posterior subluxation of the radial head and posterior bowing of the ulna.

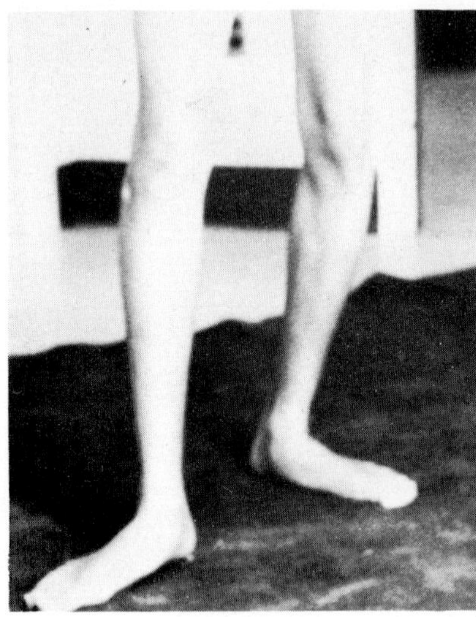

Fig. 9. Femoral anteversion, managed by twister cables. Note external rotation deformities at knees.

Pitfalls—the Lower Limb

Internal rotation deformity of the lower limb in cerebral palsy is most commonly due to persistent femoral anteversion. The use of *twister cables* in the presence of increased anteversion does not correct the deformity, but, instead, produces a compensatory external rotation at the knee joint (Fig. 9). This poses a major problem, in that surgical derotation of the femur will result in a severe external rotation deformity, which can be corrected only be derotating the tibia and fibula in the opposite direction. Therefore twister braces should be reserved for those children in whom femoral anteversion is not the cause.

In the presence of coxa valga, either true or relative due to adduction contracture or increased femoral anteversion, hip dislocation often proceeds relentlessly (Figs. 10a and b), unless a varus derotation osteotomy of the femur is performed. However, the procedure is not innocuous in the ambulatory child, since it can be expected to result in functional shortening of the operated side.

Since hip dislocation in cerebral palsy occurs at a mean age of seven years (Samilson *et al.* 1972), the acetabulum will have had a reasonable chance to develop with a femoral head in it. Thus innominate osteotomies are almost never indicated in hip dislocations in cerebral palsy, and, even if performed, the dislocation will probably recur unless a femoral varus-derotation osteotomy is performed.

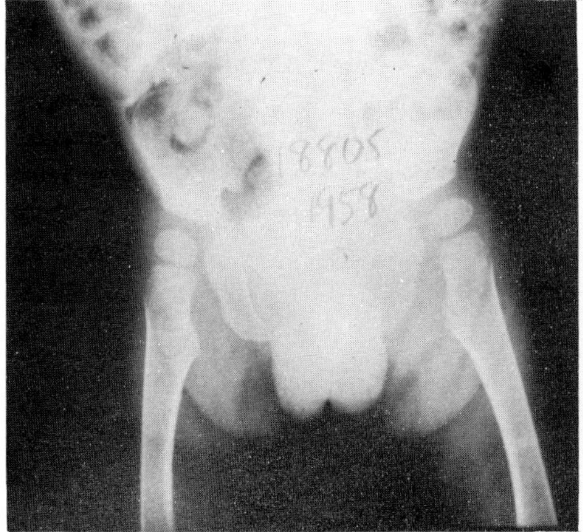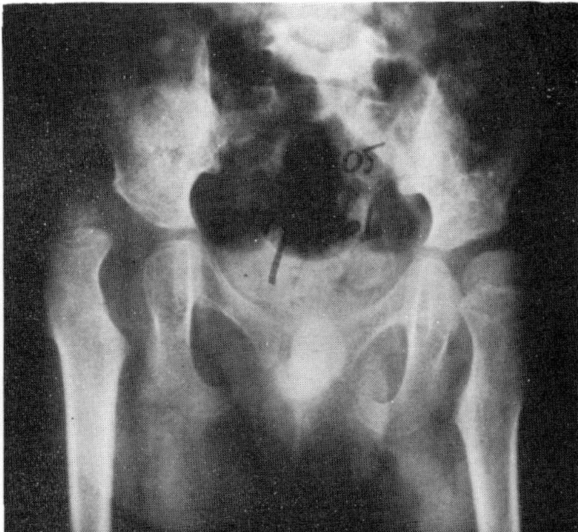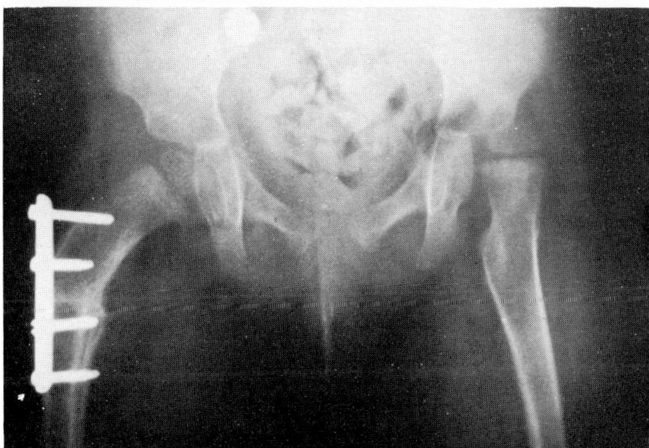

Fig. 10*a* (*top left*). Bilateral coxa valga and femoral anteversion, 1958.

Fig. 10*b* (*top right*). Same patient in 1961. Note progression to dislocation.

Fig. 11 (*left*). Varus derotation osteotomy has been performed in the upper end of the right femur. The left femur is in marked valgus and anteversion, and is proceeding to dislocation.

Unilateral adductor tenotomy and/or obturator neurectomy, especially in quadriplegic patients, has often resulted in dislocation of the contralateral hip (Samilson *et al.* 1967) (Figs. 12*a*, *b* and *c*). Post-operative 'frog' abduction casts should be avoided, since occasionally a reverse 'spread-eagle' deformity may occur (Figs. 13*a* and *b*), especially when pre-operative hip abduction power was not appreciated. When in doubt, it is helpful to perform a local block of the obturator nerve pre-operatively, and observe the posture of the child following the block. This is especially true in tension athetoids and rigid quadriplegics.

Inadequate post-operative immobilization has been felt to be a prime reason for unsatisfactory results (Evans 1966). Certainly maintenance of surgical gains requires the rational use of post-operative immobilization.

Semitendinosus transfer to the lateral femoral condyle has been described as a technique for correcting internal rotation deformity (Baker and Hill 1964). The procedure will not correct femoral anteversion, however, but will sometimes correct internal torsion due to spastic medial hamstrings.

Fig. 12*a*. Fig. 12*b*.

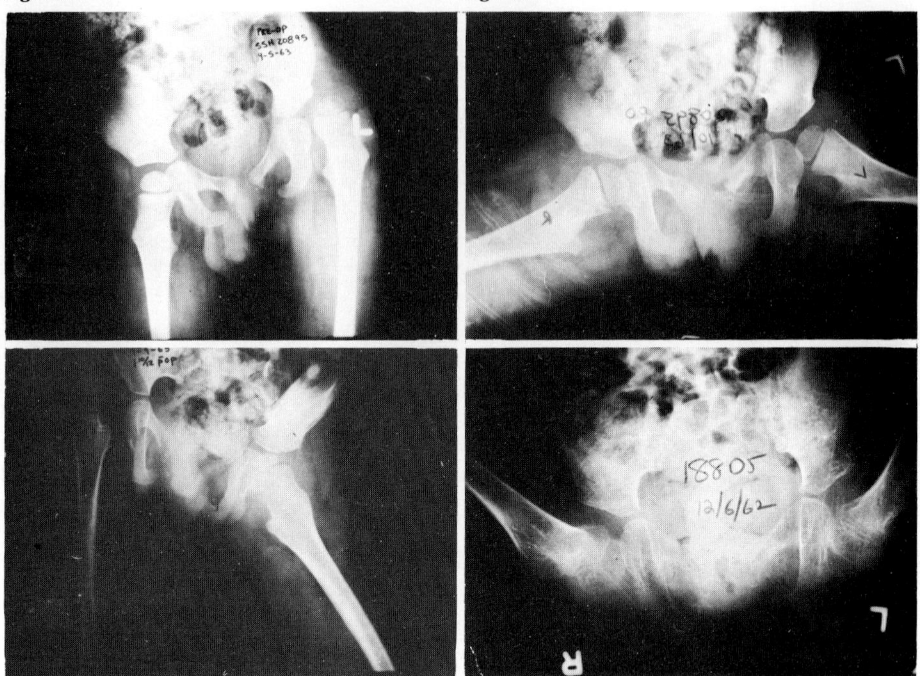

Fig. 12*c*. Fig. 13*a*.

Fig. 13*b*.

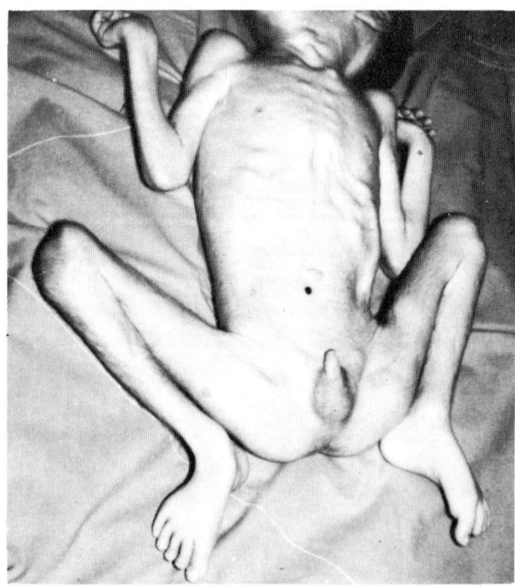

Fig. 12*a*. Spastic quadriplegia with subluxation of left hip.

Fig. 12*b*. Same patient after unilateral (left) adductor tenotomy and external obturator neurectomy.

Fig. 12*c*. Same patient 22 months later. Note dislocation of contralateral (right) hip.

Fig. 13*a*. Post-operative abduction (frog) deformity following bilateral obturator neurectomies and adductor tenotomies.

Fig. 13*b*. Same patient—note abduction (frog) deformity.

Hip flexion contracture over 25 degrees should be corrected prior to hamstring transfer to the femoral condyles to act as hip extensors. The transfers will not be efficacious in the presence of hip flexion contracture, and the ambulatory child in these circumstances will respond post-operatively by showing increased lumbar lordosis. Similarly, proximal hamstring release often results in increased lumbar lordosis and should be avoided in the presence of hip flexion deformity. After iliopsoas recession, patients often have diminished ability to climb stairs.

In the presence of hip and knee flexion, the orthopaedic surgeon should obtain X-rays of the lumbar spine, to rule out the occasional coexistent spondylolisthesis.

Before consideration of the occasional patellar tendon advancement procedure (Chandler), the surgeon must rule out rectus femoris spasticity, since it is likely to increase post-operatively and result in considerable recurvatum deformity.

If the patient has a valgus knee deformity before a proposed hamstring release or transfer, the valgus is likely to increase post-operatively.

The combination of equinus and knee flexion deformity is common in cerebral palsy (Fig. 14). If the equinus is not fixed, it may respond to correction of the knee flexion deformity. Pre-operative use of a cylinder cast in maximum knee extension, and subsequent observation of the gait, will prevent the occasional iatrogenic calcaneus deformity which may follow injudicous heel cord lengthening in this circumstance.

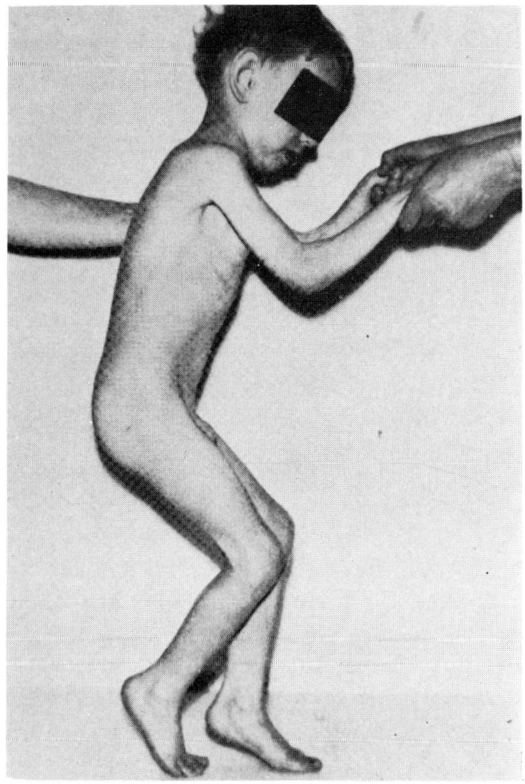

Fig. 14. 'Jump' position, with associated hip flexion, knee flexion and equinus (from Bobath).

Recurvatum (Fig. 15) following hamstring surgery may be a problem. The usual cause is either uncorrected equinus or unrecognized quadriceps (usually rectus femoris) spasticity. In addition, hamstring surgery should never by performed in association with gastrocnemius recession (Silverskiold), since, again, recurvatum will occur. In such a circumstance, soleus, acting from its distal insertion in stance phase, will pull the upper tibia posteriorly, resulting in recurvatum.

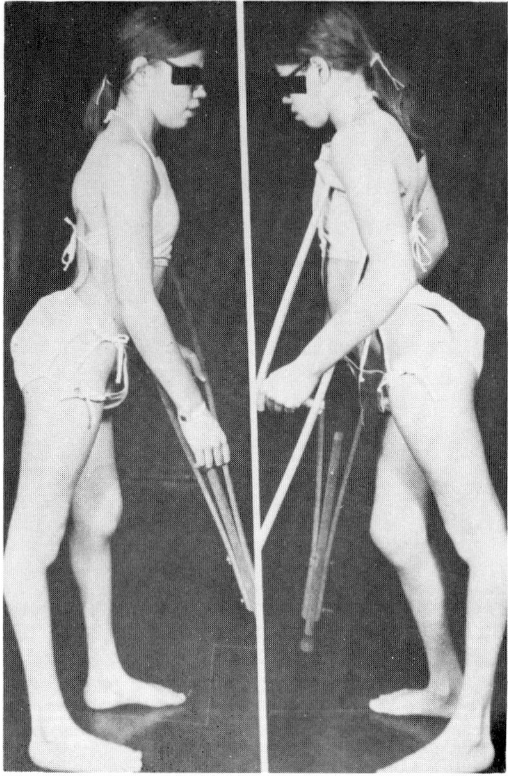

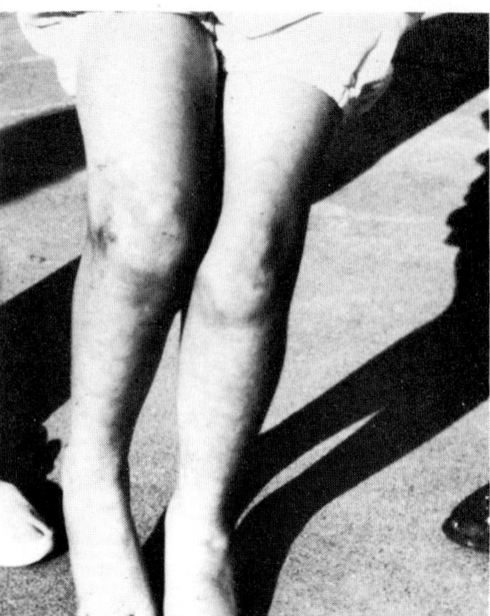

Fig. 15 (*left*). Genu recurvatum (from Banks).

Fig. 16 (*right*). Hemiplegic patient with shortening of right lower limb. Some equinus compensates for the shortening.

Obviously, limited knee flexion is a disaster in a patient who is wheelchair-bound. We must evaluate quadriceps (rectus femoris) spasticity carefully in those patients who, though assisted ambulators, may spend much of their time in a wheelchair. Pre-operative femoral nerve block may assist us in determining the efficacy of rectus femoris release in such patients.

Equinus correction is hazardous in a child who walks on tiptoes, but who will assume the plantigrade position on command. This situation is sometimes seen in mentally retarded children and in childhood schizophrenics. Failure to recognize this may result in iatrogenic calcaneus following injudicious heel cord lengthenings.

In children with hemiplegia and shortening on the hemiplegic side, it is unwise to correct all the equinus on that side because some equinus is necessary to compensate for the shortening (Fig. 16).

Following correction of equinus, toe flexor spasticity frequently increases, and occasionally it is necessary to correct this by toe flexor lengthening.

Rocker-bottom deformity (Fig. 17) may result from improper heel cord stretching performed without first locking the subtalar joint in inversion so that all passive dorsiflexion occurs at the ankle, rather than at the mid-tarsal joints. Similarly, rocker-bottom deformity may be seen when the peroneals dislocate anteriorly over the fibular malleolus. The peroneals then serve as dorsiflexors and evertors of the forefoot, and contribute to rocker-bottom deformity.

When the posterior tibial muscle contributes to equinovarus deformity (Fig. 18) (see Chapter 5), and when ankle dorsiflexors are weak, posterior tibial tendon transfer through the interosseous membrane to the middle cuneiform has proved helpful. It should never be done in the presence of triceps surae contracture, and the transfer should never be placed into the lateral cuneiform or severe valgus of the foot will result. Intramuscular posterior tibial tendon lengthening as advocated by Frost (1972) has proved efficacious on occasion, without leading to valgus deformity (Figs. 19a and b).

Never re-route both the peroneals and the posterior tibial, or calcaneus deformity will occur in cerebral palsied patients.

Peroneus longus transfer in the presence of a strong anterior tibial will result in dorsal bunion deformity (Fig. 20) due to elevation of the first metatarsal, unless the stump of the peroneus longus is inserted into the peroneus brevis.

Excessive valgus deformities of the feet (Fig. 21) may be corrected by Grice operations. Caution is necessary, however, since over-correction into varus may accrue if the graft is too long, or if there is unrecognized valgus talar tilt in the ankle mortise. Pre-operative standing antero-posterior views of the ankle are helpful in this regard.

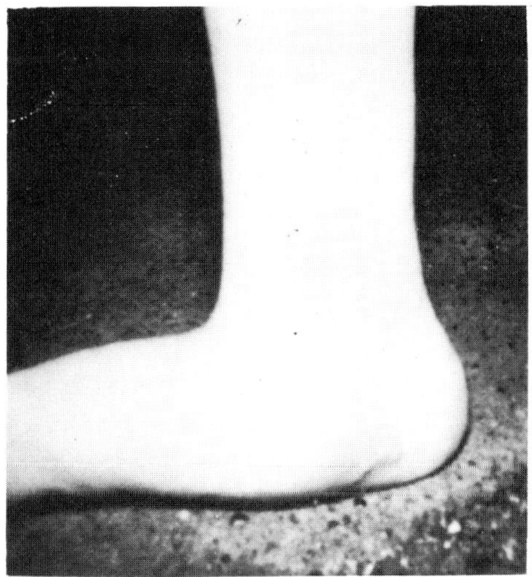

Fig. 17. Rocker-bottom foot.

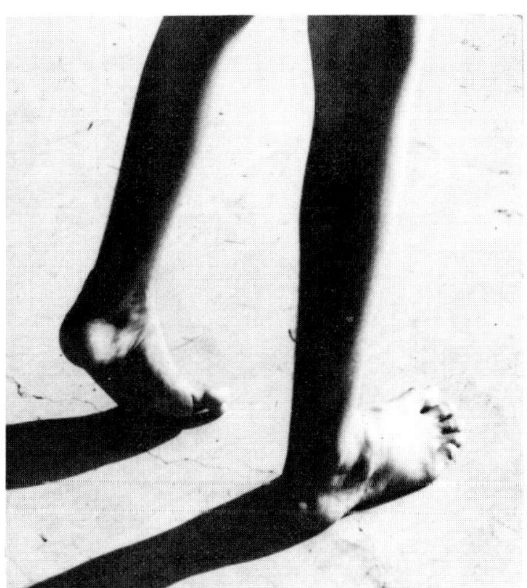

Fig. 18. Posterior tibial over-activity.

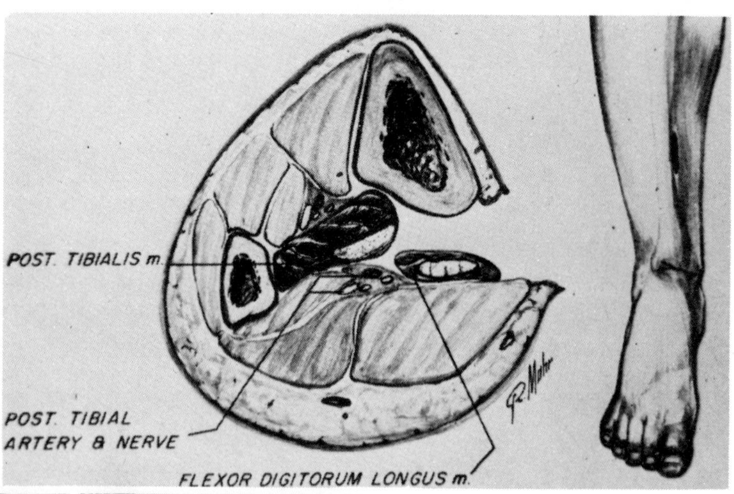

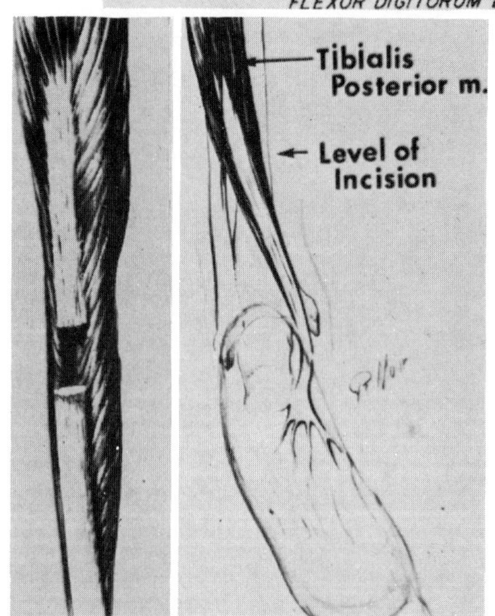

Fig. 19a (*above*). Intramuscular posterior tibial tendon lengthening, incision and approach (from Frost).

Fig. 19b (*left*). Intramuscular posterior tibial tendon lengthening (from Frost).

Fig. 20 (*below left*). Dorsal bunion deformity.

Fig. 21 (*below right*). Excessive valgus feet.

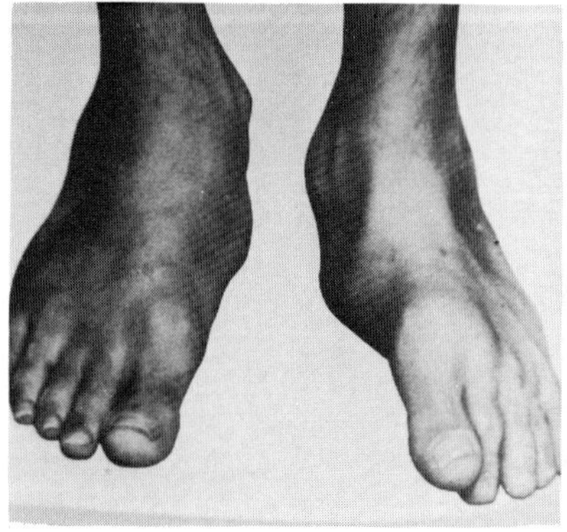

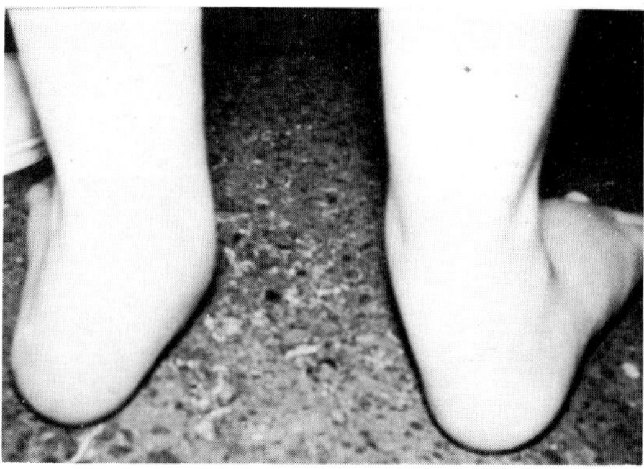

Ball and socket ankle joints have occasionally been observed following Grice procedures and triple arthrodeses (Fig. 22). As yet, there is no way to predict whether or not this will occur, but the wary will keep it in mind.

Triple arthrodesis should be reserved for a suitable age (see Chapter 4A); if done too early, excessive shortening of the foot may be anticipated and talar avascular necrosis may occur.

Excessive valgus of the foot is frequently accompanied by hallus valgus, which becomes sypmtomatic (Fig. 23). The use of the Uc-BL os calcis insert (see Chapter 4A) has proved helpful in preventing excessive valgus, prior to the age suitable for Grice operation or triple arthrodesis.

Hallux flexus (Fig. 24) is disabling to the cerebral palsied patient because the small tolerance for toe clearance in the swing phase of gait is lost. The deformity should be corrected whenever possible. Spastic abductor hallucis may be released to correct the occasional spastic hallux varus (Fig. 25).

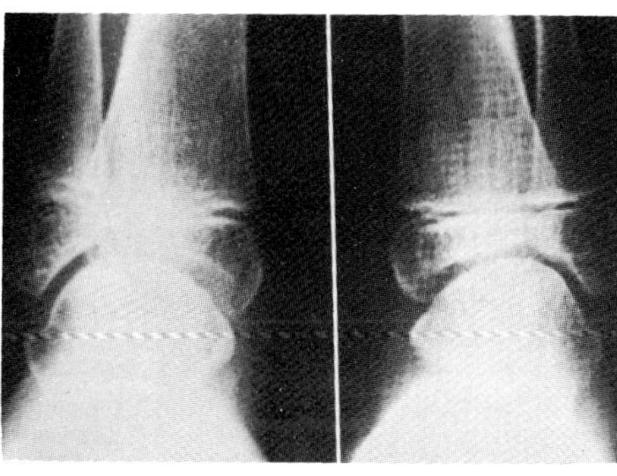

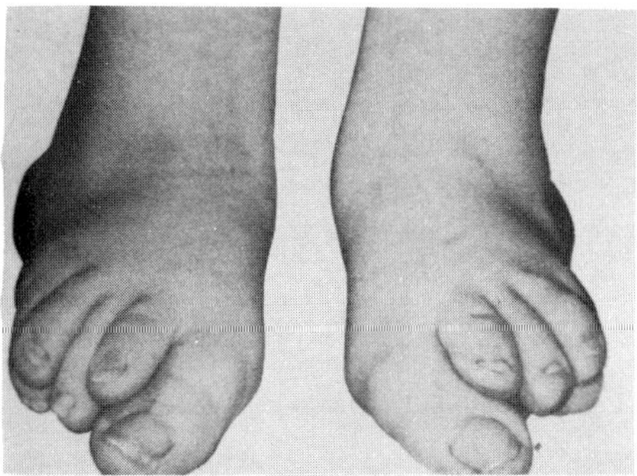

Fig. 22 (*above left*). Ball and socket ankles.

Fig. 23 (*above right*). Hallux valgus with pronated feet.

Fig. 24 (*below left*). Hallux flexus. Difficulty with toe clearance may be anticipated.

Fig. 25 (*right*). Bilateral hallux varus due to spastic abductor hallucis.

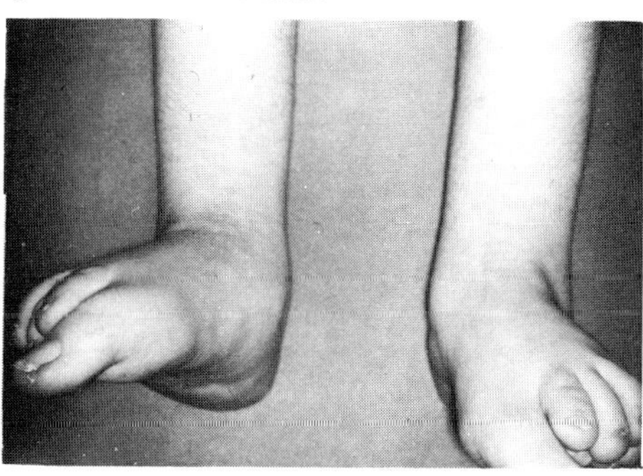

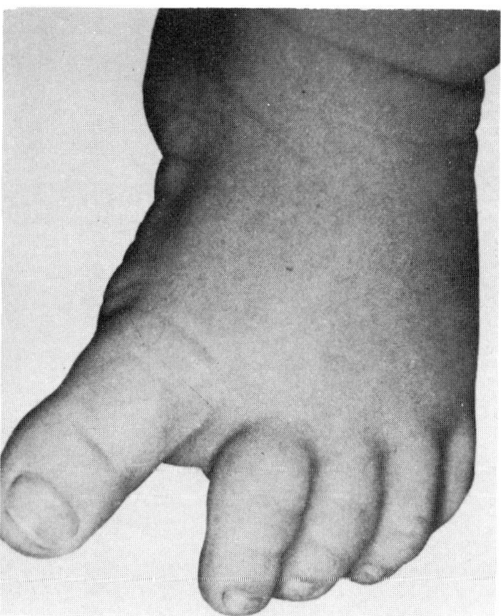

Cold, blue feet, indicative of vasomotor dysfunction, are sometimes seen in patients with cerebral palsy. Before performing elective orthopaedic surgical procedures on such feet, the surgeons should first carry out a diagnostic lumbar sympathetic block, followed by lumbar sympathectomy if the block is successful (Holmes *et al.* 1967).

Pitfalls—Spine and Pelvis

The use of Milwaukee braces in the prevention and/or correction of scoliosis in the cerebral palsied has been ineffectual and poorly tolerated by our patients. Risser jackets, Surcingle jackets and turnbuckle jackets are also poorly tolerated. For this reason, we believe that Harrington or Dwyer instrumentation is indicated in the surgical correction and maintenance of correction of scoliosis in the cerebral palsied child.

The problem of the co-existence of hip dislocation and scoliosis in the cerebral palsied patient is an onerous one. Since the scoliotic curves become fixed fairly early, and since the mean age for hip dislocation in these children is seven years (with a good resultant acetabulum), it is sometimes wiser to perform the scoliotic correction first, and correct the hip problem during the convalescence from this operation.

Early mobilization of cerebral palsied children on a tilt table following major complicated spine or hip reconstructive procedures speeds the recovery process, and seems to diminish the incidence of fractures during the convalescence.

In the very occasional instance in which acetabular reconstruction is necessary (*e.g.* a *congenital* dislocated hip in association with cerebral palsy), the innominate osteotomy should never be done in a child who has been on prolonged bed rest during the pre-operative period. The ilium will be too soft to retain the altered position induced by a bone wedge, and position will be lost. We insist that the child be ambulatory for at least three months prior to an innominate osteotomy in cerebral palsy. Further, rather than using a single Kirschner wire or Steinman pin to transfix the wedge of bone used to change the direction of the acetabulum, we use at least one wire or pin on either side of of the graft, so that it 'sits in a cage' and has very little chance of extruding.

The caution needed when contemplating unilateral hip surgery in the quadriplegic or diplegic patient is again brought to mind. Beware of the unoperated contralateral hip dislocation (see Pitfalls—Lower Limbs).

Pitfalls—Psychological

Too often, and usually unintentionally, we do not truly listen to patients or their parents. How often have you asked a cerebral palsied child for whom you have prescribed years of physical therapy, whether or not that therapy hurts? How often has the school child been frustrated by the therapist taking him out of class for his therapy session to the detriment of his intellectual development? Is your relationship with patients such that they are likely to reveal such frustrations to you? Are you sensitive enough to do something about them?

Even the cerebral palsied child with mental retardation does far better in an environment where he is a partner and not a pawn. The complete orthopaedic surgeon will include the child and his family as partners in the rehabilitation process. Patients will do far better in this relationship.

Discussion with patients and their families will help them understand what is planned and why it is planned. They should play an integral part in long-term planning. Their expectations will be realistic ones, rather than fantasies. They will be less likely to become accusatory.

Reynell (1965) has outlined the disturbances which may follow operations in children with cerebral palsy. She considers four levels of patient response. Uncommonly, there is 'overt behaviour disorganization which calls for comment from all those who have dealings with the child.' Home disturbances in behavior are seldom mentioned by parents, unless given an opportunity to do so. Less obvious behavioral disturbances, detected only by close observation, is more commonly seen, as are disturbances at deeper levels calling for more intensive study of individual children.

After surgery there is very often a depression of response level, a disturbance of attention, an increase in pain, fatigue and fear. This 'operation effect' was evident in 88 per cent of the children studied. This lasts for three to four months post-operatively. Following the initial negative emotional shift, there is usually an euphoric overswing before stabilization occurs. Fear and increased pain are often noticed when ambulation is first started after surgery. There was a close relationship between severity of operation and the emotional disturbance. Neither length of hospital stay nor age and intelligence of the child could be correlated to the severity of the emotional disturbance.

So-called 'adolescent deterioration' in cerebral palsied patients is frequently noticed. Some have related this to gain in weight. Others have discussed the possibility of rapidly growing bones increasing the stretch of muscles, with a resultant increase in spasticity (this seems highly unlikely, since spasticity is velocity sensitive, and *no* bone grows *that* fast!). The sexual identity in cerebral-palsied adolescents may be very disturbing to them, since they are likely to have very real concerns about their future functioning. Architectural barriers to their ever-widening world of experience may be most frustrating. Anxiety about their economic future may be formidable.

All of these factors should be considered by the treating orthopaedic surgeon. He shouldn't dodge the issue but encourage open communication!

REFERENCES

Baker, L. D. Hill, L. M. (1964) 'Foot alignment in the cerebral palsied patient.' *Journal of Bone and Joint Surgery*, **46A**, 1.

Beals, R. K. (1971) 'Cerebral palsy—elements for decision making.' *Instructional Course. American Academy of Orthopedic Surgeons.*

—— Dent, C. E. (1970) 'Osteomalacia with long-term anticonvulsant therapy and epilepsy.' *British Medical Journal*, **4**, 69.

Evans, E. B. (1966) 'The status of surgery of the lower extremities in cerebral palsy.' *Clinical Orthopedics and Related Research*, **47**, 127.

Frost, H. M. (1972) *Orthopedic Surgery in Spasticity.* Springfield, Ill.: C. C. Thomas.

Holmes, T. W., Gilfillan, R. S., Cuthbertson, E. M. (1967) 'Sympathectomy in the release of vasoconstriction of reponse in cerebral palsy and poliomyelitis.' *Surgery,* **61,** 129.

Lesch, M., Nylan, W. L. (1964) 'A familial disorder of uric acid metabolism and central nervous system function.' *American Journal of Medicine,* **36,** 561.

McIvor, W. C., Samilson, R. L. (1966) 'Fractures in patients with cerebral palsy.' *Journal of Bone and Joint Surgery,* **48A,** 858.

Paine, R. S., Oppé, T. E. (1966) *Neurological Examination of Children. Clinics in Developmental Medicine, Nos. 20/21.* Spastics Society with Heinemann.

Reynell, J. (1965) 'Disturbances following operations in children with cerebral palsy.' *Paper presented at a Study Group, National Spastics Society, Bristol.*

Samilson, R. L., Carson, J. J., James, P., Raney, F. L. (1967) 'Results and complications of adductor tenotomy and obturator neurectomy in cerebral palsy.' *Clinical Orthopedics and Related Research,* **54,** 61.

—— Green, W. L. (1972) 'Long-term results of upper limb surgery in cerebral palsy.' Reconstructive Surgery Chapter 5, S. Karger Switzerland.

—— Tsou, P., Aamoth, G., Green, W. L. (1972) 'Dislocation and subluxation of the hip in cerebral palsy: pathogenesis, natural history and management.' *Journal of Bone and Joint Surgery,* **54A,** 863.

CHAPTER 13

Assessment of the Results of Surgery in Cerebral Palsy

GEORGE POLLOCK

At a meeting of the Terminology Committee of the World Commission for Cerebral Palsy, cerebral palsy was described as 'a persistent but not unchanging disorder of movement and of posture due to dysfunction of the brain, excepting that caused by progressive disease, present before its growth and development are completed. Many other clinical signs may also be present.'

Cerebral palsy is, therefore, a dysfunction of the brain for which there is no cure, a fact which must be borne in mind, and which must have its reflection in the terms we use and in the conclusions we draw, when the results of conservative care or surgical treatment are assessed.

It is standard medical practice to review regularly patients who have been treated medically or upon whom surgical operations have been performed, to determine to what degree, if any, they have benefited from surgery, and to what extent treatment has enabled them to assume a reasonably normal life. This is even more necessary when judgement is passed on the influence of surgery in the habilitation of the patient suffering from cerebral palsy.

It is axiomatic that there can be no justification for operative treatment if similar benefits can be achieved by conservative means within a reasonable period of time. Thus the decision to operate is made only when the whole position has been considered by the screening panel, and the opinion formed that no further immediate benefit to the patient can be expected from continuing conservative care.

An accurate assessment of the post-operative result is possible only if a detailed report of the pre-operative state is available to the independent assessment panel for comparison. Furthermore, it is desirable in the interests of accuracy that, whenever possible, the pre-operative and post-operative examinations should be undertaken by the same independent body of assessors. The surgical team responsible for the operative procedures and for the subsequent habilitative care should not be a party to the final appraisal, lest even an involuntary bias influence decisions favourably.

Since the rate of recovery varies with the degree and extent of the physical disability present, and with the patient's intelligence, psychological state and 'drive', cognisance must be taken of these factors when the date for the post-operative assessment is set.

A simple heel cord lengthening may help to convert a patient who is chair-bound at the time of operation into an independently mobile individual within a matter of weeks, whilst a patient upon whom a hamstring transplant operation has been performed may not attain his maximum degree of improvement for one year. Similarly, a leg lengthening operation to equalise limb lengths in a hemiplegic patient may require twelve months before sound bone union and physiotherapeutic care eventually provide the patient with painless activity. An intelligent patient who co-operates in the performance of his post-operative exercises can be expected to make more rapid progress than one who is unintelligent and unco-operative. It must be appreciated, however, that some patients of relatively low intelligence may be possessed of an urge to be up and doing, sometimes to such an extraordinary degree that they show improvement far and away greater than that anticipated by even the most sanguine pre-operative assessor.* On the other hand, a patient with a high I.Q. may lack any desire to succeed, or be so emotionally attuned to his state and so apathetic and unco-operative in the performance of his post-operative exercises that a meticulously performed operation fails completely to produce improvement. Intelligence *per se* is not, therefore, the sole factor in ensuring a satisfactory post-operative course; however, all other things being equal, a fair degree of intelligence favours co-operation in post-operative care.

Thus, if the results of surgery are to be assessed on an equitable basis, adequate time must be allowed to elapse following operation before a final conclusion is drawn as to the benefits or otherwise of surgical treatment. This deliberate waiting does not, of course, preclude frequent earlier post-operative reviews.

A review at two and again at five years after the operation should meet most requirements, by allowing sufficient time to elapse for full recovery to take place within the known limits of the condition treated, or for evidence of failure or relapse to manifest themselves.

When weighing up the evidence available after any surgical operation on a cerebral palsied patient, particularly if several operations have been performed, the influences exerted by factors other than those already mentioned must be considered fully before the final conclusion is reached. Briefly these additional factors are:
    (a) the type of cerebral palsy,
    (b) the parents and home environment,
    (c) the type of surgery,
    (d) the form and type of both the pre- and the post-operative care.

The Type of Cerebral Palsy

The patient, be he child or adult, is the person most involved, and consequently it is his psychological attitude towards his disability, his acceptance of it, and his inward urge—or lack of one—to overcome his handicap which will finally influence the outcome, however good the surgical care he has received. We know from experience that the child suffering from the spastic form of cerebral palsy responds better to surgical treatment than does the athetoid, and that for the ataxic, the tremor and the rigidity cases surgery has little or nothing to offer at the present time.

A patient with widespread physical disabilities, whose condition is aggravated by low intelligence, psychological disturbance or blindness, has little chance of benefit-

---

*The author can recall such a case, where a bilateral tendo achilles lengthening and a triple arthrodesis were performed on a boy with an I.Q. of 40. An experienced assessment panel had held out no hope of surgical treatment resulting in physical progress, let alone employability, yet this young man, on his own initiative, obtained a caretaker's job and has held it, supporting himself and his widowed mother, for the last ten years.

ting from surgical treatment, but this is not to say that an operation is contra-indicated. In such a patient, surgical treatment, by rendering nursing simpler, can greatly relieve the burden placed upon parents or guardians. For example, a bed-ridden patient who, if he wishes to visit the toilet, has to be lifted and carried from his bed to the toilet and back again by ageing parents, may, after judicious surgery, be able to use a wheechair or even develop a supported walking balance. The operation may confer very little, if any, benefit on the child, but the load removed literally from the backs of his parents may be immense.

Earlier chapters in this book have emphasised that detailed study of the abnormality is essential before surgery can be planned. Equally essential is careful objective recording of the pre-operative findings. This report must describe not only the particular deformity which is going to lead to surgery, but the complete profile of the child involved, so that assessment can take into account not only specific changes resulting from the operation but also secondary changes which affect the child's general functioning.

The Parents and the Home Environment

The parents and the family enviroment are factors of considerable importance as regards both pre- and post-operative care. Intelligent, co-operative and affectionate parents can, when well instructed and supervised by the therapeutic services, play a vital rôle in the post-operative habilitation of their children. On the other hand, a home devoid of affection, with parents who are severely emotionally disturbed or scparatcd, can alienate the child and retard post-operative progress dramatically.

Selection of Type of Treatment

Surgery in cerebral palsy is not simply a question of correcting an obvious physical deformity of known cause (*e.g.* muscle imbalance, delayed bone growth, or resultant joint displacement), but presupposes a wide understanding of, and sympathy with all the underlying biological, aetiological, emotional and psychological influences affecting the child, his parents and their environment. It was a complete lack of this fuller knowledge of the background and of the basic factors involved in the assess-ment and subsequent management of cerebral palsy that discredited surgery and those who applied it, back in those early days when the success which followed the lengthening of Dr. Little's heel cord by Stromeyer held out such a glowing hope for those affected by 'spastic paralysis'.

Today, a deeper appreciation by the surgeon of the protean nature of cerebral palsy and of its many associated disorders, and a fuller appreciation of the limitations of his own art in the correction of these disorders, have done much to re-establish the reputation of the orthopedic surgeon and increase his successes. Mere surgical dexterity, unless backed by an understanding of the nature of cerebral palsy and some experience in conservative care, is not enough. Surgical operation is merely one incident in the continuing care of some cerebral palsied children, and the best surgical results tend to come to those who operate only after a sufficiently long period of personal observation and conservative care. This period may be one or even two years, but must be adequately long to enable the experienced surgeon, as a member of a team, to conclude that continued conservative care is unlikely to provide further benefit. Surgical treatment performed subject to these conditions of careful selection can open up new plateaux of progress. There are without doubt occasions when earlier surgical care is required, but these are not the rule, and the need for immediate surgery will become apparent as each case is considered individually by the team. Grossly everted feet, early subluxation of the hip and marked fixed equinus deformities are examples of deformities which may require prompt surgical intervention, but only rarely is open surgery necessary before the age of five years.

It is reasonable to accept the theory that the earlier the diagnosis is made and the habilitative programme begun, the better will the final state of the patient and the later will surgical intervention be required, if at all.

Aims of Treatment

Since cure in the real sense of the word is impossible, surgical treatment becomes merely one incident, albeit an important one, in the total programme for the habilitation of the child suffering from cerebral palsy. What do we hope to achieve by its use?

Correction of Fixed Deformity

A contractural joint deformity can be relieved by operation in a shorter period of time and more effectively than by any other method.

Reduction of Spasticity

Muscle balance cannot be restored to normal, but antagonistic muscle groups can be brought into rough equilibrium by weakening the stronger group by surgery (Crothers 1951). This effect may be the result of surgical interference with abnormal reflex pathways which cause spasticity.

Increased Stability and Posture

Fusion of joints can improve function. 'Operations do not teach the victims of cerebral palsy how to do anything when they did not know how before surgery was performed' (Terhune *et al.* 1958), but they can provide the bricks of a new foundation upon which the occupational therapist, physiotherapist and bracemaker can build, in terms of improved appearance, better function and greater skills. Keats (1970), reporting on eight years experience of fusion operations of the foot, stated that the over-all objective was to provide a 'well-balanced, painless, functional and brace-free foot in the ambulatory child'.

The importance of the post-operative programme cannot be over-emphasised. It must be well-organised, sustained and continued over a long period, if one is to prevent the recurrence of deformity due either to (a) some continuing muscle imbalance (muscle imbalance can certainly be reduced by surgery, but is rarely completely eliminated), or (b) an imbalance in the rate of growth of bone and soft tissue (Pollock and Sharrard 1958).

Cosmetic Effects

In some instances, no functional improvement can be achieved, but the patient

can be made to look more normal, and this may have important social implications
for him.

Relief for Caretakers

As has already been mentioned, in some severely handicapped patients, while the
patient's own performance is not improved, the task of those who care for him can be
made easier.

Function

Cerebral palsy is incurable. Nevertheless, certain skilfully performed orthopaedic operations on carefully selected patients, by correcting deformity, reducing
spasticity and stabilising joints, will enhance the effect of conservative care to improve
posture and function.

Assessment of Results

For clinical and humanitarian reasons, surgery in cerebral palsy has never been
submitted to the controlled trial which is now felt necessary before a new drug is
introduced into general use. What are the problems of assessing the results of surgery
in cerebral palsy?

Controls

Ideally, as with drug therapy, a new surgical technique for patients with cerebral
palsy could be explored by carrying out the operation on one group of children, while
another group is left unoperated, and then charting the progress of the two groups.
However, due to the protean manifestations of cerebral palsy, it is practically
impossible to find two groups of children whose involvement is sufficiently similar for
one to act as a control for the other. In most centres, the number of children
presenting even for one particular type of procedure over a period of time is relatively
small, and it is not possible, therefore, to develop a control group, even if this were
desirable, within a reasonable period of time.

For these reasons, most researchers fall back on using the child as his own
control, *i.e.* they assess the child fully before surgery, and assume that any improvement in his performance after surgery is a consequence of this. There are two dangers
in this approach: (a) it is never possible to know to what extent the changes are the
result of the natural history of the disease process; and (b) it is difficult to be certain
how much improvement is specific to the operation and how much is a 'halo' effect,
due to other factors not specific to the operation—in particular the degree of improvement resulting from the normal processes of maturation. Surgery involves 'admission
to hospital', 'a traumatic procedure', 'separation experience', and changes in physiotherapy techniques, to mention but the more obvious factors which could affect a
child's functioning.

These two dangers should be borne in mind particularly when studying the
results of complex procedures (such as bilateral hip and knee surgery), which may
well have involved major changes in the way the patients were managed. With more
limited procedures, such as wrist arthrodesis, it is easier to eliminate other variables
and relate changes specifically to the surgical procedure.

Who Makes the Assessment?

In a classic drug trial, where a double blind technique is used, the assessor does not know which patients have been treated, and ideally he is not part of the therapeutic team involved with the management of the patient. Again, as far as cerebral palsy programmes are concerned, these ideals are hard to sustain. It is hardly possible to achieve a blind trial, as tell-tale scars indicate that surgery has taken place; again due to the size of patient populations and the limited number of trained and experienced personnel available, it is often difficult to have the child assessed by an observer who has not been involved in the treatment programme.

Another biased assessor who features in some reports is the patient. Patients (a) want to improve, and (b) like to encourage their doctor, and will collude with him in considering themselves improved.

Where and How to Assess

The assessment of the patient customarily takes place in the clinic, and is based on procedures in which the workers in the clinic have been patiently training the child. Thus, improvement in the number of steps achieved between parallel bars may have little carry-over into the everyday situation. Measurements of motor behaviour should wherever possible be made in the child's natural environment, *i.e.* in the home and in the school.

Assessment should be (a) clinical (including investigative) and (b) functional. Clinical assessment may show that the range of movement at a knee joint has increased, but functional assessment may show that this may not have improved the child's kicking and walking.

It is not necessary here to go into the details of either the clinical and investigative or the functional techniques used in the assessment, as these are discussed elsewhere in this book. Probably the best account of functional asssessment of the child with cerebral palsy is given in Holt and Reynell's (1967) valuable book.

Some comments about scoring are perhaps appropriate here. Grading the results of surgery as 'worse', 'no change', 'good' and 'excellent' is not adequate, and the procedures adopted must allow some scorable assessment of the results. Some more objective procedure should be used which allows a scorable result. Wright and Nicholson (1973) provide an exemplary account of such a procedure in their study of the effects of physiotherapy.

Failure Rates

Detailed results of specific operations are discussed in other chapters in this book. Some general results of the author's experience may be quoted here. In a review of 466 operations it was found that the recurrence or failure rate amongst patients subjected to soft-tissue procedures was 39.4 per cent. The over-all failure rate, soft tissue, bone and joint procedures included, was 26.3 per cent. A number of these poor results in the early days were probably due to a failure to provide adequate and prolonged post-operative care.

The benefits of a good pre- and post-operative programme become evident in the results of a more recent and somewhat smaller series of 181 patients, in whom 264 operations were performed with an over-all failure rate of 17.4 per cent. This figure includes lost cases and those who died. If these cases are excluded, the failure rate is reduced to 11.7 per cent.

Many more operations are performed on the lower than the upper limbs in cerebral palsy, and the post-operative results are better. Of the 466 operations performed on the patients in the first of the two series described above, only 66 were for upper limb defects. Of the 264 operations performed on the second group of 181 patients, only 15 were on the upper extremity, and of these 36.8 per cent were failures. The failure rate for operations of the lower extremity was 16.3 per cent.

Conclusions

The deformities in cerebral palsy develop as a sequel to imbalance in the power of the antagonistic muscle groups, principally of the upper and lower limbs, although those of the trunk and neck may be affected also. Most orthopaedic surgeons classify their surgical results according to the effect these operations have had on the function as well as on the appearance of the upper or lower extremity. Few orthopaedic surgeons would fail to agree with Green and McDermott's (1942) conclusions that these 'surgical procedures, by reducing deformity, establishing better balance of motor power, decreasing the spasticity of muscles and simplifying the problems of control, are often an indispensible part of the process of habilitation'.

An observation orginally made by Carlson (personal communication), that surgical correction of a peripheral deformity frequently has a beneficial influence on a quite unrelated activity has been observed since by many workers (*e.g.* Silver and Simon 1957). An operation on the lower extremity may improve the movement and co-ordination of the trunk and upper extremities. An arthrodesis of an ankle, in a boy who was previously completely unco-operative, has led not only to mobility, but to a desire to train, and to the discovery of an educational talent not previously suspected.

This last example emphasises the importance of the assessment of the whole patient in cerebral palsy. The orthopaedic surgeon must invite colleagues—and not only those strictly involved with the child's motor activities but also those concerned with other aspects of the child's functioning—to play a part in assessing the results of surgery, and so encourage him to continue and extend his efforts to provide effective surgical treatment for those who suffer from cerebral palsy.

REFERENCES

Crothers, B. (1951) 'Clinical aspects of cerebral palsy. Life history of disease.' *Quarterly Review of Paediatrics,* **6,** 142.
Green, W. T., McDermott, L. J. (1942) 'Operative treatment of cerebral palsy of the spastic type.' *Journal of the American Medical Association,* **118,** 434.
Holt, K. S., Reynell, J. K. (1967) *Assessment of Cerebral Palsy II Vision, Hearing, Speech, Language, Communication and Psychological Function.* London: Lloyd-Luke.
Keats, S. (1970) *Operative Orthopaedics in Cerebral Palsy.* Springfield, Ill.: C. C. Thomas.
Pollock, G. A., Sharrard, W. J. W. (1958) 'Orthopaedic treatment in the treatment of cerebral palsy.' *In* Illingworth, R. S. (Ed.) *Recent Advances in Cerebral Palsy.* London: J. & A. Churchill, p. 286.
Silver, C M., Simon, S. D. (1957) 'Operative treatment of cerebral palsy involving the lower extremities.' *Journal of the International College of Surgeons,* **27,** 457.
Terhune, S. R., Shannon, P. W., DeVane, F. H., Denton, J. C. (1958) 'The role of the orthopaedic surgeon in the management of cerebral palsy.' *Clinical Orthopaedics,* **11,** 132.
Wright, T., Nicholson, J. (1973) 'Physiotherapy for the spastic child: an evaluation.' *Developmental Medicine and Child Neurology,* **15,** 146.

CHAPTER 14

Prospects for the Future

M. MARK HOFFER and JACQUELIN PERRY

Many needs of patients with cerebral palsy are now largely unmet. This book is concerned with the work of the orthopaedists, whose therapeutic aim is naturally related to the motor aspect of the disorder. It is, of course, important to realise that this is only one aspect of these disorders. Even their etiology and their objective documentation need better definition. In this chapter we will draw attention to some of the most difficult problems, before going on to discuss 'prospects' which relate particularly to the orthopaedist's interest.

Etiology

The etiology of cerebral palsy still puzzles us. Some studies suggest viral and perinatal causes (Muller *et al.* 1971, Rowlands *et al.* 1971).

Most recent articles continue to imply that anoxia is the principal cause of cerebral palsy. Recent pathological studies have indicated that there is generalized necrosis and elective parenchymal necrosis, especially in the pyramidal areas of the cerebral cortex. Vasospasm due to anoxia may be the mechanism of local necrosis.

Transabdominal amniocentesis at the fourteenth week of pregnancy has produced fluid that can determine whether kernicterus will occur. In addition, desquamated amniotic cells can be cultured by sex and analysed for sex determination and chromosomal analysis. These analyses are of importance in suspected cases of hemophilia, muscular dystrophy or chromosomal disorders such as Down's syndrome. Biochemical studies of amniotic cells in tissue culture allow early recognition of such disorders as galactosemia, hyperuricemia, Tay-Sachs' disease, Pompe's glycogen disease and Hunter's or Hurler's mucopolysaccharidosis (Kline and Gillis 1971).

As more specific causes for developmental arrest and spasticity are clearly defined, patients may be removed from that vague category of 'cerebral palsy'; families may be appropriately counselled, and we may be left with more homogeneous groups of patients (with well-defined patterns of disease) to work with.

Communication Disorders

Communication problems, which exist in many patients, constitute one of the most troublesome aspects of cerebral palsy. They tend to be most serious in the totally involved and in the dyskinetic (athetoid). Such patients are often unable to talk or write. They have poor control of their extremities and facial muscles, so it is most difficult for them to use alternative methods of communication. Some children with communication difficulties of this type are thought to be retarded because ordinary intellectual testing is impossible. Non-verbal communication systems must be designed for speechless children with poor head, mouth and extremity control. Fig. 1 shows how a buzzer communication device helped an eight-year-old apparently retarded, totally involved child communicate his wants. His intelligence was then tested objectively, and found to be within normal range. Non-verbal communication systems have been designed for attachment to modified typewriting machines. For the future, they may be combined with systems of taped phrases to develop computerized speech (Hagen and Brink 1972).

Another, often related serious oral problem in many dyskinetic patients is drooling. This annoying electrolyte depriving process is amenable to appropriate physical therapy in most cases. Some patients, however, have failed to respond to these methods. Parotid duct transfer to the esophagus has been performed with good results in some of the refractory patients (Brody, G., personal communication).

Social Problems

Even if all the disorders of cerebral palsy have been ameliorated by treatment to as great an extent as possible, the individual with cerebral palsy may still be handicapped. Inevitably his condition means that he is brought up under exceptional circumstances. As a young baby, he may spend months in hospital; the whole of his pre-school development may be slow, and he may never have those opportunities for 'growth through play' which occur for the normal nursery school child. Schooling will often be in a special facility, where the cerebral palsied child is cut off among children of his own kind and sees little of normal school life. It is not surprising that many studies have shown that the child handicapped with cerebral palsy, when he reaches adult life, is emotionally and socially in great difficulties in the outside world.

When one couples this emotional and social handicap with the attitude of many people in society today towards handicap, one realises that social difficulties may, in

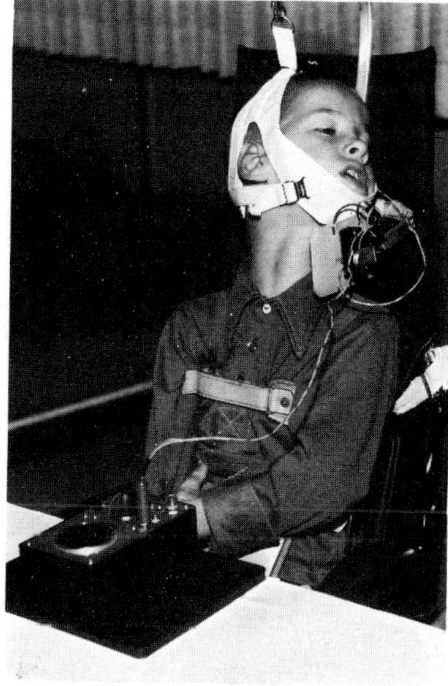

Fig. 1. An eight-year-old child utilizing a buzzer system for non-verbal communication.

fact, prove to be the most difficult to overcome. There are still many business concerns which legislate that handicapped people should not be employed, even when it can be shown that they are quite able to carry out their work as well as a normal person. If jobs cannot be found which the handicapped can do as well as a normal person, then finding some place for them in our working society is very, very difficult. Facilities for the employment of handicapped people lag far behind the needs.

For the more severely handicapped person, for whom independent existence is impossible, the needs are even greater. Many such persons now live on the wards of big institutions because no more appropriate facilities have been provided. Recently, much more emphasis has been given to the provision of small hostel accommodation where handicapped people can live reasonably independent lives, but with such assistance as they need readily available. The Scandinavians have been ahead in paying particular attention to these social needs of the handicapped, and setting up facilities where handicapped people can live, marry and lead as full lives as possible.

There is a need for many people in our society to think more seriously about the requirements of the handicapped. For example, there is a need for architects to design appropriate buildings, and car manufacturers to design suitable cars. Indeed, it is up to everybody in all aspects of social life to show more awareness of those less fortunate than themselves, and to see that adequate provision is made for their needs.

The Motor Disorder
Documentation and Analysis

Documentation of the patterns of neuromuscular balance is now best performed by a series of stress tests during physical examination. It is difficult to observe specific muscle participation in upper extremity function and in gait. Recent electromyographic studies strongly suggest that electromyography may be a more valid approach to the functional evaluation of the cerebral palsied patient. Electromyographic studies of upper extremity function before and after tendon transfers have been performed in 128 patients and suggest that some transfers may function appropriately in patterns (Samilson and Morris 1963). Electromyographic studies of hamstring muscles suggest that these muscles may be major deforming factors in patients with an internally rotated scissoring gait (Sutherland *et al.* 1969).

For many years, the posterior tibial muscle has been considered the main varus-deforming hindfoot force in cerebral palsy. Gait electromyography has shown that in some cases overactivity and phase distortion are more marked in the anterior tibial muscle. Fig. 2 is the electromyograph of a 16-year-old boy with bilateral varus hind-feet. Clinically, posterior tibial spasticity was thought to be the cause of the deformity. The electromyograph shows anterior tibial muscle hyperactivity and phase distortion.

In cases of triceps surae spasticity, the problem of whether to perform gastrocnemius recessions or Achilles tendon lengthenings has been debated. Gait electromyography has been helpful in distinguishing gastrocnemius from soleus spasticity. Fig. 3 is an electromyograph of a six-year-old girl with clinical evidence of triceps surae spasticity. The phase distortion and hyperactivity of the soleus is more impressive than that of the gastrocnemius. Fig. 4 is a quick stretch electromyograph

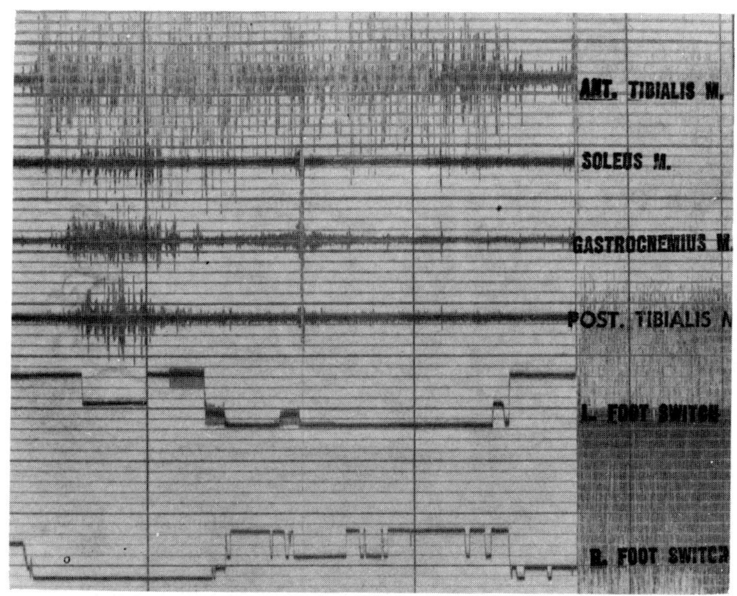

Fig. 2. Electromyograph of a 16-year-old boy with bilateral varus hindfeet, showing anterior tibial muscle hyperactivity with phase distortion.

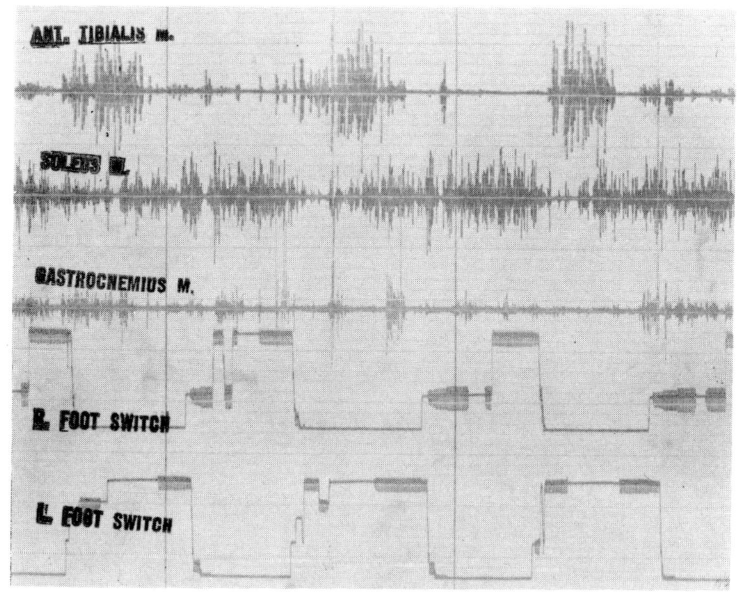

Fig. 3. Electromyograph of a six-year-old girl with triceps surae spasticity clinically. Phase distortion and hyperactivity of the soleus is more impressive than the gastrocnemius. (A study carried out by Dr. Peter Giovan.)

performed with the knees extended. It demonstrates clonus of the anterior tibial muscle, soleus, and gastrocnemius in an eight-year-old boy. Fig. 5 is a similar quick stretch electromyograph with the knee extended. It shows clonus only in the soleus of this ten-year-old boy.

Sutherland *et al.* (1969) have described a method of analysing the pathological gait, using photo instrumentation engineering and other techniques borrowed from the space industry. They have described femoral and pelvic rotation, and knee and foot motions, utilizing this technique in normals.

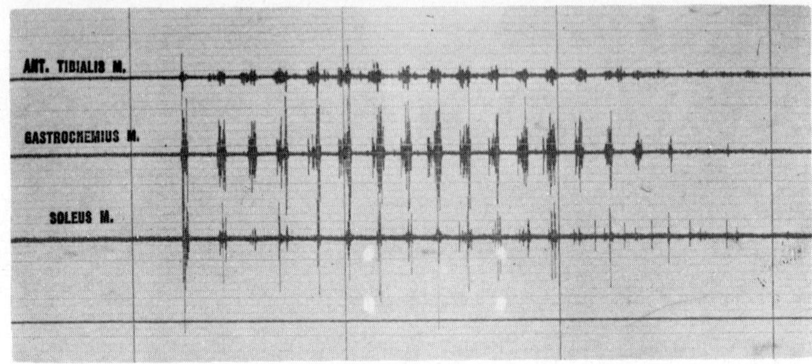

Fig. 4. A quick stretch electromyograph with knee extended showing clonus in the anterior tibial, soleus and gastrocnemius muscles in an eight-year-old boy. (A study carried out by Dr. Peter Giovan.)

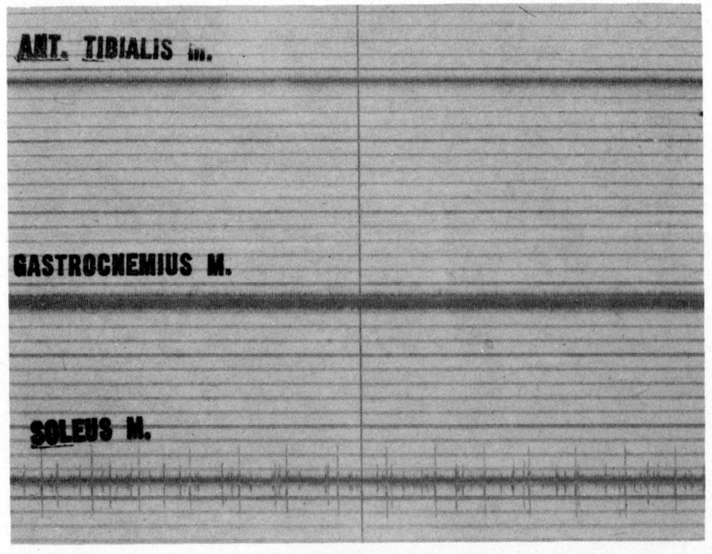

Fig. 5. A quick stretch electromyograph with knee extended shows clonus in only the soleus of this ten-year-old boy. (A study carried out by Dr. Peter Giovan.)

Drugs

Medications, including diazepam ('Valium') and L Dopa, are currently utilized and under investigation (Rosenthal *et al.* 1972, Soboloff *et al.* 1972). However, enough is known to say that we do not have a drug at the moment which can satisfactorily relieve spasticity without side effects.

Neurosurgical Procedures

Neurosurgical procedures for selected ablation of portions of the basal ganglia and for motion disorders have been devised, and are utilized in selected cases.

Motor nerve blocks for pre-operative evaluation and then selected neuro-ectomies have been utilized to improve function in some patients with motion disorders. This approach has been most helpful in the analysis of upper extremity function (Wilemon *et al.* 1971).

Devices

Hydraulically damped braces have been utilized in many centers for control of untoward upper extremity motion. These devices are now used for training purposes. It is in the schoolroom and during feeding tasks that they find their best application. The controls on all current systems are much too cumbersome to find practical widespread application. In the future, some control systems should be evolved that are lightweight, cosmetic and dependable. Fig. 6 shows a ten-year-old dyskinetic boy who utilizes his hydraulically damped brace for feeding and writing activities.

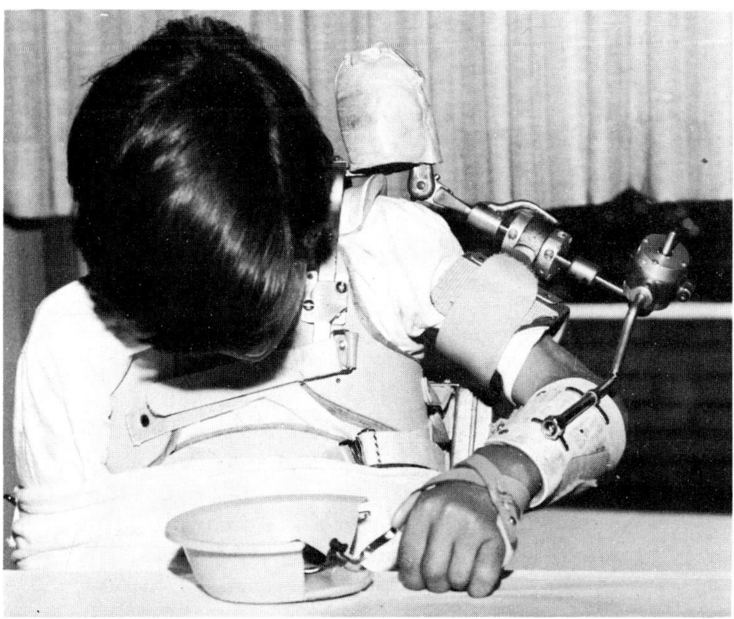

Fig. 6. A ten-year-old dyskinetic boy who uses his hydraulically damped brace for feeding and writing activities.

James Reswick, a bio-engineer closely involved with the aerospace industry suggests an alternative bio-engineering approach (Reswick 1972, personal communication).

Reswick and his team of bio-engineers view the lower motor neuron system of each muscle in the body with its spindle efferents and afferents, the muscle efferents and the golgi afferents, as a reflex arc, a dynamic system in the human being, which is analagous in many ways to the electro-mechanical servo-mechanisms used in many aerospace and industrial applications. Under certain conditions, these servo-mechanisms can become unstable, exhibiting oscillatory and uncontrolled movements. Such gyrations of the machine seem to an observer to be markedly similar to the uncontrolled movements of the dyskinetic child, and are, in fact, capable of being viewed from the same mathematical concepts or models.

Reswick views our current attempts by mechanical means as inherently inefficient. He suggests that an alternative method to damping servo-mechanisms is to alter the electrical signals which flow in the machine, in such a way that those which control power are reduced in proportion to the velocity of movements. The result of this is the same as if an energy absorber, whose action is proportional to velocity, is attached to the shaft of the servo-mechanism; but by attenuating the electrical signals the undesired movements and resulting kinetic energy are prevented from occurring, and power loss is avoided. Bulkly mechanical devices are also avoided. Furthermore, the bio-engineers suggest that there is an intriguing possibility that the signals flowing in reflex loops of cerebral palsy patients may be attenuated by electrical stimulation or inhibition.

Spinal Deformity

Spinal deformity is a major problem of the cerebral palsied patient, requiring new approaches. Application of the Dwyer approach and fixation devices may be the answer to lordoscoliosis of the thoraco-lumbar area in some of these children (Dwyer *et al.* 1969). Figs. 7*a* and 7*b* show the X-rays of an eighteen-year-old girl with cerebral palsy and thoraco-lumbar lordoscoliosis, preoperatively (Fig. 7*a*) and after Dwyer anterior fusion (Fig. 7*b*).

Neural Implants

The present state of the art of orthopaedic surgery in cerebral palsy can be described as 'selective ablative acts or some muscle trade'. Systems of neuro-stimulation developed for stroke and brain-injured patients might be applied to cerebral palsied patients in the future as a positive approach to restore muscle balance. Fig. 8 shows a 68-year-old man who suffered a cerebral vascular accident two years ago. This resulted in complete foot drop. With the use of an implanted peroneal nerve stimulator, triggered on and off by a shoe heel switch, he is able to lift his foot in gait. Fig. 9 illustrates the system of peroneal nerve implant.

Conclusions

The study of cerebral palsy involves an understanding of practically all aspects of the functioning of the human nervous system. The study of the patient with cerebral palsy not only brings reward for the sufferer himself, but provides new insight into the function of ordinary people. The orthopaedist who struggles to understand the disorders of his patient with cerebral palsy will find, therefore, that he gains reward not only from being able to help the cerebral palsied patient, but also from adding to the sum total of knowledge about human posture and movement. There are many unanswered problems, as this brief survey has indicated, and there are no more stimulating intellectual challenges within orthopaedics than that of cerebral palsy.

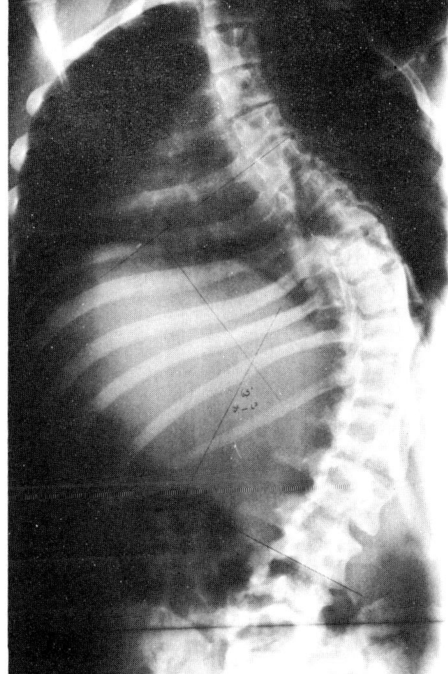

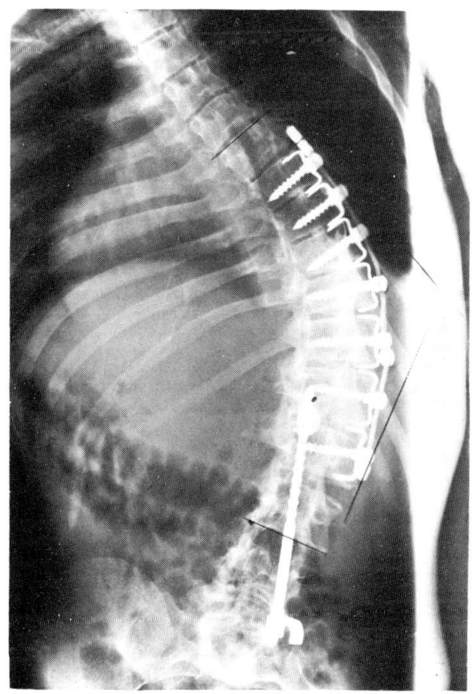

Fig. 7*a*. Pre-operative X-ray of 11-year-old girl with cerebral palsy and thoraco-lumbar lordoscoliosis.

Fig. 7*b*. X-ray of ten-year old girl with cerebral palsy and thoraco-lumbar lordoscoliosis after Dwyer anterior fusion.

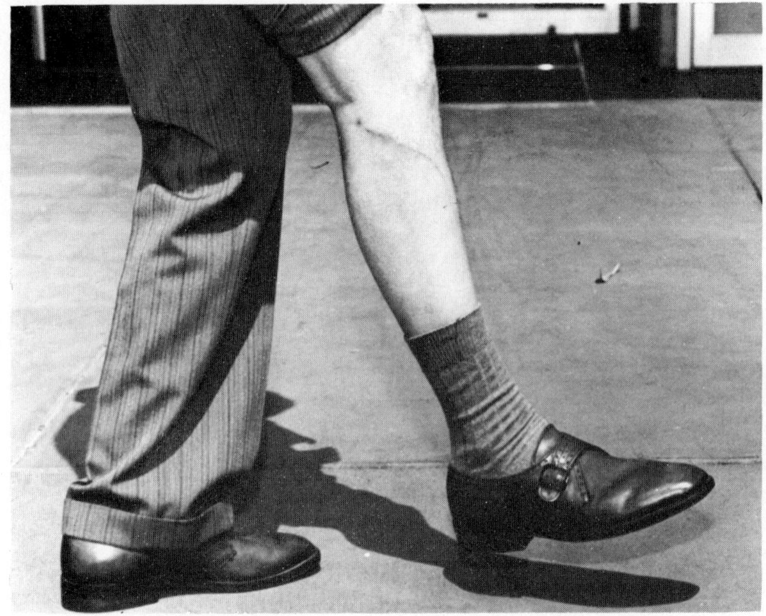

Fig. 8. A 68-year-old man two years after cerebral vascular accident utilizes an implanted peroneal nerve stimulator to enable him to use his foot in gait.

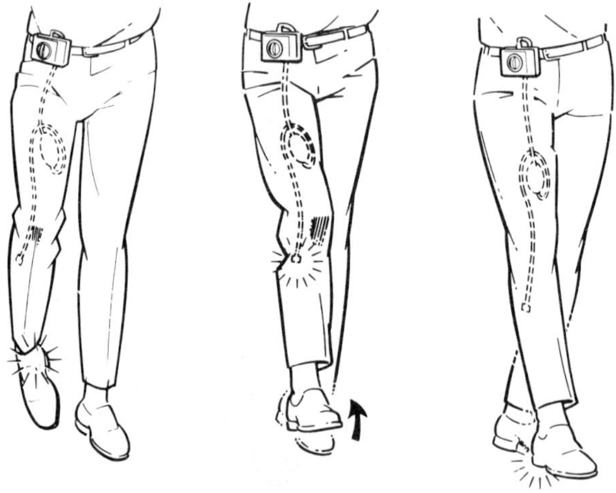

Fig. 9. Diagram showing technique of peroneal nerve implant. Lifting heel causes heel switch system to activate belt-suspended transmitter (*left*); antenna delivers pulse train through skin to implant, stimulating peroneal nerve and dorsiflexing foot (*middle*); heel strike deactivates heel switch system to terminate stimulus (*right*).

REFERENCES

Dwyer, A. F., Newton, V. C., Sherwood, A. A. (1969) 'An anterior approach to scoliosis.' *Clinical Orthopedics and Related Research,* **62,** 192.

Hagen, C., Brink, J. D. (1972) 'Non-verbal communication: a mode of communication for the severe athetoid cerebral palsy patient.' *Developmental Medicine and Child Neurology, (Abstract),* **14,** 111.

Kline, J., Gillis, S. (1971) 'Diagnostic needle aspiration in pediatrics practice?' *Pediatric Clinics of North America,* **18,** 219.

Muller, P. F., Campbell, H. E., Graham, W. E., Brittain, H., Fitzgerald, J. A., Hogan, M. A., Muller, V. H., Rittenhouse, A. H. (1971) 'Perinatal factors and their relationship to mental retardation and other perimeters of development.' *American Journal of Obstetrics and Gynecology,* **109,** 1205.

Reswick, J. (1972) Personal Communication.

Rosenthal, R. K., McDowell, F. H., Cooper, W. (1972) 'Levodopa therapy in athetoid cerebral palsy.' *Developmental Medicine and Child Neurology,* **14,** 113.

Rowlands, G., Reynolds, E. O. R., Stewart, A., Strong, L. B. (1971) 'Changing prognosis for infants of low birth weight.' *Lancet,* **1,** 516.

Samilson, R. L., Morris, J. M. (1963) 'Surgical improvement of the cerebral palsied upper limb.' *Journal of Bone and Joint Surgery,* **46A,** 1203.

Soboloff, H. F., Dias, J., Cary, G. R. (1972) 'Preliminary study of the use of L-dopa on athetoid cerebral palsied patients.' *Developmental Medicine and Child Neurology, (Abstract),* **14,** 113.

Sutherland, D. H., Schottstaedt, E. R., Larson, L. J., Ashley, R. K., Callander, J. N., James, P. N. (1969) 'Clinical and electromyographic study of seven spastic children with internal rotation gait.' *Journal of Bone and Joint Surgery,* **51A,** 1070.

Wilemon, W. K., De Paoli, F. J., Caldwell, C., Perry, J. (1971) 'Hemiplegic upper extremity posture, tone and analysis.' *Paper presented at the American Academy of Orthopaedic Surgeons Meeting, San Francisco.*

ACKNOWLEDGEMENTS

Thanks are due to the following authors and publishers for permission to reproduce their material.

CHAPTER 2

Table VI: Gillette, H. E. (1969) *Systems of Therapy in Cerebral Palsy.* Springfield, Ill., C. C. Thomas.
Figs. 2 and 4: Holt, K. S. (1966) 'Facts and fallacies about neuromuscular function in cerebral palsy as revealed by electromyography.' *Developmental Medicine and Child Neurology,* 8, 255.
Table VII: Smith, D. W. (1970) *Recognizable Human Malformations.* Philadelphia, W. B. Saunders.

CHAPTER 4A

Figs. 1, 7, 8, 11, 12, 13: Fiorentino, M. R. (1973) *Reflex Testing Methods for Evaluating C.N.S. Development.* Springfield, Ill., C. C. Thomas.
Figs. 3, 4, 22: Holt, K. S. (1965) *Assessment of Cerebral Palsy.* London, Lloyd-luke.
Fig. 14: Peiper, A. (1963) *Cerebral Function in Infancy and Childhood.* New York, Consultants Bureau.
Fig. 20: Chapchal, G. (1972) *Reconstructive Surgery and Traumatology,* Vol. XIII. Basel, S. Karger Ag.
Fig. 35: Bassett, F. H., Baker, L. D. (1966) 'Equinus Deformity in Cerebral Palsy.' *In* Adams, J. P. (Ed) *Current Practice in Orthopaedic Surgery,* Vol. 3. St. Louis, Mo., C. V. Mosby Co.
Figs. 40 and 42b: Samilson, R. L. (1973) 'Neuromuscular diseases affecting the foot.' *In* Inman, V. T. (Ed) *Du Vries' Surgery of the Foot.* St. Louis, Mo., C. V. Mosby Co.

CHAPTER 10

Fig. 1: Ingram, A. J. (1963) 'Miscellaneous affectations of the nervous system.' *In* Crenshaw, A. H. (Ed) *Campbell's Operative Orthopaedics,* 4th edn. St. Louis, Mo., C. V. Mosby Co.
Fig. 2: Eggers, G. W. N. (1952) 'Transplantation of hamstring tendons to femoral condyles....' *Journal of Bone and Joint Surgery,* 34A, 827.
Table I: Bassett, F. H., Baker, L. D. (1966) 'Equinus deformity in cerebral palsy.' *In* Adams, J. P. (Ed) *Current Practice in Orthopedic Surgery,* Vol. 3. St. Louis, Mo., C. V. Mosby Co.
Fig. 3: Baker, L. D. (1956) 'A rational approach to the surgical needs....' *Journal of Bone and Joint Surgery,* 40A, 1359.
Fig. 4: Strayer, L. M. (1950) 'Recession of the gastrocnemius.' *Journal of Bone and Joint Surgery,* 32A, 671.
Tables II and III, Figs. 5a and b, 8a-d, 9, 10a-d, 16a-f: Banks, H. H., Green, W. T. (1958) 'The correction of equinus deformity in cerebral palsy.' *Journal of Bone and Joint Surgery,* 40A, 1359.
Fig. 6: Baker, L. D. (1954) 'Triceps surae syndrome in cerebral palsy.' *Archives of Surgery,* 63, 216.
Figs. 7a and b: Silver, C. M., Simon, S. D. (1959) 'Gastrocnemius muscle recession for spastic equinus deformity in cerebral palsy.' *Journal of Bone and Joint Surgery,* 41A, 1021.
Fig. 11: Grice, D. S. (1952) 'Extra-articular arthrodesis of the subastragalar joint.....' *Journal of Bone and Joint Surgery,* 34A, 927.
Figs. 12a-j, 15a-d: Banks, H. H., Panagakos, P. (1966) 'Orthopedic evaluation of the lower extremity in cerebral palsy.' *Journal of Bone and Joint Surgery,* 40A, 1359.
Fig. 13: Baker, L. D., Hill, L. M. (1964) 'Foot alignment in the cerebral palsy patient.' *Journal of Bone and Joint Surgery,* 46A, 1.
Fig. 14: Dwyer, F. C. (1960) 'Osteotomy of the calcaneum....' In *Proceedings of the 8th Congress of Orthopedic Surgeons and Trauma,* New York. Brussels, Imprimerie Medicale et Scientifique.
Fig. 20: Edmondson, A. S. (1963) 'Postural Deformities.' *In* Crenshaw, A. H. (Ed) *Campbell's Operative Orthopedics,* 4th edn. St. Louis, Mo., C. V. Mosby Co.

Contributors

HENRY H. BANKS	Professor and Chairman, Division of Orthopaedic Surgery, Tufts University School of Medicine, Boston, Massachusetts. Past President, American Society for Surgery of the Hand.
MARTIN C. O. BAX	Research Paediatrician, Coram Research Unit, London WC1. Honorary Consultant Paediatrician, St. Mary's Hospital Medical School, London W2.
EUGENE E. BLECK	Clinical Associate Professor of Orthopaedic Surgery, Stanford University School of Medicine, Palo Alto, California. Chief, Orthopaedic Service, Children's Hospital at Stanford, California.
E. BURKE EVANS	Professor and Chairman, Division of Orthopaedic Surgery, University of Texas Medical Branch, Galveston, Texas. Orthopaedic Consultant, Moody State School for Cerebral Palsied Children, Galveston, Texas.
ERIC DENHOFF	Clinical Professor of Paediatrics, Brown University School of Medicine, Providence, Rhode Island. Past President, American Academy for Cerebral Palsy.
MOYNA GILBERTSON	Group Superintendent Physiotherapist, Hospital for Sick Children, Great Ormond Street, London WC1. Chairman of the Association of Paediatric Chartered Physiotherapists.
WILLIAM T. GREEN	Emeritus Harriet M. Peabody Professor of Orthopaedic Surgery, Harvard University School of Medicine, Boston, Massachusetts. Past President, American Academy for Cerebral Palsy.
J. LEONARD GOLDNER	Professor and Chairman, Division of Orthopaedic Surgery, Duke University School of Medicine, Durham, North Carolina. Past President, American Society for Surgery of the Hand.

M. MARK HOFFER — Assistant Professor of Orthopaedic Surgery, University of Southern California School of Medicine, Los Angeles, California.
Chief, Cerebral Palsy and Children's Reconstructive Service, Rancho Los Amigos Hospital, Downey, California.

MARGARET H. JONES — Emeritus Professor of Paediatrics, University of California at Los Angeles School of Medicine, California.
Past President, American Academy for Cerebral Palsy.

RONALD MAC KEITH — Emeritus Director, Newcomen Clinic, Guy's Hospital, London SE1.
Editor, Developmental Medicine and Child Neurology.

JACQUELIN PERRY — Professor of Orthopaedic Surgery, University of Southern California School of Medicine, Los Angeles, California.
Chief, Kinesiology Service, Rancho Los Amigos Hospital, Downey, California.

GEORGE POLLOCK — Past Chairman, World Commission for Cerebral Palsy.
Previous Consultant Orthopaedic Surgeon, Princess Margaret Rose Hospital, Edinburgh, Scotland.

ROBERT L. SAMILSON — Clinical Professor of Orthopaedic Surgery, University of California School of Medicine, San Francisco, California.
Past President, American Academy for Cerebral Palsy.

DAVID SCRUTTON — Superintendent Physiotherapist, Newcomen Centre, Guy's Hospital, London SE1.
Physiotherapy Adviser to the Special Care Units of the Inner London Education Authority's Schools for the Educationally Subnormal.

W. J. W. SHARRARD — Consultant Orthopaedic Surgeon, Sheffield Children's Hospital and Sheffield Royal Infirmary, Derbyshire.
Honorary Clinical Lecturer in Orthopaedic Surgery, University of Sheffield, Derbyshire.

SAMUEL B. THOMPSON — Clinical Professor of Orthopaedic Surgery, University of Arkansas School of Medicine, Little Rock, Arkansas.
Past President, American Academy for Cerebral Palsy.